Transdisciplinary
Public Health

Transdisciplinary Public Health

Research, Education, and Practice

Debra Haire-Joshu and
Timothy D. McBride

EDITORS

FOREWORD BY EDWARD F. LAWLOR

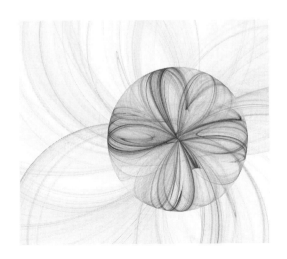

JB JOSSEY-BASS™
A Wiley Brand

Library of Congress Cataloging-in-Publication Data

Transdisciplinary public health : research, education, and practice / [edited by]
Debra Haire-Joshu and Timothy D. McBride. – 1st ed.
　　　p. ; cm.
　Includes bibliographical references and index.
　ISBN 978-0-470-62199-8 (pbk.); ISBN 978-1-118-41534-4 (ebk.); ISBN 978-1-118-41802-4 (ebk.);
ISBN 978-1-118-55295-7 (ebk.)
　I. Haire-Joshu, Debra.　II. McBride, Timothy D.
　[DNLM: 1. Public Health.　2. Evidence-Based Practice.　3. Interdisciplinary
Communication.　4. Public Policy.　5. Socioeconomic Factors. WA 100]
　362.1–dc23
　　　　　　　　2012046802

Printed in the United States of America
FIRST EDITION
PB Printing　10 9 8 7 6 5 4 3 2 1

Contents

For Corrie, Joel, and Chris

For Shirley L. Porterfield

Figures and Tables

Figures

Tables

Foreword

Transdisciplinarity has become the academic and policy word of our time in public health. Research initiatives, teaching and degree programs, public health interventions, service delivery systems, even ideas about architecture, are being defined by the promise of this new approach to framing problems and solutions across disciplinary lines.

We are still at the beginning of this project, the hopeful stage. We still have more rhetoric than we have useful examples and evidence of the payoffs of this approach. This book makes a great leap in the conceptualization of transdisciplinary approaches and also provides concrete examples in practice, teaching, policy, and research.

There are many barriers between us and the ultimate success of this enterprise. Scholars select a particular discipline for deep personal and professional reasons, and they are socialized and reinforced early in their careers to achieve excellence within a relatively narrow band of research. Incentives, from funding to academic promotion, reinforce these boundaries. Organizations—from academic departmental structures to research institutes to public sector agencies to professional societies—define a certain scope of interaction and discourse. Outlets like professional journals and conferences by and large line up along traditional lines of disciplines and program interventions. More subtle barriers—like language, psychology, culture, status differences within the sciences, "town and gown" tensions between potential community and academic partners, and academic prejudices—also get in the way of the free flow of ideas and academic traffic that is envisioned by this field.

The good news is these barriers are breaking down at a furious pace. Funding is starting to reward transdisciplinary work in a serious way. Pioneer academics and practitioners—such as those contributing to this book—are conceptualizing the field, creating methods of transdisciplinary work, and training the next generation of scholars and practitioners. Organizational innovation and true partnerships are lagging behind, but the right relationships and conversations are emerging.

So I cannot help but think what the next generation, the second edition of this book, will look like. Let's imagine that transdisciplinary time is like Internet time, and the pace of innovation and change in the field will occur at warp speed. The next edition of this book will not be a collection of individual chapters by individual authors, but rather team written, using a common language and replete with the kinds of innovative models, practice solutions, pedagogies, policy breakthroughs, and organizational inventions that are the promise of the transdisciplinary field. The teams will operationalize the kinds of scholarly, practice, and translational collaborations that are the vision of this book. As Daniel Stokols and his colleagues state in chapter 1 of this first edition in their definition of the field, "scholars *and practitioners* from both academic disciplines *and nonacademic fields work jointly* . . . to yield innovative solutions to particular scientific and societal problems" [emphasis added]. The next generation book will have evidence and evaluation not only of process approaches to transdisciplinarity but also of effective interventions, solutions, and outcomes.

In the meantime this book, *Transdisciplinary Public Health*, has given us the wherewithal to make great and rapid progress in advancing this field. We have new conceptual and definitional clarity and a roadmap for some of our intellectual and practice development, such as in systems science and cross-sector service delivery approaches. We have examples of early success and early innovations across teaching, research, and service delivery applications. Perhaps most important, the book conveys the sense of excitement and energy that this vanguard of academics and practitioners is bringing to this new field.

Edward F. Lawlor

Preface

As public health and social problems have become more complex, the understanding of these problems and the design of solutions to these problems requires both perspectives from multiple disciplines and fields and cross-disciplinary research and practice teams. This need to blur the boundaries between disciplines and between fields, to bring in scholars and perspectives from a range of disciplines, has led to the development of the field of transdisciplinary public health. Transdisciplinary collaborations require the creation of fundamentally new conceptual frameworks, hypotheses, and research strategies that synthesize diverse approaches and ultimately extend beyond them to *transcend* preexisting disciplinary boundaries and ultimately to translate research findings into practical solutions to real-world social problems.

In two path-breaking reports,[1,2] in 2003 and 2006, that respond to the growth of the literature on transdisciplinary methods, the Institute of Medicine reviewed this literature and spoke to the need to expand beyond traditional educational methods that favor unidisciplinary approaches (focusing, for example, on epidemiology, behavioral science, or economics) and that teach students to focus on individual pieces of population health puzzles. These traditional approaches maintain the existing scientific knowledge "silos" that can limit the understanding of complex systems that affect population health. In contrast, transdisciplinary methods hold promise as an effective tool set for problem solving in public health research and practice. However, effective use of these methods requires the development of public health professionals who can understand the interactions among the biological, behavioral, social, and public health sciences; use this knowledge in the development of shared disciplinary frameworks for analyzing health problems; and then improve practice by integrating and evaluating transdisciplinary solutions. Thus, as with any new public health methodology, this approach requires the development of new knowledge and skills and their integration into public health education programs and schools. In the words of the reports:

> The most striking change in public health research in the coming decades is the transition from research dominated by single disciplines, or a small number, to transdisciplinary research. . . . The practical ramifications of the transdisciplinary approach to education are that schools of public health may need to rethink their structure and modes of instruction in

order to develop professionals that can interact synergistically when confronting health concerns. . . . Schools of public health have a primary responsibility for educating faculty, researchers, and senior-level practice professionals. The challenges of the 21st century require an educational approach that is ecological in nature, an approach that emphasizes the determinants of health and their interaction. Education for public health in the 21st century requires cultural competence, and broad new competencies in information technology, communication, and genomics, and a vast reemphasis on practical aspects of training.[1]

Through transdisciplinary research, we can achieve a far greater understanding of how the interactions of social, behavioral, and genetic factors affect health and illness. This knowledge, in turn, will enable major improvements in the well-being of individuals and populations. . . . Many intermediate steps are required, including the training of investigators in transdisciplinary research.[2]

Organization of This Book

Transdisciplinary Public Health: Research, Education, and Practice, provides a roadmap for educating students in public health programs in ways that develop competency in transdisciplinary research and practice. The book is divided into three sections.

Part 1 provides an overview of the concepts and practices involved in designing a public health education program. It begins with a chapter by Daniel Stokols, Kara Hall, and Amanda Vogel titled "Transdisciplinary Public Health: Definitions, Core Characteristics, and Strategies for Success." This chapter provides a foundation by describing transdisciplinary research and practice as it is conceptualized in this book (and currently in the public health research community). The conceptualization reflects the unique characteristics of the approach. This is followed by a description of the four phases that make up a transdisciplinary initiative and the goals and processes that define each phase. This discussion takes into account the roles of individuals, teams, and organizations in carrying out an initiative. Finally, the important factors and characteristics specific to transdisciplinary public health are presented.

In chapter 2, Sarah Gehlert and Teri Browne describe best practices for training a new generation of scholars to function in a transdisciplinary way. They also provide a review of the literature on the components of successful transdisciplinary teams, discuss how this literature is incorporated into model transdisciplinary training programs, and offer recommendations for training.

Designing transdisciplinary education and training requires specific attention to the transdisciplinary competencies and skills needed by students, a subject explored by Lauren Arnold, J. Aaron Hipp, Anne Sebert Kuhlmann, and Elizabeth Budd in chapter 3. Building on the foundations of the previous chapters, they describe transdisciplinary competencies as important guiding principles for public health, and provide steps for ensuring that appropriate transdisciplinary skills are integrated into public health degree programs.

Chapter 4 presents an innovative evaluation framework, created by chapter authors Douglas Luke, Sarah Moreland-Russell, and Stephanie Herbers, that is useful for planning and implementing evaluations of transdisciplinary training programs in public health. This framework can be applied to the evaluation of transdisciplinary initiatives across any institution; it offers objective indices for assessing transdisciplinary training programs and institutional transdisciplinary integration in an academic setting. The chapter also provides an example of one such initiative and recommendations for future evaluations.

The chapters in part 2 address cross-cutting themes underlying transdisciplinary research and practice. They offer readers the opportunity to reorganize individual, team, and organizational thinking and practice around transdisciplinary research and practice, as a means of promoting long-lasting solutions to complex problems in human health. In addition, they present four diverse perspectives on transdisciplinary methods as applied to several public health issues.

In chapter 5, Timothy McBride, Lisa Pollack, Abigail Barker, and Leah Kemper focus on the issue of the social determinants of health, and particularly the role of economic inequality, from a transdisciplinary point of view. They present examples of innovative transdisciplinary theories from public health and economics that are being used to understand the impact of inequality on health, and then they offer a range of new empirical methods, drawn from the burgeoning field of simulation models, that mirror these transdisciplinary theoretical methods in order to illustrate how these methods can be used to understand complex public health problems. Finally, these authors explore how such methods are translated into policy, the final action step of transdisciplinary practice.

The use of law and public policy as prime tools for implementing transdisciplinary research is explored by Sidney Watson in chapter 6. Though such use is not widely understood or explored, Watson argues that law and public policy are at the core of transdisciplinary public health research and practice, and she describes methods that allow lawyers to work more effectively as part of transdisciplinary teams using public policy and law.

Chapter 7, by Bradley Stoner, describes ways in which anthropologists and other social scientists, working as members of transdisciplinary teams, examine cultural perspectives on health and integrate these cultural approaches into interventions designed to minimize health risks.

Finally, Ross Brownson describes integrating evidence-based public health practice into transdisciplinary methods, in chapter 8. He notes that the hallmark of transdisciplinary problem solving is its emphasis on the translation of research findings into practical solutions to social problems—that is, transdisciplinary action research. This requires using evidence-based methods to inform transdisciplinary approaches and translate scientific outcomes into practical applications. This chapter comprehensively addresses the transdisciplinary aspects of each part of the process of acquiring and applying scientific evidence, and the importance of this process to public health education and training.

Parts 3 and 4 introduce six case studies of transdisciplinary methods; these cases were designed to solve real-world problems through classroom learning. The chapters are divided between domestic and international experiences. The three chapters in part 3 focus on current domestic public health issues. In chapter 9, Debra Haire-Joshu explores integrating transdisciplinary methods into an inventive course on the prevention of maternal-child obesity, a major focus of current public health policy. The course demonstrates how to employ transdisciplinary methods while working with home-visiting organizations to prevent obesity, thus operating in a real-world setting.

Chapter 10, by Melissa Jonson-Reid, Nancy Weaver, Brett Drake, and John Constantino, describes a transdisciplinary course on developing approaches to violence and injury prevention in youth. This innovative course incorporates the use of theoretical perspectives from numerous disciplines in solving child maltreatment problems and explores how this learning can lead to new solutions.

Matthew Kreuter and Debbie Pfeiffer then offer, in chapter 11, a description of another innovative course, one that uses transdisciplinary skills to link public health and social service systems in order to promote tobacco control and treatment. Collaborations involving both food stamp offices and tobacco quitlines (telephone counseling) result in a real-world illustration of transdisciplinary problem solving.

The final three chapters, in part 4, present internationally focused courses on malnutrition, water sanitation, and air pollution. First, Lora Iannotti discusses a course that reviews the critical disciplines that should serve as a foundation to transdisciplinary problem solving in relation to global hunger and undernutrition in developing countries. In chapter 12, she shows how students can use these transdisciplinary methods to track the progress of three action domain working groups (in research, programming, and policy), and she offers methods to critically evaluate student performance.

In chapter 13, Ramesh Raghavan, Ravikumar Chockalingam, and Zeena Johar present a fascinating case study of a course implemented in rural India, where students using a transdisciplinary framework developed an understanding of real-life health problems facing communities and found ways to assist these communities in overcoming the problems. Students worked on transdisciplinary teams on one of five assigned public health challenges and integrated insights from a variety of disciplines into solutions, learning how the concepts of social ecology in public health and differing worldviews can be reconciled with the realities of life in the developing world.

Finally, Gautam Yadama, Kenneth Schechtman, Pratim Biswas, Mario Castro, and Nishesh Chalise add a unique perspective to transdisciplinary public health through their description of another intriguing case study, this one focused on the evolving and interlinking trajectories of household energy choices, local ecologies, and rural livelihoods in India. Using this real-world example, the authors offer examples of the transdisciplinary training of the next generation of public health practitioners so that they can effectively address environmental issues affecting the very poor.

Conclusion

This book combines an introduction to transdisciplinary methods and practice with new perspectives on transdisciplinary public health, and applies all this to a description of how these methods can be applied and implemented in public health education and training. The chapter authors offer a range of disciplinary perspectives and contributions, providing real-world examples of the importance of transdisciplinary approaches to public health practice and training.

A challenge to date in the public health profession has been how to effectively and practically apply transdisciplinary concepts to public health education and training. This book presents numerous case studies that address this challenge, along with evaluation of the approaches presented and methods for implementing these approaches. It is intended that readers will discover how to engage in education, policy, and practice that recognize the linkages between and across multiple aspects of our society and its environment, and that they will then be able to integrate these findings across multiple social perspectives and fields of knowledge into solutions that lead to the betterment of the public's health. Transdisciplinary methods represent our best hope for solving complex public health and social problems, and it is crucial that our education programs, now focused largely on unidisciplinary approaches, be developed to incorporate these methods.

Acknowledgments

We would like to acknowledge the invaluable assistance of Lisa Pollack, Kimberly Freels, and Jamie Adkisson. Karen Emmons, Vincent Francisco, Laura

Rasar King, Lynne MacLean, Kenneth R. McLeroy, Robin Lin Miller, and Daniel Stokols provided valuable feedback on the original book proposal. Lynne MacLean and Kenneth R. McLeroy also provided thoughtful and constructive comments on the complete draft manuscript. Thank you to all of these reviewers.

Debra Haire-Joshu and Timothy D. McBride

Notes

1. Gebbie K, Rosenstock L, Hernandez LM; Institute of Medicine, Committee on Educating Public Health Professionals for the 21st Century, eds. Who Will Keep the Public Healthy?: Educating Public Health Professionals for the 21st Century. Washington, DC: National Academies Press; 2003.
2. Hernandez LM, Blazer, DG, eds.; Committee on Assessing Interactions among Social, Behavioral, and Genetic Factors in Health, Board on Health Sciences Policy. Genes, Behavior, and the Social Environment: Moving beyond the Nature/Nurture Debate. Washington, DC: National Academies Press; 2006.

The Editors

Debra Haire-Joshu, PhD, is the Joyce Wood Professor and associate dean for research in the Brown School at Washington University in St. Louis, and holds a secondary appointment with the School of Medicine. She is an internationally renowned scholar of health behavior who develops population-wide interventions to reduce obesity and prevent diabetes, particularly among underserved youth. She directs the Center for Obesity Prevention and Policy Research and the Center for Diabetes Translation Research. Her current research is supported by a number of National Institutes of Health (NIH) agencies—including the National Cancer Institute, the National Institute of Diabetes and Digestive and Kidney Diseases, and the Centers for Disease Control and Prevention—and the Missouri Foundation for Health. Her studies include translation of evidence-based obesity prevention approaches through national organizations. Her work includes the development of a model statewide database for evaluating obesity-related policies in Missouri. This system is now being disseminated to other states across the country. She was recently a member of the Institute of Medicine Committee on Obesity Prevention Policies for Young Children, aged zero to five years. She served as a Health Policy Fellow in the office of Senator Barack Obama and as a Robert Wood Johnson Health Policy Fellow for the Committee on Health, Education, Labor and Pensions when it was chaired by Senator Edward Kennedy. Her work as chair of the Health Policy Committee of the Society of Behavioral Medicine led to her appointment as a Distinguished Fellow of that society. She is also a member of Delta Omega, the honorary society for public health. She has published and presented her research extensively, and reviews for numerous professional journals and NIH research review groups.

  Timothy D. McBride, PhD, is a professor in the Brown School at Washington University in St. Louis, and a health policy analyst and leading health economist shaping the national agenda in rural health care, health insurance, Medicare policy, health economics, and access to health care. He is currently studying the uninsured, Medicare Advantage and Medicare Part D in rural areas, health reform at the state and national levels, access to care for children with special health care needs, and long-term Social Security and Medicare reform. In addition to his scholarly publications in leading journals, he has produced a collection of reports, white papers, and other policy products that have contributed to the national policy debate. He has testified before Congress and consulted with important policy constituents on Medicare and rural health policy. He is a member of the Rural Policy Research Institute Health Panel that provides expert advice on rural health issues to Congress and other policy-makers. He serves as a member of several national committees and boards, including the advisory board of the American Society of Health Economists (ASHE), the editorial boards for the Health Administration Press and the *Journal of Rural Health*, and the methods council for AcademyHealth, and is cochair of the Health Policy Faculty Forum for the Association of University Programs in Health Administration.

The Contributors

Lauren D. Arnold, PhD, MPH, is assistant professor of epidemiology at Saint Louis University, St. Louis, Missouri. Trained in epidemiology, she has a long-standing interest in women's health, chronic disease, and survey research and has conducted work in osteoporosis, vulvodynia, and breast cancer. She seeks to use biomarkers and genomic medicine to add to the understanding of risk stratification and health disparities and to direct prevention and control efforts on the screening, health communication, and policy levels. Her current research involves biomarker studies in multiple myeloma, HPV/cervical cancer vaccination survey work, and an examination of cancer health disparities using data from the American Cancer Society's Cancer Prevention Study II cohort. She also works in health communication, focusing on an exploration of knowledge and perceptions of genomic medicine and how these play a role in community public health and ultimately policy.

Abigail R. Barker, PhD, is a statistical analyst for the Center for Rural Health Policy Analysis, Rural Policy Research Institute at Washington University in St. Louis. She received her PhD degree in economics at the University of Minnesota. Her past work includes econometric modeling of intergenerational poverty, studies of the US- and foreign-born science and technology workforce, and analysis of school-level data on racial and socioeconomic achievement gaps. Her current work focuses on understanding how markets can be successfully integrated into the health care sector, using Medicare Advantage and related data to analyze behavior and simulate outcomes and also incorporating insights from behavioral economics into the modeling process.

Pratim Biswas, PhD, is chairman of the Department of Energy, Environmental and Chemical Engineering at Washington University in St. Louis. He has expertise in aerosol science and engineering, with applications in environmental and energy nanotechnologies. He is interested in technological interventions that eventually lead to protection of public health and also greatly interested in environmental public health—both in terms of the engineered work environment and the natural environment. He has more than twenty-five years of teaching and research experience in this field.

Teri Browne, PhD, is assistant professor of social work at the University of South Carolina. Her research expertise and interests include nephrology social work and the understanding of kidney disease; kidney transplantation, especially in terms of social networks and racial disparity; social work and health care settings; patient navigation; oral medication self-management; African Americans' knowledge and behavior regarding early detection of kidney disease; psychosocial issues of chronic illness, health, and disability; and clinical social work practice and skills.

Ross C. Brownson, PhD, is a professor in the Brown School and School of Medicine at Washington University in St. Louis. A leading expert in chronic disease prevention and an expert in the area of applied epidemiology, he is an intellectual, educational, and practice leader in the field of evidence-based public health. Brownson serves as a member of the faculty advisory council of Washington University's Institute for Public Health, and codirects the Prevention Research Center—a major, CDC-funded center jointly led by Washington University and Saint Louis University—which develops innovative approaches to chronic disease prevention. He leads a large number of other major research and training projects funded by a broad array of federal and foundation sources, including the National Institutes of Health and the Robert Wood Johnson Foundation. He is an associate editor of the *Annual Review of Public Health*, serves on the editorial board of five other journals, and is a board member of the American College of Epidemiology. Active in the American Public Health Association and the Missouri Public Health Association, he is the editor or author of the books *Chronic Disease Epidemiology and Control, Applied Epidemiology, Evidence-Based Public Health*, and *Community-Based Prevention*.

Elizabeth Budd, MPH, is a doctoral student in the Brown School at Washington University in St. Louis.

Mario Castro, MD, MPH, is professor of pediatrics at the Washington University School of Medicine. With a background in research and public health, he is tackling the problem of respiratory disease from two angles. On the research side, he is following children from very early in life and looking at how their genetic, biological, and immune responses and their environment are coming together to cause some of them to develop asthma (NIH RSV Bronchiolitis in Early Life study). He is also studying causes of asthma (through an NIH Specialized Center of Research grant) and what makes severe asthma different from milder forms (Severe Asthma Research Program). He is the lead investigator for two major asthma networks—the NIH Asthma Clinical Research Network and the American Lung Association Asthma Clinical Research Center network—that are studying better ways to treat asthma. On the public health side, he is involved in a number of community-based efforts in St. Louis to improve delivery of asthma care, and to boost awareness of smoking's health effects and respiratory diseases. Through a grant from the CDC, he is leading the Controlling Asthma in St. Louis project. This project aims to build on the collaborations and community-based participatory approach of the St. Louis Regional Asthma Consortium to improve asthma management in a defined urban population with a large and unmet asthma control need. Castro has spent the last seventeen years examining mechanisms of asthma and translating these results to clinical and public applications. This has resulted in ninety scientific articles, reviews, and book chapters.

Nishesh Chalise, BS, is a doctoral candidate and a research assistant in the Social Systems Design Laboratory in the Brown School at Washington University in St. Louis, where he assists with the qualitative data collection and analysis for the National Science Foundation and the Institute of Physics. In an independent study, he is working on a coupled natural and human systems (CNH) project, developing and administering household surveys, analyzing data, and building system dynamic models. He plans to continue conducting research in the CNH field and creating models of these complex interactions.

Ravikumar Chockalingam, MD, MPH, is one of the founders of a community health worker program in rural India, and uses his public health training to help improve health systems in India and beyond. He began working with the IKP Centre for Technologies in Public Health (ICTPH) in the rural Thanjavur district in India, serving as an associate vice president for ICTPH's rural health system. Currently, he is a research assistant at Washington University in St. Louis. He continues to serve ICTPH from St. Louis in an advisory role.

John Constantino, MD, is the Blanche F. Ittleson Professor of Psychiatry and Pediatrics, Washington University in St. Louis, where he conducts a longstanding research program involving the primary prevention of child maltreatment, a program linked to a public home visitation program supported by the State of Missouri. The goal is to develop a feasible and effective public health program for the prevention of child abuse and neglect and also to link it to public mental health and social service systems. Constantino served on and chaired the Missouri Mental Health Commission for four years following his appointment by the state governor in 2004. In his clinical work he has emphasized the mental health care of children in public health settings; this work includes eight years at a psychiatric hospital for children (serving the eastern third of Missouri), and current consulting efforts at Grace Hill and the Family Support Network in St. Louis. Constantino also has a large autism research program in Missouri, where he is involved with public health efforts to improve early identification and appropriate intervention for affected children and their families and directs an ongoing autism prevalence surveillance program funded by the CDC.

Brett Drake, PhD, is a professor in the Brown School at Washington University in St. Louis. He researches matters of child welfare, focusing on early intervention cases of child neglect and the connections between socioenvironmental conditions and child neglect. His current research analyzes census and child protective data to assess the efficacy of protective and preventive services. His research focus and his many years of child welfare practice, at the direct and clinical levels, inform the master's degree–level classes he teaches, which address topics ranging from diversity and human behavior to analysis of practice.

Sarah Gehlert, PhD, is the E. Desmond Lee Professor of Racial and Ethnic Diversity in the Brown School at Washington University in St. Louis; the principal investigator and director of the university's NIH-funded Center for Interdisciplinary Health Disparities Research; and project leader of one of the center's four interdependent research projects. She is also core leader of the Health Disparities and Communities Core of the CDC-funded Chicago Center for Excellence in Health Promotion Economics. She directed the University of Chicago's Maternal and Child Health Training Program from 1992 to 1998 and was principal investigator on a National Institute of Mental Health–funded, community-based study of rural and urban women's health and mental health from 1997 to 2001. She serves on the internal advisory committee of the University of Chicago's Cancer Research Center and on the external advisory committee of the center's Specialized Program of Research Excellence in Breast Cancer, the strategy team of the California Breast Cancer Research Program's Special Research Initiatives, and the Metropolitan Chicago Breast Cancer Mortality Reduction Task Force. Her professional activities also include memberships on the site visit committee of the Social and Behavioral Research Branch of the National Human Genome Research Institute, the professional advisory board of the Epilepsy Foundation of Greater Chicago, the research advisory council of the Epilepsy Foundation of America, and the steering committee of the Washington Park Children's Free Clinic in Chicago. She was chair of the 2007 NIH Summer Institute on Community-Based Participatory Research. Gehlert serves as president-elect of the Society for Social Work and Research, a member of the editorial board of *Research in Social Work Practice*, and a consulting editor for *Social Work Research*.

Kara L. Hall, PhD, is a health scientist, director of the Science of Team Science (SciTS) Team, and codirector of the Theories Project in the Science of Research and Technology Branch, Behavioral Research Program, Division of Cancer

Control and Population Sciences at the National Cancer Institute (NCI). During her career she has participated in a variety of interdisciplinary clinical and research endeavors. Her research has focused on the development of behavioral science methodologies such as the design of survey protocols, meta-analytic techniques for health behavior theory testing, and applications of health behavior theory to multiple content areas and the development of computerized, tailored interventions to foster health promotion and disease prevention behaviors.

Stephanie Herbers, MPH, MSW, is assistant director of evaluation in the Center for Public Health Systems Science, Washington University in St. Louis. She currently serves as an evaluation lead on several projects, including the Missouri Foundation for Health's nine-year Tobacco Prevention and Cessation Initiative and a multistate evaluation of the use of evidence-based guidelines by tobacco control programs. Her research and evaluation interests include mixed-method approaches, program sustainability, capacity building for evaluation, and translation and dissemination of results. In addition to her experience in tobacco prevention and control, she has been involved in the implementation and evaluation of community-based programs for older adults.

J. Aaron Hipp, PhD, is assistant professor in the Brown School at Washington University in St. Louis. His research, teaching, and service are grounded in the theories and scholarship of social ecology, environmental health, and social work and the inherently transdisciplinary investigation of people-in-environment. His novel interests and approach lie with how place, specifically public built environments, affects the people-environment interaction. His research asks how public built environments (parks, communities, streets) both promote and constrain healthy community behaviors and health outcomes. His teaching in geographic information systems, environmental health, public health and the built environment, and research methods focuses on local and global case studies, methodologies, and applications of material to advance student pedagogy. Much of his coursework uses a community-based learning model of applying in-class knowledge and skills to real-world challenges and opportunities.

Lora Iannotti, PhD, is assistant professor in the Brown School at Washington University in St. Louis. Her current research focuses on evaluation and impact modeling of programs addressing undernutrition, infectious diseases, and poverty. In two project sites in Haiti and East Africa, she is studying the combined effects of interventions designed to prevent undernutrition, improve water and sanitation, and foster economic development. She has expertise in the areas of infant and young child nutrition and micronutrient deficiencies (zinc, iron, and vitamin A) affecting resource-poor populations. She is actively involved in developing the global health components of the MPH program at Washington University's Brown School and within the Institute for Public Health.

Zeena Johar, PhD, is president of the IKP Centre for Technologies in Public Health (ICTPH). She obtained her PhD degree from the Swiss Federal Institute of Technology (ETH Zurich) in molecular modeling and design, following receipt of a master's degree in chemistry with a specialization in quantum chemistry from Panjab University. She joined the IKP Trust in 2007 to pursue her passion of translating basic science research into population-based applied research, and she is one of the founding members of ICTPH, a research institute working toward innovating sustainable, replicable, and scalable health care delivery models for rural India. As president she has played an instrumental role in conceptualizing the strategic alignment of ICTPH with the overall mission of the IKP Trust. Johar is currently spearheading the Tanjore Health Systems Pilot, a network of nurse-managed, rural, micro health centers facilitating diagnostic and curative services with a focus on community-based preventive care in conjunction with hamlet-based community health workers. Through supplying primary care coupled with relevant financing that supports critical referral networks and by pricing end-to-end health care delivery, ICTPH aims to provide optimal health outcomes with minimal health expenditure for rural beneficiaries.

Melissa Jonson-Reid, PhD, is a professor in the Brown School at Washington University in St. Louis, where she is coordinator of the school's children, youth, and families concentration and teaches master's degree–level courses on social work in the public school setting, the evaluation of programs and services, and the joint practice of social work and law. She studies outcomes associated with child and adolescent abuse and neglect and is particularly interested in how the relationship between child maltreatment and later educational, health, and sociobehavioral outcomes may be moderated by child welfare and educational services. She also has interests in school social work, early intervention with maltreating families, long-term service use patterns across systems, and the integration of theory with services research. She has practice experience in domestic violence counseling and also school social work, having been a school social worker and administrator with the California public school system, and is active in policy and professional development in school social work on regional and national levels. She currently serves as a program evaluation consultant for school social workers in three school districts, a children's advocacy unit at Legal Services of Eastern Missouri, and various regional child welfare initiatives.

Leah M. Kemper, MPH, is a research analyst at Washington University in St. Louis and a statistical and policy analyst for the Rural Policy Research Institute's Center for Rural Health Policy Analysis. Her research interests include Medicare and Medicaid policy, health reform, the uninsured, and access to health care services and health insurance for rural Americans. She regularly produces policy briefs and papers in these areas and her experience of working with policymakers in multiple states also serves to inform her research. Previously, she held a position as a research coordinator at the Center for Health Policy at Washington University.

Matthew W. Kreuter, PhD, is a professor in the Brown School and director of the Center for Cancer Communication Research, Washington University in St. Louis. A nationally known public health expert in the field of health communications, he also serves as a member of the faculty advisory council of the Institute for Public Health at the university and holds a secondary appointment at the Washington University School of Medicine. Founder and director of the Health Communication Research Laboratory, Kreuter has developed and evaluated a wide range of health communication programs to promote health, modify behavior, and prevent and manage disease. His book *Tailoring Health Messages* is the first comprehensive book on tailored health communication. He currently serves on the Institute of Medicine's Board on Population Health and Public Health Practice. Other funders of his work include the National Institute of Child Health and Human Development, National Institute of Nursing Research, the CDC, the Office of Disease Prevention and Health Promotion, and the Susan G. Komen Breast Cancer Foundation.

Anne Sebert Kuhlmann, PhD, MPH, is assistant dean of public health in the Brown School at Washington University in St. Louis. She teaches public health and social work research methods and program planning and evaluation, as well as an undergraduate course in international public health. She has published on a wide range of issues related to health behavior, including family planning, injury prevention, weight management for pregnant and postpartum women, and HIV prevention in international settings. She also consults on the development, implementation, and evaluation of HIV/AIDS-related behavior change projects.

Edward F. Lawlor is the William E. Gordon Distinguished Professor and dean of the Brown School at Washington University in St. Louis, and founding director of the University's Institute for Public Health. Lawlor's academic and research interests are in access to health care, health care reform, policy analysis, and aging. A national Medicare expert, he is the author of *Redesigning the Medicare Contract: Politics, Markets, and Agency*. Prior to joining the Brown

School in 2004 he served as dean of the School of Social Service Administration and director of both the Center for Health Administration Studies and the graduate program in health administration and policy at the University of Chicago. He is founding editor of the *Public Policy and Aging Report*. For ten years Lawlor was a member and secretary of the Chicago Board of Health, and he has served on numerous policy and advisory bodies in the fields of health care and aging.

Douglas A. Luke, PhD, is professor in the Brown School at Washington University in St. Louis. A leading researcher in the areas of health behavior, organizations, policy, and tobacco control and a top biostatistician and social science methodologist, he has made significant contributions to the evaluation of public health programs, tobacco control and prevention policy, and the application of new methods to community health interventions. He has expanded the repertoire of statistical methods, particularly in the use of social network analysis and hierarchical linear models, in the field of public health. He directs Washington University's Center for Public Health Systems Science, has led the doctoral program at the Saint Louis University School of Public Health, and participates in key community health behavior study decisions at the National Institutes of Health. In addition to advancing the Brown School's public health work, he supervises the work of doctoral students. He is active in the American Statistical Association, the International Network for Social Network Analysts, and the Society for Community Research and Action.

Sarah Moreland-Russell, PhD, is associate director of the Center for Public Health Systems Science, Washington University in St. Louis. She serves as the evaluation lead for Washington University's Institute for Clinical and Translational Science project and the St. Louis County Department of Health's Communities Putting Prevention to Work initiative. She also serves as principal investigator on the User Guide Project, an effort supported by the CDC and designed to translate guidelines from the CDC's *Best Practices for Comprehensive Tobacco Control Programs—2007* into practices and policies to be implemented at state and local levels. Her primary research interests include health policy analysis and evaluation, organizational and systems science and evaluation, and dissemination and implementation of public health policies, research ethics, and health communication among minority and non-English-speaking populations.

Debbie Pfeiffer, MA, is a project manager in the Health Communication Research Laboratory, Washington University in St. Louis. She also serves as project coordinator for the CDC- and NCI-funded Cancer Prevention and

Control Research Network (CPCRN) at the university's Brown School. She has been involved with the CPCRN project and other related projects in the Health Communication Research Laboratory since 2004. Over the past six years, she has been responsible for establishing and developing relationships with community organizations; working collaboratively with community and public health organizations to develop, implement, and evaluate programs that increase cancer awareness among minority and medically underserved populations; and developing and delivering evidence-based training for community organizations. Her research interests focus on cancer prevention and control in the St. Louis Hispanic community and in building community campus partnerships for health.

Lisa M. Pollack, MPT, MPH, is a doctoral student at Washington University in St. Louis. She previously worked as a statistical data analyst for the Rural Policy Research Institute's Center for Rural Health Policy Analysis. Her experience includes measuring and understanding how lack of access to health care adversely affects low-income, underserved populations; examining the impact of health policy on the accessibility and organization of health services; and exploring ways to change policy to improve access to health care. She has coauthored several policy briefs, has made original contributions to the field through peer-reviewed presentations at academic conferences, and has several papers in progress for peer-review publications.

Ramesh Raghavan, MD, PhD, is associate professor in the Brown School and School of Medicine at Washington University in St. Louis, where he teaches courses on mental health policy and advanced statistics in the master's degree program. A psychiatrist and health services researcher by training, he also serves as a faculty associate at the Brown School's Center for Mental Health Services Research and the Washington University Center for Applied Statistics. Previously, he was policy director for the National Child Traumatic Stress Network, and before that he was a Public Health Fellow at the UCLA/RAND Center for Adolescent Health Promotion. His research focuses on mental health services and policies for vulnerable children, especially those in the child welfare system. He has studied the effects of Medicaid and Medicaid managed care on mental health service use, the longitudinal stability of health insurance coverage, and access to mental health care consistent with national standards among children in the child welfare system. His current work focuses on the economics of implementation of evidence-based mental health interventions and on the costs of child maltreatment. His work has received financial support from the Agency for Healthcare Research and Quality, the Administration for Children and Families, the National Institute of Mental Health, and the state of Missouri.

Kenneth B. Schechtman, PhD, is associate professor of biostatistics at the Washington University School of Medicine. An applied statistician with expertise in the design and analysis of clinical trials and with broad experience in the conduct of both small clinical trials and large multicenter clinical trials, especially in the areas of cardiology and exercise physiology, he currently directs all consulting activities in the division of biostatistics. He is director of the biostatistics core of Washington University's Pepper Center, a multifaceted program project studying the effects of exercise and hormone replacement therapy in older adults. In collaboration with the School of Public Health at Saint Louis University, he also directs the biostatistics subcontracts of two NIH-funded randomized trials focused on improving the diet of inner-city youth and on encouraging women to have mammograms. He is actively associated with the data coordinating centers for several multicenter clinical trials and observational studies. Thus he has served as director of biostatistics and data management for the Diltiazem Reinfarction Study and as an investigator or coprincipal investigator at the data coordinating center of the HERITAGE Family Study, the Frailty and Injuries: Cooperative Study of Intervention Techniques, and the Collaborative Longitudinal Evaluation of Keratoconus Study. Schechtman is also the biostatistician for the Protocol Review and Monitoring Committee of the Alvin J. Siteman Cancer Center, directs the biostatistics core of an asthma program project, and is an investigator in a randomized clinical trial focused on exercise following hip fracture.

Daniel Stokols, PhD, is Chancellor's Professor of Social Ecology in the Department of Psychology and Social Behavior and the Department of Planning, Policy and Design and dean emeritus of the School of Social Ecology at the University of California, Irvine. His research interests include the design and evaluation of community and worksite health promotion programs; factors that influence the success of transdisciplinary research and training programs; the health and behavioral impacts of environmental stressors such as traffic congestion, crowding, and information overload; and the application of environmental design research to urban planning and facilities design.

Bradley P. Stoner, MD, PhD, is associate professor of anthropology in Arts & Sciences and associate professor in the Division of Infectious Diseases, School of Medicine, Washington University in St. Louis. His research addresses issues at the interface of anthropology, public health, and medicine. Most recently his work has focused on social and behavioral aspects of sexually transmitted diseases (STDs). Other areas of interest include the study of health care access and decision making, biomedicine as a cultural system, alternative or heterodox medical systems, culture-bound syndromes, and the role of anthropology in clinical and public health research. He is currently conducting research on sociocultural aspects of STD control in developed countries, including analysis of sex partner networks, perception of symptoms and health-seeking responses, concordance and discordance in sexual partnerships, and the ethnography of community risk, and is working with colleagues in medicine and public health using ethnographic approaches to specific issues in STD/HIV transmission. This research has indicated that choice of sex partners within STD networks is not a random occurrence but rather a highly patterned phenomenon that varies by disease. This work draws from advances in epidemiology and mathematical modeling as well as medical anthropology.

Amanda L. Vogel, PhD, MHS, is a behavioral scientist with SAIC-Frederick, Inc., where she provides support to the office of the associate director in the Behavioral Research Program of the National Cancer Institute (NCI) at Frederick. Her research interests lie in three areas: program evaluation related to the implementation and outcomes of both large federal grant programs and community-based health interventions; the science of team science, including interdisciplinary collaborations and community-academic partnerships; and community-engaged scholarship, including community-based participatory research and community-engaged training of health professions students. She has expertise in the use of qualitative methods, including case study, interview, document review, and expert panel methods.

Sidney D. Watson, JD, is professor of health law at Saint Louis University. A specialist in health law and health care access for the poor, she has spent her legal career advocating on behalf of low-income people, both as a legal services lawyer and as a law professor. From 1977 to 1981, she was director of clinical education at Tulane University School of Law, where she founded both Tulane's law clinic and its trial advocacy program. From 1980 to 1987, she was a legal services lawyer in Louisiana and Alaska. In Louisiana she served as managing and senior attorney in the health, welfare, and elderly units of the New Orleans Legal Assistance Corporation and also directed the Farmworkers Legal Assistance Project for migrant and seasonal farmworkers. In Dillingham, Alaska, she was the supervising attorney of the Alaska Legal Services Corporation Bristol Bay office, which served thirty-two native villages. Currently, Watson is advocating for improved access to Medicaid services for people with disabilities and others. A frequent speaker to consumer, disability rights, and children's groups about Medicaid and access to care, she has also written extensively on racial and ethnic disparities in health care, health reform, physicians and charity care, and health care for the homeless. She is the editor of *Representing the Poor and Homeless: Innovations in Advocacy*, and the author of *A Georgia Advocate's Guide to Health Care*, now in its third edition. She is a former member of the American Bar Association's Commission on

Homelessness and Poverty and also served on the National Health Law Program Task Force on Civil Rights and Health Care Reform during the Clinton-era health reform initiative.

Nancy Weaver, PhD, is associate professor of public health at Saint Louis University. She has been active in the areas of injury prevention, physical activity, and health communication for the past fifteen years and formerly directed the research methods and biostatistics core of a National Cancer Institute Center of Excellence in Cancer Communication Research. She has extensive expertise in combining qualitative and quantitative methods, developing measurement tools, and providing technical and training assistance to public health practitioners. Her work is largely multidisciplinary and involves partnerships with state and national agencies, community organizations, and various academic disciplines.

Gautam Yadama, PhD, is associate professor and director of international programs in the Brown School at Washington University in St. Louis. His research interests include micro-institutional strategies of development, social and economic development, international development, and the role of nongovernmental organizations in development. He helps train students to build new research and policy initiatives in order to foster greater participation of underserved populations throughout the world. He also serves as the Brown School's liaison with the Open Society Institute, helping to educate social work professionals and to develop social policy infrastructure in Central Asia and the Caucasus. In addition he is actively engaged with the university community as a member of the steering committee for the McDonnell International Scholars Academy, and he is also the academy's ambassador to Chulalongkorn University in Thailand.

Transdisciplinary
Public Health

Part 1

Defining Transdisciplinary Research and Education

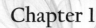
Transdisciplinary Public Health
Definitions, Core Characteristics, and Strategies for Success

Daniel Stokols
Kara L. Hall
Amanda L. Vogel

Learning Objectives

- Understand transdisciplinary approaches in public health.
- Define public health problems using a transdisciplinary approach.
- Describe why and when a transdisciplinary approach is needed.
- Explain how a team-based approach to public health works.
- Explain why working collaboratively with diverse communities and constituencies is important in public health.

•••

The publication of this book reflects the burgeoning interest and investment in cross-disciplinary approaches to scientific questions and societal problems

This work was supported by contract number HHSN-276-2007-00235U. This project was funded, in whole or in part, with federal funds from the National Cancer Institute, National Institutes of Health, under Contract No. HHSN261200800001E. The content of this chapter does not necessarily reflect the views or policies of the Department of Health and Human Services, nor does mention of trade names, commercial products, or organizations imply endorsement by the US government.

in several research domains in recent decades.[1-5] As social problems are inherently complex and multifaceted, their resolution or amelioration often calls for cross-disciplinary research that integrates perspectives from multiple disciplines and fields. Moreover, the translation of science into new and effective programs and policies typically requires the creation of partnerships spanning diverse groups, including academic groups, governmental agencies, nongovernmental organizations (NGOs), and community groups.[6-10] Reflecting these realities, the boundaries between disciplines and fields have become increasingly blurred as scholars and practitioners representing diverse perspectives form scientific and translational teams to work collaboratively at the nexus of their knowledge domains.[11-14] These trends have given rise to a new interdisciplinary field, the *science of team science* (SciTS), which aims to better understand the circumstances that facilitate or hinder effective team-based research and practice and to identify the unique outcomes of these approaches in the areas of productivity, innovation, and translation.[15,16]

The SciTS field includes a special focus on cross-disciplinary, team-based approaches. These approaches aim to draw together the most appropriate conceptual frameworks, theories, and methodological approaches from a variety of disciplines in order to address complex scientific and societal problems most effectively. Disciplines are socially constructed in the sense that large numbers of scholars working in various domains have come to agree over time that particular substantive foci, levels of analysis, and conceptual and methodological tools are associated with particular disciplines (such as physics, biology, sociology, or economics) and professional fields (such as law, business, or medicine). Thus these disciplines emphasize different kinds of knowledge in their subject matter, including particular sets of life, physical, or social science "facts"; their analytical levels range from nano, molecular, and cellular to intrapersonal, organizational, and community perspectives; and each is uniquely associated with particular theoretical and methodological exemplars—for instance, Newtonian and Einsteinian conceptualizations of energy and matter or Freudian and radical behaviorist paradigms or functionalist versus conflict theories of organizations and societies.[17,18]

In this chapter, the term *field* is differentiated from the term *discipline* as defined earlier. A field is a cross-disciplinary area of scientific inquiry or professional practice that focuses on a particular research topic or societal problem. Fields of inquiry and practice encompass multiple disciplinary perspectives that are deemed relevant for understanding a particular research question or societal problem. Examples of fields spanning multiple disciplinary perspectives include public health, urban planning, sustainability studies, and SciTS. The recent growth of cross-disciplinary, team-based research and practice stems from the recognition that whereas disciplines provide useful tools for framing research and practice, approaches derived from a single discipline may not provide the necessary tools to fully understand and address complex scientific and societal problems, particularly when it comes to identifying and understanding multiple interacting causal factors and developing innovative solutions. Thus a variety of new cross-disciplinary fields have arisen in recent decades to provide more integrative, broad-gauged analyses of complex scientific and societal problems.

Scholars have distinguished various forms of cross-disciplinary collaborative research and practice, with the three most commonly identified forms being *multidisciplinary* (MD), *interdisciplinary* (ID), and *transdisciplinary* (TD) collaborations. Some conceptualize MD, ID, and TD modes of research and problem solving as subtypes of cross-disciplinarity that are arrayed along a continuum ranging from lower to higher levels of integration and potential for innovation.[19-22] Accordingly, the MD approach is typically understood as the sequential or additive *combination* of ideas or methods drawn from two or more disciplines or fields to address a problem; the ID approach involves the *integration* of perspectives, concepts, theories, and methods from two or more disciplines or fields to address a problem; and the TD approach entails not only the *integration* of approaches but also the *creation* of fundamentally new conceptual frameworks, hypotheses, and research strategies that synthesize diverse approaches and ultimately extend beyond them to *transcend* preexisting disciplinary boundaries.[2,5,23,24] Another hallmark of a TD approach that distinguishes it from other cross-disciplinary approaches is the emphasis on translation of research findings into practical solutions to social problems, which Hadorn and Pohl[2] refer to as *problems of the life world* and Stokols[8] characterizes as *transdisciplinary action research*.

These proposed distinctions, however, belie some of the complexities involved in differentiating among the MD, ID, and TD modes of inquiry and problem solving. First, each of these forms of cross-disciplinary research and practice can be pursued by individuals working on their own or collaborating with others on a team. Second, MD, ID, and TD approaches rarely occur in isolation from each other. More often, individual scholars or teams of scientists and practitioners transition among them and also engage in unidisciplinary (UD) modes of inquiry during different phases of a single project.[5,25] It may be a challenge to determine when, exactly, an initiative has transitioned from coordination to integration (from MD to ID) or from integration to synthesis, extension, and transcendence (from ID to TD). Third, among scholars of cross-disciplinary research, there is continuing discussion about whether TD is descriptive of a research process or whether it best describes the research outcomes that eventually emerge from projects that may include some blend of MD, ID, and TD processes. Reflecting the blurred boundaries between areas of specialization in cross-disciplinary collaboration, there is a great deal of overlap in the definitions of ID and TD put forward in various federal government funding announcements and guidance documents (see, for example, materials from the National Academy of Sciences,[26] the National Institutes of Health,[27] the National Science Foundation,[28] and the US Department of Health and Human Services[29]).

Despite these definitional complexities, we believe there are practical and scientific benefits to conceptualizing transdisciplinary research and practice as distinct from ID research and practice. First, TD approaches emphasize the generation of novel, often paradigm-expanding or -creating, conceptual frameworks, hypotheses, research designs, and translations of scientific outcomes into solutions to social problems.[21,30] These products may have transformational effects in the realms of theory development, research, and community practice. Introducing students, scholars, and community practitioners to TD approaches inspires high aspirations and offers a frame of reference for encouraging scientists and professionals to achieve the most innovative intellectual and translational advances possible (see, for example, Glass and McAtee;[31] Frumkin[32]). In addition, framing TD research and practice as offering the greatest potential for innovation of all cross-disciplinary methods highlights this method's increased likelihood of producing highly significant and effective scientific outcomes and practical applications.[33,34] For instance, by including the term *transdisciplinary* in the title of its request for applications to establish cancer research and training centers (in tobacco use research, energetics and cancer, health disparities, and cancer communications), the National Cancer Institute conveyed to applicant teams the importance of striving to achieve transformative innovations in the field of cancer prevention and control.[35-39]

Second, the distinctive focus of TD approaches on translating scientific outcomes into practical applications leads to unique team compositions and outcomes. TD teams may include not only scientists from multiple disciplines and fields but also practitioners, policymakers, and community members who together offer a broad array of relevant knowledge and points of view useful for translating scientific findings into improved practices and policies. The goal of translation and the breadth of expertise brought to bear by a TD team maximize the potential for scientific and translational innovations and impact.

To reflect these unique characteristics of the TD approach, we propose the following definition of TD research and practice: *an integrative process whereby scholars and practitioners from both academic disciplines and nonacademic fields work jointly to develop and use novel conceptual and methodological approaches that synthesize and extend discipline-specific perspectives, theories, methods, and translational strategies to yield innovative solutions to particular scientific and societal problems.*

This definition highlights the emphasis on integration and innovation in TD initiatives. There are two main forms of TD integration: horizontal and vertical. *Horizontal integrations* involve the linkage of disciplines at similar levels of analysis, such as an integration of the genetic perspective of biology and the molecular perspective of chemistry. *Vertical integrations* bridge knowledge domains associated with different analytical levels, such as an integration of the intrapersonal perspective of psychology and the societal perspective of urban planning. TD integration can occur in a variety of ways over the course of a TD collaboration, based on the specific needs that emerge in that collaboration given its target problem, team membership, and goals. For example, integration might be reflected in novel conceptual frameworks, research goals, or translational advances. It might result in methodological innovations as well, such as the application of research approaches and methods from one discipline to address research questions grounded in a very different discipline. In sum, TD integration can occur in both the substantive content and methodological approaches of a collaborative initiative, and in both the research and translational phases. We will return to these forms of TD integration later in this chapter, in the section outlining strategic guidelines for TD public health.

In this section we defined TD research and practice and identified key features that distinguish the TD approach from other cross-disciplinary approaches. In the next section we describe the distinctive processes involved in implementing TD collaborations. In the subsequent section, we describe characteristics of the TD approach that are specific to the public health context. Finally, we close with a discussion of key challenges and emerging directions related to the pursuit of TD public health and with our developing understanding of the value of this approach.

The Four Phases of a TD Initiative

We conceptualize TD research and practice as having four relatively distinct phases—*development, conceptualization, implementation,* and *translation* (figure 1.1). This proposed conceptualization builds on and extends conceptualizations of TD offered by other scholars (Aboelela et al.,[19] Hadorn et al.,[2] Kessel et al.,[20] Lawrence and Despres,[23] TD-Net,[40] Wagner et al.,[22] and Wickson et al.[24]). Briefly, the development phase involves the formation of a team of collaborators and the initial steps toward developing a joint research initiative, including establishing a shared understanding of the problem definition and the mission of the group. The conceptualization phase involves collaborative teamwork to develop research questions or hypotheses and a research design that reflect the integrative nature of the initiative. The implementation phase involves the execution of the planned research, and the translation phase applies research findings toward the development of an innovative solution to the real-world problem.

These four phases of a TD initiative are generally sequential, and the processes and outcomes generated during each phase influence those that

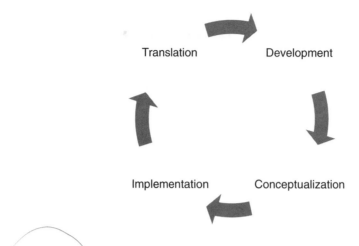

Figure 1.1. Four phases of a transdisciplinary initiative

occur in subsequent phases. However, the four phases also may be recursive, or iterative. For example, insights that emerge during the second through fourth phases may lead to midproject changes in the composition of the TD team formed during the first phase, in order to bring in additional areas of expertise. In addition, preliminary outcomes in the third phase may lead to the production of new research questions and hypotheses, expanding the conceptual work done in the second phase. This recursive process also applies to multiple related scientific and practical initiatives.[8,41] For example, once new knowledge is generated or a novel conceptual framework is developed, it serves as the state-of-the-science example for subsequent research, training, and translational innovations. In addition, findings from community problem-solving efforts may prompt refinements in existing theoretical frameworks and occasionally give rise to entirely new frameworks[13,42] as well as new research endeavors. This occurs, for example, when a city council's or non-governmental organization's efforts to address a particular social or health problem prompt subsequent scientific research in collaboration with university-based scholars.

Goals and Processes in Each TD Initiative Phase

Each of the phases of a TD initiative has specific goals and distinctive team processes (table 1.1). During the development phase, key goals are to identify the scientific or societal problem of interest as well as the disciplines, fields, and areas of practice relevant to addressing the problem. This work may be done by a core group of collaborators, who then work to recruit additional team members with expertise in the necessary knowledge domains and with

Very GOOD incorporate into team project

Table 1.1. Goals and processes of the four phases of a transdisciplinary initiative

	Development	Conceptualization	Implementation	Translation
Goals	Identify the scientific or societal problem and the disciplines, fields, and areas of practice relevant to understanding and addressing it. Form a diverse team of scientists, professionals, and community members possessing these areas of expertise.	Develop novel research questions, hypotheses, a conceptual framework, and research methods that integrate and extend approaches from multiple disciplines and fields.	Execute the planned research. Create refinements and additions to the research questions, hypotheses, and methodological approaches as needed to maximize the effectiveness and innovative nature of the initiative.	Apply research findings to develop innovative solutions to real-world problems.
Processes	Develop a shared understanding of the target problem and team mission. Learn the relevance of all team members' expertise to the target problem, and begin to develop a shared vocabulary.	Use team processes and the institutional environment to promote innovation and integration.	Engage in a reflective process to intermittently assess and enhance activities, retaining an integrative approach.	Support sustained participation of the broad team of collaborators, including both scientists and practitioners.

a diverse array of substantive, methodological, and practical knowledge. A TD team's developmental processes are likely to benefit when members include not only scientists but also professionals and members of local stakeholder groups—including practitioners, policymakers, and citizens—who represent several spheres of community practice and whose diverse perspectives can enrich the development of translational applications to particular community problems.[7,43]

Once assembled, team members begin the initial processes that will move them toward collaborative integration and cohesion. Key processes in this phase include developing a shared mission and goals for the particular collaboration and devoting time as a group to establishing an understanding of each member's unique knowledge sets, based on his or her disciplinary or professional training and scientific and practice experiences.[44] To be successful, team members must first understand and acknowledge differences in their perspectives and values, and then they can move on to find common ground and shared values that can be a foundation for their ongoing collaboration.

Another critical process during this phase is to develop a shared vocabulary that spans or transcends team members' unique backgrounds and can be used by members to communicate with one another about their joint initiative. This shared vocabulary begins to emerge during conversations to develop shared goals and learn about one another's areas of expertise. Communication strategies such as the use of analogies and lay language in lieu of discipline-specific jargon help to bridge the gaps between disciplines and fields, as well as the gap between scientists and practitioners, during this early phase of collaboration.[45] As the team moves into the next phase, members may develop new language for key concepts in their collaborative endeavor.

The goals of the conceptual phase are to develop novel ideas, hypotheses, research questions, and research methods that integrate the perspectives and knowledge domains of the team members, enabling them to address the target problem in innovative ways. A hallmark of success in this phase is the development of a conceptual framework that integrates approaches from a variety of disciplines and fields, potentially extending beyond them to introduce previously unthought-of associations and hypotheses.

Processes involved in this phase focus on integrating team members' perspectives and knowledge domains relevant to the target problem in order to develop novel research approaches. The involvement of team members with diverse perspectives is essential to producing TD innovations. Members with varying expertise introduce a breadth of perspectives, and when integrated, these diverse views are more likely to produce new research directions than are the views produced by more homogeneous teams. During the dialogue that is necessary to produce a research program that reflects the integration of multiple disciplinary perspectives, more diverse teams are more likely to engage in debate.[46] Debate can best lead to creative outcomes when premature consensus is avoided.[47]

Team processes are crucial to the success of the conceptual phase. The presence of multiple effective avenues for communication encourages and supports freedom of expression, promotes creativity, actively encourages the integration of perspectives and approaches, and is critical to supporting the challenging work of synthesizing knowledge domains.[47] Also critical are team and institutional environments that explicitly support integrative approaches, risk taking, and cross talk among colleagues from different departments, institutions, and agencies. Outcomes of this phase may include the creation of novel ideas, hypotheses, and conceptual models; new research programs with innovative integrative designs; and related grant proposals (see, for example, Northwestern University Clinical and Translational Sciences Institute[48]).[8]

During the implementation phase, the focus is on executing the planned research. During this time, team members also, ideally, engage in a reflective process in which they intermittently assess and refine their approaches. This enables the team to revise or create additional research questions and hypotheses and refine data collection and analysis approaches. It is optimal if, during this process, team members retain an integrative perspective. As the collaboration continues and participants both deepen their understanding of the target problem and learn more about one another's areas of expertise and how this knowledge applies to the problem, they may begin to see new research avenues and translational opportunities. They may also identify a need to bring in new team members with different areas of expertise in order to pursue these new research and translational opportunities. New team members who join during this phase may help to refine existing research questions and methods or add new ones, thereby leading to additional innovations in the team's approaches. Outcomes of the implementation phase include shared databases; completed data collection, analysis, and interpretation; empirical discoveries; inventions in research and practice; scholarly publications; and the integration of new knowledge into TD curricula and training resources.

Finally, the goals of the translation phase are to apply research findings to develop innovative approaches to effectively addressing real-world problems. This phase involves the sustained participation of the broad team of collaborators, as the participation of both scientists and practitioners is needed to maximize the success of translational activities. TD scholars and practitioners often have divergent opinions and expectations of each other's status as team members and about the goals and intended outcomes of translational research.[6] Consequently, it is essential that TD researchers and scholars develop shared understandings about these and other issues at the outset of their collaboration. These conditions are necessary to produce the intervention designs, timetables, and action plans that are intended near-term outcomes of the translational phase of TD collaboration. Also, depending on the specific goals and intended deliverables of their partnership, team members may need to work together to establish evaluative criteria and methodologies for assessing the near- or longer-term societal impacts of their proposed programs and policies. Possible outcomes of this phase include the emergence of new structures of multisector collaboration that are sustained even after a funded research project has ended (see, for example, Shen[49]); innovations in existing programs and policies enacted at state, national, and international levels; or entirely new programs and policies; and more distally, demonstrable improvements in the social conditions affected by these innovations, such as positive changes in population health, social justice, or environmental quality (see, for example, Breslow and Johnson[50]).

Influence of Individual, Team-Based, and Organizational Factors

Each phase of a TD initiative influences all the others, and at the same time, the TD process as a whole is influenced by multiple overlapping conditions—including individual team members' characteristics, team-based traits, and organizational contexts—each of which can exert substantial influences on the way that collaboration plays out and, as a result, on the ultimate success of the TD initiative.

At the individual level, team members' values and perspectives, assumptions about the validity of research methods and findings, attitudes about individual versus team pursuits, and opinions of and experiences with cross-disciplinary approaches all influence their activities within the team and, as a result, team dynamics.[51]

Team-based traits, including team structures (for example, hierarchical versus nonhierarchical), work routines and processes, group attributes, and available infrastructure and resources (such as shared databases or shared work space and facilities), shape the ultimate effectiveness of the team in working through the four phases and achieving the ultimate goals of integration, innovation, and transformative solutions (see, for example, Fiore,[52] Katzenbach and Smith[53]). Team-based work routines and processes include the frequency of in-person versus distance interactions among team members, as well as the availability and quality of the cyber-infrastructure and the frequency with which it is used for electronic collaboration.[25,54-56] Team attributes such as leadership structures and styles, shared goals and norms, decision-making strategies, and individualized versus interdependent incentive structures for collaboration and performance have also been found to exert strong influences on the effectiveness of TD teams (see, for example, Paletz and Schunn,[57] Stokols et al.[58]).

TD teams often include members from different organizational units, such as different departments or research centers within a university, or from different organizations entirely, such as universities, businesses, not-for-profit organizations, and governmental agencies. Each of these organizational contexts brings to bear its own set of expectations and priorities, which may support or impair an individual's participation in a TD team.[59,60] In addition, TD teams may be nested within consortia or networks, such as those created through grant initiatives, which introduce another layer of influences on team processes. Additional aspects of the organizational context that strongly influence collaborative dynamics include factors such as organizational leaders' support or lack of support for team-based and cross-disciplinary initiatives,[61] and formal policies, such as tenure and promotion policies, that do or do not reward team-based work in a manner equivalent to individual work.[30]

Emergent States Important to TD Success

The aforementioned team-based factors affect most collaborative research and practice initiatives. There are specific qualities or states of collaborative teams, however, that are particularly relevant to TD collaborations because of the influence they have over the processes necessary to achieve syntheses and extensions of preexisting discipline- and field-based approaches and to produce innovative research and practice outcomes. Emergent states arise in teams when representative dynamic attitudes, values, cognitions and motivations, or other particular team qualities *emerge* through the team experience.[62] Three particularly potent emergent states in TD research and practice are critical awareness, psychological safety, and transactive memory systems.

Critical awareness describes an understanding among team members that all disciplines and fields, including their own, have substantive and methodological strengths and limitations.[63-65] It also describes an awareness of the strengths and limitations of integration, given these circumstances. Ideally, critical awareness is combined with a strong grounding in one or more disciplinary traditions, including familiarity with those traditions' theoretical and methodological approaches as well as their overall strengths, limitations, and blind spots.[63,65] The combination of these abilities enables team members to consider and identify the potential contributions of other disciplines, fields, and areas of practice in order to effectively address the target problem.[65] It also helps to eliminate bias toward a particular disciplinary approach, which can limit the quality and novelty of new research and translational directions. Ultimately, these abilities empower the team to produce the highest quality, most innovative approach to the target problem.[64] Critical awareness also enables team members to stay goal oriented, remaining focused on solving the research or practical problem at hand using the variety of available approaches, rather than becoming deadlocked over the disciplinary approach that should be pursued.[63]

Critical awareness among most or all of the members of a TD team enables processes necessary to integrative approaches, such as discussions that weigh the relative merits and weaknesses of various discipline- and field-based approaches that explicitly address the challenges and processes involved in the task of integration and also potentially collaborative benefits and synergies.[64] By recognizing the limitations of their own customary approaches, team members may be better able to work integratively to produce an approach that transcends the limitations of the participating disciplines and fields.

Psychological safety within the team,[66] also called intragroup safety,[67] is what team members experience when they believe that the team environment is a safe place to express independent thoughts and opinions and even divergent assumptions about the nature of varied research approaches[14] and that they need not fear embarrassment, rejection, or punishment. In teams representing particularly different areas of expertise and knowledge—such as teams that include scientists from both the social and biological sciences along with practitioners, policymakers, and community members—team members may feel their expertise is not understood, acknowledged, or valued. In addition, members of diverse teams may fear that they may appear uninformed or that their ideas may be misinterpreted by colleagues with different disciplinary values and terminologies. All these factors may affect team members' ability to engage in the group processes needed to produce integration and innovation.

Psychological safety in the team helps support the same collaborative processes that are supported by critical awareness and that are necessary to achieve the integrative and innovative outcomes that distinguish TD initiatives, including weighing the relative merits of different disciplinary approaches to the target problem. Psychologically safe team environments promote active listening and discussions that are characterized by open sharing of ideas and mutual respect. These characteristics, in turn, foster co-learning and productive work toward developing novel, integrative ideas.

Finally, *transactive memory systems* refer to team members' shared awareness of each individual member's expertise, knowledge, and skills.[68] Teams begin to develop these transactive memory systems in the developmental phase of the TD initiative, as members learn about one another's areas of expertise and the relevance of these areas to the joint endeavor. Transactive memory systems continue to deepen and expand as teams progress through the four phases of the initiative. These systems can enhance team performance throughout these phases[44] by supporting the interactive processes that lead to the generation of integrative conceptual models, research questions, hypotheses, and research methods. In addition, transactive memory systems may facilitate team coordination activities, including division of responsibilities and knowledge transfer, which can lead to more successful research outcomes.[69] These coordination activities also reinforce transactive memory systems by formalizing knowledge about the expertise and skill sets possessed by each team member and making that knowledge more visible. The addition or departure of team members and the development of new expertise by existing team members require that transactive memory systems be updated. Regular interaction among group members, including planned opportunities to learn about existing and new expertise on the team, can ensure that team members' transactive memory systems remain up to date and include the unique characteristics, roles, and knowledge recently acquired.

Characteristics of TD Public Health

As other scholars have noted (see, for example, Hadorn et al.,[2] Klein,[5] Lawrence and Despres,[23] Neuhauser et al.,[43] Carew and Wickson[70]), the conceptualization of TD research and practice is enriched when it is contextualized; that is, when it is related to a particular set of scientific questions and societal problems, such as those addressed by a particular discipline or field. In this section, we discuss TD approaches within the specific context of public health.

An important characteristic of public health is the field's inherently multidisciplinary structure, which is reflected in the five areas of emphasis required of all accredited training programs in public health: biostatistics, epidemiology, environmental health science, health policy and management, and social and behavioral sciences.[71] MD fields such as urban planning and urban studies similarly encompass several disciplines within their scholarly, educational, and problem-solving missions. Much of the training and research in those fields reflects interdisciplinary and transdisciplinary as well as multidisciplinary approaches.[72,73] Moreover, many public health graduate courses and also research and translational programs emphasize ID integration of concepts, methods, and data among, but not limited to, the five core areas of emphasis included in accredited training programs. This overarching emphasis on MD and ID approaches establishes a reference point for scholars' and practitioners' work to achieve solutions to public health problems.

Added Value of a TD Public Health Approach

Given the highly integrative nature of the field of public health, it seems reasonable to ask what added value there is in encouraging public health scientists to move beyond the already prevalent MD and ID approaches to achieve TD approaches. In this section, we attempt to answer this question. We start by invoking the analogy of a geographical landscape. The current landscape of public health research and practice is defined by varied methodological and knowledge domains drawn from different disciplines and fields. These diverse domains, comparable to the varied regions of a country, can perhaps provide fertile ground for building collaborative partnerships and projects spanning several health-related disciplines. The diversity of this public health landscape provides opportunities for cross-disciplinary research and practice that are considerably greater than those found in fields that are more *discipline-centric*, such as the field of sociology, which faces interdisciplinary challenges.[74]

The potential for moving from ID integration to TD innovations that transform public health research and practice increases when scholars and practitioners begin to envision, and to actively pursue, new regions and more transformative forms of partnerships within the public health landscape. It is the divergence or tension between the *existing landscape* comprising prior and ongoing public health scholarship on the one hand and the *futurescape* comprising potential integrative opportunities envisioned by scholars and practitioners on the other that fuels transformative TD innovations in science and translation. In the field of landscape ecology, the term *futurescape* refers to "landscapes of the future that may be so far from our current landscape visions that they seem fantasy."[75] TD approaches are distinct from ID approaches owing to their potential not only to synthesize but also to extend current conceptualizations and thus to lead scholars and practitioners into unexplored terrain that may redefine the map of the public health landscape and transform public health research and practice. As these new regions of the public health landscape are discovered, they establish new understandings of what cutting-edge or highly innovative research and practice is, and they act as reference points for judging subsequent innovations. As a result, the leading edge of both research and practice continues to be pushed forward, while past innovations are gradually adopted and institutionalized. TD approaches have the potential to accelerate the pace of this forward progress in both research and practice.

Examples of TD Public Health Research and Practice

Over the last two decades, conceptualizations of public health research and practice have become increasingly interdisciplinary, and in some cases, transdisciplinary. Exemplifying this trend are the *social ecological models* of public health problems that have emerged in recent years (see, for example, Green et al.[76]).[77-80] These models offer a *broad conceptual scope* and *holistic, integrative orientation*, often combining concepts from multiple fields and disciplines in ways that address multiple levels of analysis and create previously unexplored intersections of widely varied knowledge domains. For example, ecological theorists have drawn connections among societal conditions of urban sprawl, physical activity patterns, and population health.[9,81-83] Other scholars have documented the separate and joint influences of environmental racism, air pollution, substandard housing, lack of social cohesion in neighborhoods, and the psychological sequelae of poverty to explain the ways in which health disparities and low socioeconomic status "get under the skin" to engender a wide range of health problems.[84-90] Still others have investigated the influences of the natural (nonbuilt) environment on population health,[32,91,92] as well as the joint impacts of psychological, sociocultural, economic, and biological factors on the etiology of chronic and infectious diseases (see, for example, Cassel[93]).[94-96] Some of the ecological analyses and empirical studies noted here have included in a single conceptual model individuals' genetic heritage and health behaviors; family, neighborhood, and community-level circumstances; population health characteristics; and health care expenditures. The social ecological models underlying these and many other studies have created numerous new opportunities for TD collaborations in public health research and practice.

Overview and Strategic Guidelines for TD Public Health

In this section, we return to the major themes presented in this chapter in order to highlight their practical implications, specifically as related to strategies for successful TD initiatives and lessons for the evaluation of TD initiatives. We then envision the broad outcomes of TD approaches for the advancement of research and practice. Finally, we consider emerging directions and challenges for TD public health, including the specification of criteria for gauging the novelty and assessing the outcomes of TD research and translational innovations.

Strategies for Successful TD Initiatives

We began this chapter by defining TD public health and highlighting the attributes that distinguish TD approaches from other cross-disciplinary approaches. TD approaches include unique goals for both the processes and outcomes of research, namely to transcend the boundaries among disciplines and fields in order to create innovative approaches that integrate and build upon the most promising approaches, wherever they may have originated, with the ultimate goal of producing practical solutions to real-world problems. This three-part emphasis on integration, innovation, and practical solutions sums up the essence of the TD approach and is also at the root of the four interrelated phases of a TD initiative that we have described in this chapter.

Each of the four phases of a TD initiative is crucial to its overall success. For instance, the development phase is vital to ensure that the right team members are included in order to maximize the innovative potential of a research and practice initiative. The absence of team members with knowledge in areas of science and practice particularly relevant to the target problem can produce an initiative that more closely resembles a UD approach. Alternatively, the absence of team members with skills specific to integrating approaches from multiple domains—such as strong knowledge in two or more disciplines and the critical awareness necessary to consider the strengths and weaknesses of approaches from varied disciplines—can hinder integration and produce an initiative that resembles an MD or ID approach. In a reflection of the importance of team building, universities are increasingly investing in faculty members and organizational units dedicated to supporting the development of research teams.[26,97] In addition, in 2010 the National Organization of Research Development Professionals was established to develop and operate programs that facilitate cross-disciplinary, team-based research and reduce administrative and institutional constraints on these scientific approaches.[98]

The conceptual phase affords team members dedicated time to collaborate in developing novel ideas, hypotheses, research questions, and methodological approaches. Recognizing the importance of this phase, funding agencies have created dedicated financial support for the formation of teams and the team processes necessary to develop integrative research questions, hypotheses, and conceptual frameworks.[99,100] For the success of the implementation phase, adequate support is needed—at the levels of the team, academic institution, and funding institution—for continued team collaboration to implement the research plan, revise it as needed, and pursue emerging research directions. Finally, the translation phase is crucial to achieving the ultimate goal of a TD initiative—to create solutions to real-world problems. Only by including practitioners in the TD team, from the early stages of the initiative, can this goal be fully realized within the initiative's context. Although research findings can be translated into practice by other teams, at other times, and at other geographical locations, TD initiatives aim to incorporate immediate application to real-world problem solving, and the inclusion of practitioners in the team enables this final phase.

It is important to recognize that each of the four phases of a TD project requires team members to invest considerable time and other resources if they are to fully engage in key processes within each phase to achieve the most collaborative outcomes. The recent emergence of funding to support the first two phases of a TD initiative—which supplements longer-standing funding for TD research implementation—is now enabling teams to dedicate the necessary time to these foundational phases of a TD initiative.

As described earlier in this chapter, multiple overlapping factors influence the likelihood that TD initiatives will engage successfully in processes essential to developing integrative, innovative approaches and achieving the team's major scientific and translational goals. These include both scientific challenges and practical factors, such as characteristics of TD team members, team processes, conditions in the organizational and institutional environments where team members are located, and infrastructure and support—or lack thereof—in related funding. Each of these influences has the potential to introduce challenges or barriers to engaging in TD processes or to provide support for these processes.

A scientific challenge for all efforts at integration, whether horizontal or vertical, is how to balance concerns of breadth versus depth. Teams should strive to identify the key goals they hope to achieve through integration and synthesis of concepts, and work toward them while also retaining the integrity of the original discipline- or field-based approaches and promoting the synthesis necessary to innovate. Concerns about potentially superficial results from trying to address and integrate highly disparate knowledge domains spanning scholarly and community practice contexts can best be addressed by keeping a dual focus, seeking both to create innovative and practical outcomes and to retain the integrity of the approaches that are synthesized.

With regard to nonscientific influences on success, challenges at one level often can be addressed successfully at another level. For example, although it sometimes is the case that members of a TD team have competing rather than complementary goals related to their participation, team processes can help to accommodate these discrepancies so that teams are still able to meet their collective goals. Also, whereas a larger number of participating institutions and organizations can impose a wider array of bureaucratic and administrative challenges, institutional policies and procedures that support collaboration across institutions and organizations can facilitate TD team science. Furthermore, these multi-institutional collaborations have the capacity to integrate a broader range of intellectual, material, and financial resources, which can better support success in TD initiatives. If care is taken—by team leaders and members, participating institutions and organizations, and funders of TD initiatives—to develop team processes and institutional environments that support the processes central to each of the four phases of TD research, success is more likely.[69]

Lessons for Evaluation of TD Initiatives

The overall goals of a TD initiative not only lay the foundation for the goals and processes in each of its four phases but also provide benchmarks and indicators of success that can structure process and outcome evaluations of that initiative. The goals and process we identified in each of the four phases of a TD initiative also provide reference points for evaluation efforts. They can be used for process evaluations, ideally with feedback loops that can support quality improvement during the course of the initiative. Evaluation that examines processes and outcomes within each phase can help to identify whether a team is engaging in all the processes necessary to fully realize the goals of its TD initiative, identify areas where the team could benefit from technical assistance, and support obtaining enhanced quality of assistance. Toward the end of a TD initiative, evaluation can help to explain potential reasons why particular initiative goals were met. For example, process evaluations may be able to assess whether or not team members effectively implemented the core phases and processes of a TD initiative and achieved the phase-specific outcomes over the course of their collaboration, or whether their teamwork might be more accurately characterized as a UD, MD, or ID effort.

In addition to process factors, evaluations of TD initiatives can assess a wide variety of near- and far-term scientific and translational outcomes, which may occur over years or decades and at multiple scientific and societal levels. Outcomes to be examined include integration, innovation, and the ultimate scientific or societal value of an initiative, as measured by its varied impacts on programs, policies, and ultimately the public's health.

Assessments of such varied and complex outcomes introduce certain conceptual and methodological complexities, such as how to establish criteria for both defining and measuring success in each of these outcomes. A helpful rule of thumb in evaluations of innovation is to compare outcomes to such elements of the preexisting research or practice context as conceptualizations and theories, methodological approaches, empirical knowledge, and best practices, as well as to emergent opportunities for conceptual, methodological, and translational advances that have not yet been fully achieved.[70]

Multimethod evaluation approaches that use a wide variety of quantitative and qualitative data sources reflecting different discipline- and field-based perspectives to assess outcomes at varying points in time are most likely to thoroughly capture and characterize results of a TD initiative. Multimethod approaches may include, for example, observations and reports of team processes; objective indices of team productivity such as number of papers published, the caliber of the journals publishing these papers, and number of additional grants obtained to build on the research or practice endeavor; and peer-experts' subjective appraisals of the degree of cross-disciplinary integration and the level of innovation and possible transformative impact, as demonstrated in team products such as publications, research proposals, and community problem-solving strategies.

Multimethod approaches have been used in recent evaluation studies to measure TD processes and outcomes and to compare them to their UD, MD, or ID counterparts.[51,101] Criteria for gauging the degree of TD innovation and conceptual departures from the existing landscape of public health research and practice include (1) the number of analytical levels vertically bridged through a particular collaboration and reflected in the products of that work,[102] (2) the number of distinct disciplinary or epistemological perspectives integrated in a particular research or translational project,[25,103] (3) peer subjective appraisals of the novelty and transformative impact on science and society associated with a TD innovation,[104] and (4) evidence for the creation of fundamentally new concepts, research methods, or translational best practices that depart from and improve on the current landscape of public health research and practice, as discussed earlier in this chapter. These multiple criteria can be applied to both processes and outcomes of a TD collaboration as they emerge during the conceptual, research, and translational phases of TD action research.

The articulation of criteria for judging the novelty and translational value of TD innovations is a key challenge that must be addressed by each team in the context of its research and translational goals and the state of the art in its particular area of inquiry. The evaluation of translational outcomes of TD collaboration, in particular, poses a distinctive set of challenges relative to assessing outcomes associated with TD development, conceptualization, and implementation. First, long timelines are typically required to assess the value and impacts of translational innovations (for example, new community programs, clinical practices, or public policies). Moreover, securing multiyear funding to assess both mid- and longer-term outcomes of TD translations is becoming increasingly difficult, particularly during an era of budgetary constraints. One strategy for evaluating the outcomes of TD collaborations is to incorporate annual archival data (pertaining, for example, to team publication rates and changes in public health outcomes in particular communities) into longitudinal, time series designs that assess changes in community outcomes.[101] These extended time series research designs that incorporate publicly available data on scientific, community, and societal outcomes have the added advantages of being unobtrusive (for example, by avoiding direct surveys and interviews of community members) and, in many cases, anchored in substantial data sets that are gathered routinely by research, governmental, and community organizations.

Envisioning the Broader Outcomes of TD Approaches

In addition to the focus on creating practical solutions to real-world problems, one outcome of collaborative, interdisciplinary TD processes is that TD initiatives typically take a holistic, systems approach. Systems thinking is an approach to problem solving that situates problems in holistic systems with complex interacting factors that exert influences on one another.[105] It proposes that efforts to solve a complex problem require identifying and considering the array of factors that may interact in a complete system to produce the problem, factors that may in turn be subjected to interventions to solve the problem. In the field of public health, system approaches consider factors from multiple areas of science, including biological, behavioral, environmental, and socioeconomic factors, in attempts to identify the causes of and solutions to public health problems. TD approaches are ideally suited to supporting systems-level research and solutions to public health problems.

These approaches are also one means of speeding progress toward practical solutions to public health problems, as they produce scientific inquiries that consider and include interacting factors from a wider range of disciplines and fields than are typically examined in other approaches. These inquiries can therefore produce findings with implications for a range of fields and produce expansive applications to practice that address a variety of factors in the system of interest. In contrast to UD research, which involves a slow, iterative approach that remains bounded within a single disciplinary area, TD research initiatives with a systems perspective can produce dramatic advances in a shorter period of time. They can also identify potential needs to explore entirely new and fruitful research directions that may be outside of the realm of any one discipline, and thus test new relationships, pathways, and paradigms.

Different areas of science and practice are typically dissimilar in their development and maturation. For established areas of inquiry, the systematic boundaries and dynamics of the target phenomena may be clearly delimited and defined, along with the particular disciplines and fields that are deemed to be the essential for understanding the scientific or societal problems at hand. In other newly emerging areas of science and practice, potential causal factors that influence and explain the major target problems and those disciplines most relevant to their analysis and resolution have yet to be identified. Clearly defining the problem to be addressed and understanding the state of the science related to that problem can help a TD team to identify the next set of research questions, or the next set of practical goals, that should be pursued and also the disciplines and fields that should be engaged in that pursuit. For instance, problem domains in which challenges still exist related to basic measurement or in which knowledge is still highly limited may not be ready for the development of translational solutions. For example, although there is burgeoning interest in personalized medicine, which tailors treatments to individuals based on their unique genetic and demographic profiles, knowledge must first be gained about the genetic markers that would be of most benefit in this approach. TD public health research and practice cannot circumvent fundamental gaps in the knowledge about a particular problem area, but they can facilitate progress toward practical solutions by creating more holistic, comprehensive analyses of and solutions to complex health problems at community, national, and global levels.

Summary

The increase in interest in cross-disciplinary approaches to scientific questions and the need to solve societal problems is leading to a demand for cross-disciplinary research that integrates perspectives from multiple disciplines and fields. Reflecting this demand, scholars and practitioners are increasingly working collaboratively in scientific and translational teams that produce team-based research and practice. The recent growth of cross-disciplinary, team-based research and practice stems from the recognition that single disciplines may not provide the necessary tools to fully understand and address complex scientific and societal problems, particularly as related to identifying and understanding multiple interacting causal factors and developing innovative solutions. This chapter has outlined the practical and scientific benefits of the transdisciplinary approach to research and practice. It has also described the distinctive processes involved in implementing transdisciplinary collaborations, the unique characteristics of the TD approach in the public health context, the emerging directions for pursuing this approach in public health, and the scientific and societal benefits associated with this scientific approach.

Key Terms

four phases of a TD initiative	Development, conceptualization, implementation, and translation
interdisciplinary	Integrating two or more academic disciplines or fields of study in research or practice.
multidisciplinary	Combining several academic disciplines or fields of study in research or practice.
science of team science	A field focused on conceptual and methodological strategies aimed at understanding and enhancing the processes and outcomes of collaborative, team-based research.
transdisciplinary	Involving an integrative and creative process whereby scholars and practitioners from both academic disciplines and nonacademic fields work jointly to develop and use novel conceptual and methodological approaches that synthesize and extend discipline-specific perspectives, theories, methods, and translational strategies to yield innovative solutions to particular scientific and societal problems.

Review Questions

1. What are the important differences among the unidisciplinary, multidisciplinary, interdisciplinary, and transdisciplinary approaches?

2. Why has the demand for transdisciplinary approaches to public health grown so much in recent years?

3. Describe a current public health problem that is well suited to a transdisciplinary approach. Why is it a good candidate for this approach?

4. Why is it necessary to use a team-based approach when studying problems using transdisciplinary methods?

References

1. Frodeman R, Klein JT, Mitcham C, eds. The Oxford Handbook of Interdisciplinarity. New York: Oxford University Press; 2010.

2. Hadorn GH, Hoffman-Riem H, Biber-Klemm S, Grossenbacher-Mansuy W, Joye D, Wiesmann U, et al., eds. Handbook of Transdisciplinary Research. London: Springer; 2008.

3. Repko AF. Interdisciplinary Research: Process and Theory. Los Angeles, CA: Sage; 2008.

4. Crow MM. Organizing teaching and research to address the grand challenges of sustainable development. BioScience. 2010;60(7):488–489.

5. Klein JT. Creating Interdisciplinary Campus Cultures: A Model for Strength and Sustainability. San Francisco: Jossey-Bass; 2010.

6. Altman DG. Sustaining interventions in community systems: on the relationship between researchers and communities. Health Psychology. 1995;14:526–536.

7. National Institute of Environmental Health Sciences. Partnerships for Environmental Public Health. Research Triangle Park, NC: National Institute of Environmental Health Sciences; 2010.

8. Stokols D. Toward a science of transdisciplinary action research. American Journal of Community Psychology. 2006;38(1):63–77.

9. Frumkin H, Frank L, Jackson R. Urban Sprawl and Public Health: Designing, Planning, and Building for Healthy Communities. Washington, DC: Island Press; 2004.

10. Best A, Stokols D, Green LW, Leischow S, Holmes B, Buchholz K. An integrative framework for community partnering to translate theory into effective health promotion strategy. American Journal of Health Promotion. 2003;18(2): 168–176.

11. Miller TR, Baird TD, Littlefield CM, Kofinas G, Chapin FSI, Redman CL. Epistemological pluralism: reorganizing interdisciplinary research. Ecology and Society [online serial]. 2008;13(2):46. Available at: http://www.ecologyandsociety.org/vol13/iss2/art46.

12. Wuchty S, Jones BF, Uzzi B. The increasing dominance of teams in production of knowledge. Science. 2007;316:1036–1038.

13. Brown VA, Harris JA, Russell JY, eds. Tackling Wicked Problems through the Transdisciplinary Imagination. London: Earthscan; 2010.

14. Eigenbrode SD, O'Rourke M, Wulfhorst JD, Althoff DM, Goldberg CS, Merrill K, et al. Employing philosophical dialogue in collaborative science. BioScience. 2007;57(1):55–64.

15. Borner K, Contractor N, Falk-Krzesinski HJ, Fiore SM, Hall KL, Keyton J, et al. A multi-level perspective for the science of team science. Science Translational Medicine. 2010;2(45).

16. Stokols D, Hall KL, Taylor B, Moser RP. The science of team science: overview of the field and introduction to the supplement. American Journal of Preventive Medicine. 2008;35(2 suppl):S77–S89.

17. Stokols D, Fuqua J, Gress J, Harvey R, Phillips K, Baezconde-Garbanati L, et al. Evaluating transdisciplinary science. Nicotine & Tobacco Research. 2003; 5(suppl 1):S21–S39.

18. Kuhn T. The Structure of Scientific Revolutions. Chicago: University of Chicago Press; 1970.

19. Aboelela SW, Larson E, Bakken S, Carrasquillo O, Formicola A, Glied SA, et al. Defining interdisciplinary research: conclusions from a critical review of the literature. Health Services Research. 2007;42(1 suppl):329–346.

20. Kessel FS, Rosenfield PL, Anderson NB, eds. Interdisciplinary Research: Case Studies from Health and Social Science. New York: Oxford University Press; 2008.

21. Rosenfield PL. The potential of transdisciplinary research for sustaining and extending linkages between the health and social sciences. Social Science & Medicine. 1992;35:1343–1357.

22. Wagner CS, Roessner JD, Bobb K, Klein JT, Boyack KW, Keyton J, et al. Approaches to understanding and measuring interdisciplinary scientific research (IDR): a review of the literature. Journal of Informetrics. 2011;5(1):14–26.

23. Lawrence R, Despres C. Introduction: futures of transdisciplinarity. Futures. 2004;36(4):397–405.

24. Wickson F, Carew A, Russell A. Transdisciplinary research: characteristics, quandaries and quality. Futures. 2006;38(9):1046–1059.

25. Hall K, Stokols D, Moser R, Taylor B, Thornquist M, Nebeling L, et al. The collaboration readiness of transdisciplinary research teams and centers: findings from the National Cancer Institute TREC baseline evaluation study. American Journal of Preventive Medicine. 2008;35(2 suppl):161–172.

26. Committee on Facilitating Interdisciplinary Research, National Academy of Sciences, National Academy of Engineering, Institute of Medicine. Facilitating Interdisciplinary Research. Washington, DC: National Academies Press; 2004.

27. National Institutes of Health. Interdisciplinary Research Consortium. Available at: nihroadmap.nih.gov/interdisciplinary [accessed January 7, 2010].

28. National Science Foundation. What Is Interdisciplinary Research? Available at: www.nsf.gov/od/oia/additional_resources/interdisciplinary_research/definition .jsp [accessed January 7, 2010].

29. US Department of Health and Human Services. Exploratory Centers (P20) for Interdisciplinary Research. Available at: grants.nih.gov/grants/guide/rfa-files /RFA-RM-04-004.html [accessed August 24, 2011].

30. Klein JT. A taxonomy of interdisciplinarity. In: Frodeman R, Klein JT, Mitcham C, eds. The Oxford Handbook of Interdisciplinarity. Oxford, UK: Oxford University Press; 2010:15–30.

31. Glass TA, McAtee MJ. Behavioral science at the crossroads in public health: extending horizons, envisioning the future. Social Science & Medicine. 2006;62(7):1650–1671.

32. Frumkin H. Beyond toxicity: human health and the natural environment. American Journal of Preventive Medicine. 2001;20(3):234–240.

33. Jordan GB. Factors influencing advances in basic and applied research: variation due to diversity in research profiles. In: Hage J, Meeus MTH, eds. Innovation, Science, and Institutional Change. Oxford, UK: Oxford University Press; 2006:173–195.

34. Stokols D. Toward strategic team science: reducing opportunity costs while enabling innovation. Paper presented at: First Annual International Conference on the Science of Team Science; April 2010; Chicago.

35. National Cancer Institute. Transdisciplinary Tobacco Use Research Centers. Available at: dccps.nci.nih.gov/tcrb/tturc [accessed August 19, 2010].

36. National Cancer Institute. Transdisciplinary Research on Energetics and Cancer. Available at: www.compass.fhcrc.org/trec [accessed August 19, 2010].

37. National Cancer Institute. Centers for Population Health and Health Disparities. Available at: cancercontrol.cancer.gov/populationhealthcenters [accessed August 19, 2010].

38. National Cancer Institute. Health Communication and Informatics Research: NCI Centers of Excellence in Cancer Communications Research. Available at: www.cancercontrol.cancer.gov/hcirb/ceccr/ceccr-index.html [accessed August 19, 2010].

39. Morgan G, Kobus K, Gerlach KK, Neighbors C, Lerman C, Abrams DB, et al. Facilitating transdisciplinary research: the experience of the transdisciplinary tobacco use research centers. Nicotine & Tobacco Research. 2003;5(suppl 1):S11–S19.

40. TD-Net. Transdisciplinary Research. Bern, Switzerland: Swiss Academy of Arts and Sciences; 2010.

41. Green LW. From research to "best practices" in other settings and populations. American Journal of Health Behavior. 2001;25(3):165–178.

42. Lewin K. Action research and minority problems. Journal of Social Issues. 1946;2:34–36.

43. Neuhauser L, Richardson D, Mackenzie S, Minkler M. Advancing transdisciplinary and translational research practice: issues and models of doctoral education in public health. Journal of Research Practice. 2007;3(2):1–24.

44. Moreland RL, Myaskovsky L. Exploring the performance benefits of group training: transactive memory or improved communication? Organizational Behavior and Human Decision Processes. 2000;82(1):117–133.

45. Kahn R, Prager D. Interdisciplinary collaborations are a scientific and social imperative. The Scientist. 1994;8:12.

46. Simons T, Pelled L, Smith K. Making use of difference: diversity, debate, and decision comprehensiveness in top management teams. The Academy of Management Journal. 1999;42(6):662–673.

47. Dreu CD, West M. Minority dissent and team innovation: the importance of participation in decision making. Journal of Applied Psychology. 2001;86:1191–1201.

48. Northwestern University Clinical and Translational Sciences Institute. SciTS and Team Science Resources. Chicago: Northwestern University Clinical and Translational Sciences Institute; 2010.

49. Shen B. Toward cross-sectoral team science. American Journal of Preventive Medicine 2008;35(2 suppl):S240–242.

50. Breslow L, Johnson M. California's proposition 99 on tobacco, and its impact. Annual Review of Public Health. 1993;14:585–604.

51. Stokols D, Hall K, Moser R, Feng A, Misra S, Taylor B. Evaluating cross-disciplinary team science initiatives: conceptual, methodological, and translational perspectives. In: Frodeman R, Klein J, Mitcham C, eds. Oxford Handbook on Interdisciplinarity. New York: Oxford University Press; 2010:471–493.

52. Fiore SM. Interdisciplinarity as teamwork—how the science of teams can inform team science. Small Group Research. 2008;39(3):251–277.

53. Katzenbach JR, Smith DK. The Wisdom of Teams. Boston: Harvard Business School Press; 1993.

54. Olson JS, Hofer EC, Bos N, Zimmerman A, Olson GM, Cooney D, et al. A theory of remote scientific collaboration (TORSC). In: Olson GM, Zimmerman A, Bos N, eds. Scientific Collaboration on the Internet. Cambridge, MA: MIT Press; 2008:74–97.

55. Stokols D, Harvey R, Gress J, Fuqua J, Phillips K. In vivo studies of transdisciplinary scientific collaboration: lessons learned and implications for active living research. American Journal of Preventive Medicine. 2005; 28(2 suppl 2):202–213.

56. Hesse BW. Of mice and mentors: developing cyber-infrastructures to support transdisciplinary scientific collaboration. American Journal of Preventive Medicine. 2008;35(2 suppl):S235–S239.

57. Paletz SBF, Schunn CD. A social-cognitive framework of multidisciplinary team innovation. Topics in Cognitive Science. 2010;2:73–95.

58. Stokols D, Misra S, Hall K, Taylor B, Moser R. The ecology of team science: understanding contextual influences on transdisciplinary collaboration. American Journal of Preventive Medicine. 2008;35(2 suppl):96–115.

59. Chen G, Kanfer R. Toward a systems theory of motivated behavior in work teams. Research in Organizational Behavior. 2006;27:223–267.

60. Marks MA, DeChurch LA, Mathieu JE, Panzer FJ, Alonso A. Teamwork in multiteam systems. Journal of Applied Psychology. 2005;90(5): 964–971.

61. Gray B. Enhancing transdisciplinary research through collaborative leadership. American Journal of Preventive Medicine. 2008;35(2 suppl):S124–S132.

62. Marks M, Mathieu JE, Zaccaro SJ. A temporally based framework and taxonomy of team processes. Academy of Management Review. 2001;26:356–376.

63. Mansilla VB, Duraising ED. Targeted assessment of students' interdisciplinary work: an empirically grounded framework proposed. Journal of Higher Education. 2007;78(2):23p.

64. Borrego M, Newswander L. Definitions of interdisciplinary research: toward graduate-level interdisciplinary learning outcomes. Review of Higher Education. 2010;34(1):61–84.

65. Campbell D. Ethnocentrism of disciplines and the fish-scale model of omniscience. In: Sherif M, Sherif CW, eds. Interdisciplinary Relationships in the Social Sciences. Chicago: Aldine Press; 1969:328–348.

66. Mathieu J, Travis Maynard M, Rapp T, Gilson L. Team effectiveness 1997–2007: a review of recent advancements and a glimpse into the future. Journal of Management. 2008;34:410–476.

67. Hulsheger UR, Anderson N, Salgado JF. Team-level predictors of innovation at work: a comprehensive meta-analysis spanning three decades of research. Journal of Applied Psychology. 2004;94:1128–1145.

68. Wegner DM. A computer network model of human transactive memory. Social Cognition. 1995;13:319–339.

69. Cummings J, Kiesler S. Collaborative research across disciplinary and organizational boundaries. Social Studies of Science. 2005;35(5):703–722.

70. Carew AL, Wickson F. The TD wheel: a heuristic to shape, support and evaluate transdisciplinary research. Futures. 2010;42(10):1146–1155.

71. Council on Education for Public Health. Accreditation Criteria: Public Health Programs. Washington, DC: Council on Education for Public Health; amended June 2005. Available at: www.ceph.org/pdf/PHP-Criteria.pdf.

72. Pinson D. Urban planning: an "undisciplined" discipline? Futures. 2004;36(4):503–513.

73. Ramadier T. Transdisciplinarity and its challenges: the case of urban studies. Futures. 2004;36(4):423–439.

74. Jacobs JA, Frickel S. Interdisciplinarity: a critical assessment. Annual Review of Sociology. 2009;35(1):43–65.

75. Fry GLA. Multifunctional landscapes—towards transdisciplinary research. Landscape and Urban Planning. 2001;57(3–4):159–168.

76. Green LW, Richard L, Potvin L. Ecological foundations of health promotion. American Journal of Health Promotion. 1996;10(4):270–281.

77. McLeroy KR, Norton BL, Kegler MC, Burdine JN, Sumaya CV. Community-based interventions. American Journal of Public Health. 2003;93(4):529–533.

78. Schneider M, Stokols D. Multilevel theories of behavior change: a social ecological framework. In: Shumaker SA, Ockene JK, Riekert KA, eds. The Handbook of Health Behavior Change. 3rd ed. New York: Springer; 2009:85–105.

79. Stokols D. Translating social ecological theory into guidelines for community health promotion. American Journal of Health Promotion. 1996;10(4):282–298.

80. Breslow L. Social ecological strategies for promoting healthy lifestyles. American Journal of Health Promotion. 1996;10(4):253–257.

81. Dannenberg AL, Jackson RJ, Frumkin H, Schieber RA, Pratt M, Kochtitzky C, et al. The impact of community design and land-use choices on public health: a scientific research agenda. American Journal of Public Health. 2003;93(9):1500–1508.

82. Frank LD, Engelke PO, Schmid TL. Health and Community Design: The Impact of the Built Environment on Physical Activity. Washington, DC: Island Press; 2003.

83. Sallis JF, Cervero RB, Ascher W, Henderson KA, Kraft MK, Kerr J. An ecological approach to creating active living communities. Annual Review of Public Health. 2006;27(1):297–322.

84. Adler NE, Stewart J. Using team science to address health disparities: MacArthur network as case example. Annals of the New York Academy of Sciences. 2010;1186:252–260.

85. Bullard RD. Dumping in Dixie: Race, Class, and Environmental Quality. Boulder, CO: Westview Press; 1990.

86. Evans GW. The environment of childhood poverty. American Psychologist. 2004;59(2):77–92.

87. Diez Roux AV, Mair C. Neighborhoods and health. Annals of the New York Academy of Sciences. 2010;1186:125–145.

88. Evans GW, Kim P. Multiple risk exposure as a potential explanatory mechanism for the socioeconomic status-health gradient. Annals of the New York Academy of Sciences. 2010;1186:174–189.

89. Kawachi I, Berkman LF. Neighborhoods and Health. New York: Oxford University Press; 2003.

90. Jerrett M, Burnett RT. Air pollution and cardiovascular events. New England Journal of Medicine. 2007;356(20):2104–2105. Author reply: 2105–2106.

91. Wells NM, Evans GW, Yang Y. Environments and health: planning decisions as public health decisions. Journal of Architectural and Planning Research. 2010;27(2):124–143.

92. Michell R, Popham F. Effect of exposure to natural environment on health inequalities: an observational population study. The Lancet. 2008;372:1655–1660.

93. Cassel J. The contribution of the social environment to host resistance: the fourth Wade Hampton Frost Lecture. American Journal of Epidemiology. 1976;104(2):107–123.

94. Cohen S, Tyrrell DA, Smith AP. Psychological stress and susceptibility to the common cold. New England Journal of Medicine. 1991;325(9):606–612.

95. Hiatt R, Breen N. The social determinants of cancer: a challenge for transdisciplinary science. American Journal of Preventive Medicine. 2008;35(2):S141–S150.

96. Catalano R, Goldman-Mellor S, Saxton K, Margerison-Zilco C, Subbaraman M, LeWinn K, et al. The health effects of economic decline. Annual Review of Public Health. 2011;32(1):1.1–1.20.

97. Northwestern University Clinical and Translational Sciences Institute. Research Team Support and Development. Available at: www.nucats.northwestern.edu

/collaboration-resources/research-team-support-development [accessed August 3, 2011].

98. National Organization of Research Development Professionals. [Home page.] Available at: www.nordp.org [accessed August 3, 2011].

99. National Science Foundation. Science of Learning Centers [discussion of awards]. Available at: www.nsf.gov/funding/pgm_summ.jsp?pims_id=5567 [accessed November 6, 2012].

100. National Institutes of Health. Scientific Meetings for Creating Interdisciplinary Research Teams in Basic Behavioral and Social Science Research (R13). Available at: grants.nih.gov/grants/guide/rfa-files/RFA-CA-10-017.html [accessed November 14, 2010].

101. Hall K, Stokols D, Stipelman B, Vogel A, Feng A, Masimore B, et al. Assessing the value of team science: a study comparing center and investigator-initiated grants. American Journal of Preventive Medicine. 2012;42(2):157–163.

102. Misra S, Harvey RH, Stokols D, Pine KH, Fuqua J, Shokair SM, et al. Evaluating an interdisciplinary undergraduate training program in health promotion research. American Journal of Preventive Medicine. 2009;36(4):358–365.

103. Mitrany M, Stokols D. Gauging the transdisciplinary qualities and outcomes of doctoral training programs. Journal of Planning Education and Research. 2005;24:437–449.

104. Spaapen J, Dijstelbloem H. Evaluating Research in Context: A Method for Comprehensive Assessment. The Netherlands: Consultative Committee of Sector Councils for Research and Development; 2005.

105. Mabry PL, Olster DH, Morgan GD, Abrams DB. Interdisciplinarity and systems science to improve population health—a view from the NIH Office of Behavioral and Social Sciences Research. American Journal of Preventive Medicine. 2008;35(2):S211–S224.

Chapter 2

Transdisciplinary Training and Education

Sarah Gehlert
Teri Browne

Learning Objectives

- Describe a transdisciplinary approach to training and education.
- Explain the history of transdisciplinary education and training.
- Identify the value of transdisciplinary approaches for health promotion.
- Define the attributes of successful transdisciplinary teams.
- Present examples of existing transdisciplinary education and training programs.
- Offer recommendations for future transdisciplinary educational programs.

• • •

Chapter 1 outlined the practical and scientific benefits of the transdisciplinary approach to research and practice and also considerations and techniques for implementing transdisciplinary collaborations in the public health context, especially in teams. This chapter picks up where chapter 1 left off, and its mission is to describe how best to educate a new generation of students to function as transdisciplinary scholars or practitioners. This work entails the ability to adjust boundaries to address the complexity of a problem, use the best of disciplinary knowledge and methods, and then go beyond all this to create new intellectual spaces. In order to achieve our mission, we will, first, review the knowledge base on the factors that make for successful transdisciplinary teams. Next, we will review existing transdisciplinary education and training programs. We will end with recommendations for future transdisciplinary education.

The notion of *transdisciplinarity*, while new to the field of health, has existed for over forty years in education and the social sciences. Although originally introduced by Piaget,[1] the term was first related to education by Erich Jantsch in 1972, in his argument for reshaping higher education through a government-industry-university model of societal planning. In Jantsch's model, knowledge is organized into goal-oriented systems consisting of four levels: (1) meaning values, the purposive level; (2) social systems designs, the normative level; (3) physical technology, natural ecology, and social ecology, the pragmatic level; and (4) physical technology, natural world, and human psychological world, the empirical level.[2]

Jantsch's grouping of academic disciplines in response to emerging problems is characteristic of transdisciplinarity. Hoffman-Riem et al. say that "transdisciplinary orientations to research, education, and institutions try to overcome the mismatch between knowledge production in academia, and knowledge requests for solving societal problems."[3] As was the case in Jantsch's work, mismatches between traditional academic structures and the needs of society often are addressed by configuring disciplines in new ways.

Most researchers would agree that disciplines, as the primary units of academic communities, produce specialized knowledge that is essential to education and research. Yet the most prolific researchers are often those who operate outside their own disciplines.[4] Conversely, operating strictly within the boundaries of a discipline can be restrictive and may cause a scholar to minimize the complexity of problems. Transdisciplinarity depends on the ability of disciplinary scholars to adjust their boundaries to address new problems and issues as they arise.

Value of Transdisciplinary Approaches for Health Promotion

As articulated by Nicolescu, transdisciplinary approaches are useful in any domain that exhibits complexity. He emphasizes the value of taking a holistic view of phenomena, thus allowing their complexity to be captured without reducing them to their component parts and then missing how those parts fit together to form a whole. Nicolescu speaks of different levels of reality governed by different types of logic and points out that reducing complex phenomena to "a single level governed by a single form of logic" limits the potential of researchers to successfully address social problems.[1]

An additional benefit of transdisciplinary approaches over others—such as unidisciplinary, multidisciplinary, and interdisciplinary approaches—is that they create products that are greater than the sum of their parts. Nicolescu writes about creating new meanings of complex phenomena that "traverse and lie beyond different disciplines."[1] By moving beyond the often rigid definitions of phenomena that exist within individual disciplines and challenging those definitions by considering the theories and empirical knowledge bases of other disciplines, broader definitions and understandings of those phenomena that more closely fit reality can be created, with more valid descriptors. This new approach to, or configuration of, disciplines is essential for addressing modern social problems because traditional disciplinary definitions fail to capture the complexity of the phenomena that contribute to those problems.

In a large transdisciplinary research project on health disparities, stress was identified as a pathway between what happens in the neighborhood social environment and changes in hormone expression among African American women with a particularly aggressive form of breast cancer.[5,6] The transdisciplinary team of biological, behavioral, and social scientists and community stakeholders progressed through the four stages of transdisciplinary research outlined in chapter 1. As the membership of the transdisciplinary team grew to include additional disciplines during the team's development and conceptual phases, it became clear that disciplinary scholars on the team defined stress in very different ways:

- Social and behavioral science team members used the term *stress* to mean people's perceptions of how they respond in terms of affect and behavior to what occurs in their environments. In this conception, stress might arise in response to a death in the family or the loss of a job. For these scientists, stress varied by gender, socioeconomic status, coping style, and a number of other factors.

- Endocrinologists on the team defined stress as a physiological response to a variety of stressors. This group of biological scientists did not consider differences by gender or socioeconomic status, but instead considered humans to be homogeneous in terms of their stress response.

- Biopsychologists on the team (behavioral scientists combining the disciplines of psychology and biology) took a position between the views of the social and biological scientists. Although, like the biologists, the biopsychologists focused on the physiological stress response, they at the same time acknowledged gender differences and coping styles. Unlike the social scientists on the team, however, they failed to consider socioeconomic status, which is an important consideration in health disparities research.

While there was no right or wrong definition of stress for this transdisciplinary research team, the point is that it took a diverse team of social, behavioral, and biological scientists to capture the phenomenon of stress in a way that was meaningful to health disparities research. The team discovered that definitional boundaries of key phenomena are broader and more complex and inclusive on research teams where multiple overlapping definitions are represented. Including a wide range of diverse disciplines on this team ensured a definition of stress that included social, behavioral, and biological components, thus laying the groundwork for the development of multipronged interventions (that is, complex interventions to address a complex phenomenon). Developing the interventions then allowed the team to progress to the implementation and translation phases.

Capturing complexity is crucial for ameliorating disparities in the wide range of conditions and diseases in which they occur. The determinants of health disparities occur at multiple levels,[7,8] thus requiring an approach capable of capturing their multifaceted and complex nature.[9] This approach relies on collaborations among social, behavioral, and biological scientists to identify and represent the multilevel determinants of health disparities within the same analyses, often using shared models. Efforts that focus on one level and that fail to capture all the levels of influence on health disparities may affect individual health outcomes without ever making a dent in racial and ethnic disparities.[10]

Attributes of Successful Transdisciplinary Teams

Transdisciplinary teams that are able to operate as mutually informative units create new intellectual spaces that allow them to visualize a full range of influences on health; thus "it is the mechanics or functioning of transdisciplinary teams that confers their advantage over other approaches."[9]

Transdisciplinary teams operate best in environments that do not privilege one discipline, or one way of knowing, over others. Larger schools and departments have more resources and therefore more power on university campuses. Avoiding disproportionate influence requires the creation of a level playing field on which disciplinary scholars are able to recognize one another's expertise and benefit from that expertise. This leads to the psychological safety (the belief that the team environment is a safe place to express independent thoughts and opinions) and transactive memory systems (shared awareness of the expertise, knowledge, and skills of each member of the team) mentioned in chapter 1. One way in which this environment can be achieved is to designate shared spaces for teams outside individual schools and departments. Large transdisciplinary research centers work best when they are centrally administered rather than administered through an individual school or department, to avoid the privileging of one discipline or group of disciplines over others.[11]

Institutional administrations can also help to ensure successful transdisciplinarity by recognizing and rewarding collaborations that occur across schools and departments. These collaborations diffuse a culture of collaboration across schools and departments, institutions, and the outside community. Designing a system for rewarding transdisciplinary collaborations might include developing rules for tenure and promotion that incentivize publications with multiple authors from a range of disciplines working in the same area of inquiry. Conversely, valuing publications by single authors and rewarding only the first author of a multiauthored paper works against transdisciplinary team functioning.[12]

Successful transdisciplinary teams share a number of attributes beyond strong institutional commitment. One of the most important of these is the development of a common language or lexicon unique to the research project, or projects, at hand. Part of team members' recognition of one another's expertise comes from the ability to understand the work of other team members. Although every scholar on the team will not understand the science of other disciplinary scholars on the team at the same level or in the same depth as his or her own science, it is possible to capture the essence of those other sciences in such a way as to enable each team member to explain how his or her work fits into the team's functioning as a whole. In other words, each scholar should be able to tell the team's story.

In 2002, a major impetus for transdisciplinary research was launched by Elias Zerhouni, then director of the National Institutes of Health. Titled Roadmap for 21st Century Medical Research, this initiative sets out a "vision for a more efficient and productive system of medical research,"[13] and supports novel partnerships among social, behavioral, and biological scientists to address complex health problems such as this nation's growing health disparities. The approach recognized the impossibility of adequately understanding health and well-being without taking into account their biological, behavioral, and social determinants.

The Roadmap for 21st Century Medical Research catalyzed a number of transdisciplinary research initiatives, each with its own mandate to foster transdisciplinary research and training. The Centers for Population Health and Health Disparities and the Centers of Excellence in Cancer Communication P50 initiatives were launched in 2003 and are now in their second cycle of funding. The P50 Transdisciplinary Tobacco Use Research Centers began the following year and were funded through 2009. The U54 Transdisciplinary Research on Energetics and Cancer (TREC) initiative was launched in 2007 and recently began its second cycle of funding.

For example, the TREC centers aim to reduce cancer linked with obesity, poor diet, and low levels of physical activity. Each of the four funded TRECs (at Washington University in St. Louis, Harvard University, the University of Pennsylvania, and the University of California, San Diego) has an Education, Training and Outreach Core to promote transdisciplinary research and train postdoctoral fellows to be the next generation of transdisciplinary cancer researchers. At Washington University in St. Louis, postdoctoral fellows are helped to select a primary mentor and a two- to three-person mentoring team that represents a range of disciplines and experience at various points on the project spectrum from discovery to dissemination and implementation.

Successful transdisciplinary teams develop shared, unified models to which each discipline contributes. These models help team members and outsiders to visualize each discipline's contribution to the whole and to better understand how each contributes. This fosters a feeling of unity among team members and helps them to recognize their dependence on others in addressing complex phenomena, such as health disparities.

A number of processes facilitate successful transdisciplinary functioning. It is important, for example, to maintain a continuous dialogue among team members' projects, with mutual adjustments in design and measurement of variables to foster integration of findings and ensure that information is useful for the team as a whole. This can be achieved through frequent formal and informal meetings at which scholars from different projects and disciplines present to one another. Too often, research team members present to one another only when funders make site visits. In addition, developing a plan for the resolution of conflict, which is inevitable on any team but especially an issue for teams that are transdisciplinary, helps to ensure smooth functioning. This plan might establish an internal steering committee and a chain of command for decision making.

Finally, successful transdisciplinary teams are those that have leaders who foster cooperation and the free exchange of ideas, work to build consensus, and discourage competition and defensiveness among team members. Importantly, these leaders counter the tendency of disciplinary scholars to focus entirely on their own projects and issues by continually recalling team members' attention to the bigger picture and their shared questions.

It is important to always keep an eye on developing the next generation of transdisciplinary scholars. University administrations play a key role in facilitating this effort through a variety of actions, including fostering cross-disciplinary units and courses; providing start-up funds for transdisciplinary collaborations among junior and senior disciplinary scholars; and creating shared physical spaces that foster interactions among students, postdoctoral fellows, and academic researchers from a variety of disciplines (we present further training program recommendations in the following section). The Institute for Mind and Biology at the University of Chicago, for instance, has a long-standing professional development series in which graduate students and postdoctoral fellows from different laboratories present their work to one another on a monthly, rotating basis. These students and fellows come from a variety of disciplines, such as psychology and biology, and share an interest in developmental biology and neuroscience.

The Genesis of Interdisciplinary and Transdisciplinary Training

Calls for interdisciplinary and transdisciplinary training have been heard at least since the late 1990s in the United States. A 1996 report by the Organisation for Economic Co-operation and Development, for example, encouraged universities to train across disciplines and form university-industry-government collaborations for the promotion and diffusion of knowledge.[14] This echoes the suggestion for government-industry-university models made by Jantsch twenty years earlier.[2]

In the following decade, the National Academies and Institute of Medicine produced two reports on cross-disciplinary education. The first of these reports, published in 2003, focused on public health education and recommended that graduate education programs in schools of public health include these eight content areas: informatics, genomics, communication, cultural competence, community-based participatory research, global health, policy and law, and public health ethics.[15] The report outlined six major responsibilities of schools of public health, including that schools serve as the focal point for multischool transdisciplinary research.

Then in 2004 the National Academies and Institute of Medicine drew on recommendations and feedback from university faculty and administrators, nonacademic scientists, and business leaders for a second report that addressed undergraduate, graduate, and postgraduate education across a number of fields and disciplines, recommending that undergraduate students gain a solid foundation in one discipline but also add courses from other disciplines to "understand the culture of other disciplines, gain new skills and techniques, and network with other researchers."[4] The report also suggested that graduate students should have multiple advisors from different disciplines and attend conferences on topic areas outside their primary fields. Postdoctoral fellows were encouraged to find institutions favorable to interdisciplinary research as well as mentors with histories of mentoring across departmental lines. Researchers and faculty members were encouraged to "immerse themselves in the languages, cultures, and knowledge of their collaborators."[4]

Existing Transdisciplinary Training Programs

A number of transdisciplinary training programs have appeared over the past few years in the United States. In reviewing these programs we first will outline formal academic degree programs and then consider other, less formal, training approaches.

Academic Degree Programs

In reviewing academic degree programs we found a range of approaches to exposing students to other disciplines. Some programs merely bring students from different disciplinary backgrounds together for training. Others emphasize training by instructors from various disciplines in the same curricula. Few programs, however, have instituted measures to foster and support students' ability to use these new cross-disciplinary learning environments to broaden their thinking about complex problems and translate that understanding into solutions. In this section we review three academic programs that have made strides toward this end.

Neuhauser, Richardson, Mackenzie, and Minkler[16] describe the genesis of the transdisciplinary doctor of public health program at the University of California, Berkeley, School of Public Health as the realization that focusing on traditional biomedical models without considering underlying social and ecological influences yields imperfect solutions to society's health problems. The school's first step toward transdisciplinary functioning was made in 1996, when discipline-specific doctor of public health programs were merged to form a more unified program connected to a number of disciplines. In 2004, this program took a more transdisciplinary and translational focus when a problem-solving approach to learning was implemented, built around DrPH-in-Action projects. For example, one project was built around emergency preparedness and carried out in post-Katrina New Orleans with health workers there. Another focused on youth development as students and faculty worked with the Alameda County Public Health Department to identify ways to improve the health department's services to at-risk youth. Challenges encountered included structuring team projects so that they fit within a one-semester timeline.

The transdisciplinary studies program at Claremont Graduate University in California provides resources and guidance for the larger university on how to incorporate transdisciplinarity into curricular and research efforts. The university defines *transdisciplinarity* as "the interaction of three or more disciplines, distributed across two or more schools, that produces results not likely to be obtained by any one discipline alone."[17] Since 2003, Claremont Graduate University has required all its doctoral students to take a transdisciplinary core course, called a T-course, during their second year of study. Some recent T-course titles are "The Nature of Inquiry; Evolution, Economics, & the Brain"; "Transdisciplinary Perspectives on the Age of Reform in the US, 1890–1920"; "Intensive Research Methods"; and "Working across Cultures." These courses are taught in seminar and lecture formats that combine content from a range of disciplines.[18]

In addition to offering T-courses, Claremont's transdisciplinary studies program has created reading and working groups to engage students and faculty in joint research and training. The university provides students and faculty with $500 grants to create these groups, with the proviso that each group includes students and faculty from at least three disciplines. This effort is furthered by transdisciplinary research and dissertation awards that support faculty and student research and scholarship grounded in a transdisciplinary approach. Transdisciplinary dissertation grants, for example, are awarded to doctoral students who work on research projects involving at least three disciplines, with dissertation advisors from at least two schools.[19]

The master of public health (MPH) program at the Brown School at Washington University in St. Louis held its first classes in 2009. The curriculum design was shaped by a philosophy of transdisciplinary problem solving around public health topics. Students are required to take at least two courses from a menu of "transdisciplinary problem solving in public health" (TPS) courses. Students also take courses from a "foundations in public health" sequence, a survey course called "Cross-Cutting Themes in Public Health," a series of three research methods and statistics courses, and a practicum in the field of public health, and they complete a culminating experience. The TPS courses begin in the first year, and are taken in addition to more traditional research methods courses and a number of electives, which can include other transdisciplinary courses.

The TPS courses form the cornerstone of the Washington University MPH program. In these seminar-style courses, students are exposed to a wide range of perspectives from diverse disciplines about the various causes of and potential solutions to a specific public health problem. Students work in groups to integrate these transdisciplinary perspectives into a richer understanding of the problem at hand, with the aim of developing new solutions to current public health problems that draw on the knowledge bases, theories, and methods of different disciplines. The specific public health topics covered in the courses vary from semester to semester. Some recent examples are prevention of obesity, undernutrition in developing countries, and health disparities (more detailed examples of the transdisciplinary courses offered are presented in part 3 of this book).

Other Training Approaches

A number of less formal transdisciplinary training programs exist across the country. For example, the National Public Health Training Centers Network provides funding to improve the public health of vulnerable communities through the transdisciplinary training of students, clinicians, and community stakeholders. In 2005, the program provided training to 2,057 students of allopathic and osteopathic medicine; 2,130 nursing, advanced practice nursing, and physician assistant students; 1,259 dental, pharmacy, public health, mental health, and other allied health students; and 2,020 community health workers.[20] Across the country, Area Health Education Centers, funded through Title VII of the Public Health Service Act, train students from a variety of health disciplines and provide them with opportunities to work with underserved populations.[21]

The Leadership Education in Neurodevelopmental Disabilities and Related Disorders (LEND) program is another example of transdisciplinary training for students in professional programs. In 2011, thirty-nine LEND programs were located in thirty-two US states, all of them funded by the federal Maternal and Child Health Bureau.[22] Although each LEND program has different foci and curricular elements, all make use of faculty from a variety of disciplines and offer training on the multilevel determinants of health. Students work on joint, community-engaged research projects aimed at addressing common health conditions and share coursework.

The LEND program at the University of Pittsburgh, for example, provides graduate and postgraduate mentored training to students and trainees from a range of fields and disciplines, such as medicine, psychology, education, public health, law, and social work.[22] The core faculty members who provide this training likewise represent a range of fields and disciplines, including psychology, pediatrics, public health, occupational therapy, education, physical therapy, speech and language pathology, dentistry, audiology, and social work. Students and trainees work with faculty mentors on shared research projects addressing neurodevelopmental conditions such as autism, sickle cell disease, and fragile X syndrome.

The LEND training program at the University of Washington offers training to students, health professionals, and pre- and postdoctoral fellows studying or working in audiology, pediatrics, health administration, nursing, nutrition, occupational therapy, dentistry, physical therapy, psychology, public health, social work, special education, and speech-language pathology.[23] Students and trainees receive instruction from disciplinary faculty who provide their own perspectives on neurodevelopmental disabilities as part of a specialized program that supplements the students' regular disciplinary coursework.

The University of California, Irvine, provides a few transdisciplinary opportunities for undergraduate and graduate students. The Inter-Disciplinary Summer Undergraduate Research Experience (ID-SURE) program supports undergraduate students from different disciplines in a program of training and research opportunities related to health promotion and disease prevention.[24] ID-SURE students participate in a ten-week course taught by faculty mentors from both the biological and social sciences.[25] Additionally, doctoral students at the university's School of Social Ecology often take two courses that train them in transdisciplinary theories.[26]

Some universities provide individual transdisciplinary courses rather than programs of study. The University of Toronto, for example, offers a graduate-level course titled "Transdisciplinary Studies in Infectious Disease (using Hepatitis C as a model)." This course is open to students from different disciplines and reviews scientific, medical, and social aspects of the hepatitis C virus to provide students with a holistic understanding of illnesses related to that virus.[27]

Recommendations for Future Transdisciplinary Training

In this section we offer recommendations for future transdisciplinary training, basing them on our review of existing programs. These recommendations address six training issues: program structure, socialization, content, pedagogy, evaluation, and additional resources.

Program Structure

Transdisciplinary training programs need to have the support of institutional administrations in order to achieve success, as was mentioned earlier in this chapter.[20,28,29] The transdisciplinary studies program at Claremont Graduate University, for example, is campuswide and determines policy and practice for the campus as a whole.

Support from the central administration can help to diffuse a transdisciplinary culture across the institution and, in so doing, reduce barriers to program success. These barriers might come in the form of different schedules and degree requirements for students in different areas; different expectations for tenure and promotion of faculty; and insufficient time to implement seminars and courses that expose students and trainees to a range of perspectives and that might involve community-engaged research.[7] Clark recommends that directors of transdisciplinary programs report to academic vice presidents or provosts rather than to deans, in order to "embed" the program in the culture and functioning of the larger university.[28]

Institutions can help to maximize the success of their transdisciplinary training programs by recognizing that teaching in such programs is likely to be particularly time consuming for faculty when it involves components such as problem-based learning and group projects.[29,30] Pellmar and Eisenberg suggest that universities can improve program success by sharing the overhead for such transdisciplinary efforts across departments and arranging for shared facilities. They argue that universities should create and foster new, independent transdisciplinary centers and institutes (such as the Institute for

Mind and Biology at the University of Chicago) for conducting such training, rather than housing it in existing departments.[31] Successful transdisciplinary programs also employ a wide base of faculty willing to engage in training and research, so that programs are not dependent on small cadres of faculty for all their needs.[20,29]

The National Academy of Sciences and Institute of Medicine,[4] recommend that transdisciplinary training programs have the following attributes if they are to be successful.

- Flexible departmental and school budgets and cost-sharing policies
- Financial support to start programs, and bridge funding for programs that are in between external funding opportunities
- New faculty recruitment that is shared across departments, schools, and colleges
- Faculty incentives for transdisciplinary scholarship and training
- Tenure and promotion policies and procedures that accommodate transdisciplinary work and the unconventional teaching, service, and research demands of such work

In addition to universities, Nandiwada and Dang-Vu[21] suggest that another ideal location for transdisciplinary training is teaching health centers. These centers—funded by the Health Resources and Services Administration of the US Department of Health and Human Services (www.hrsa.gov/grants/apply /assistance/teachinghealthcenters) and the 2009 American Recovery and Reinvestment Act (www.hrsa.gov/grants/apply/assistance/TeachingHealthCenters /section5508.html)—provide primary care residency programs in community-based, ambulatory patient care centers across the country to address the medical needs of underserved communities. Nandiwada and Dang-Vu suggest that these teaching health centers are ideal locations for transdisciplinary training in both rural and urban areas of the country and could provide training for a range of health disciplines and attend to the social as well as medical aspects of patient care.

Socialization

Successful transdisciplinary training programs are able to socialize trainees so that they can be more effective members of transdisciplinary teams.[32] This can be done not only through formal training at the undergraduate, graduate, doctoral, and postgraduate levels[4] but also by introducing the concepts related to transdisciplinary health as early in the continuum of education as grade school.[33]

Trainees need to learn about basic group process skills, communication, and negotiation and conflict resolution early in their education.[20,29,34] These skills are too often assumed to be intuitive when they are not. Two means of teaching these skills are group exercises, which might involve role-playing and practice, and the facilitation of interactions among the disciplines that address their different cultures and approaches.[29,35,36] For example, teams of students from different disciplines can work on a common problem across courses in the curriculum. Faculty can also "immerse themselves in the languages, cultures, and knowledge of their collaborators."[4] One way of doing this is through seminars and workshops that are attended by students, community members, and faculty. Transdisciplinary collaboration in research and teaching by faculty members can also serve as a model of this behavior for students.[37,38]

Bronstein[35] argues that transdisciplinary training programs are most successful when students are trained to be dependent on one another for completing a shared project, with each providing a different piece of the puzzle. This can be accomplished through formal and informal interactions and through the creation of program goals that emphasize collective ownership among investigators. Some have suggested the fostering of joint social interactions across disciplines.[4,31] This effort might include shared on-site cafeterias, lounges, and other more public spaces that are designed to attract students, trainees, staff, and investigators from a variety of disciplines. Each laboratory at the Institute for Mind and Biology at the University of Chicago, for example, hosts a "cookie day" on Wednesday afternoons and everyone in the building is encouraged to attend. The institute also provides building space for teams led by social and behavioral scientists.

Content

Successful transdisciplinary training programs have courses taught or cotaught by faculty from a variety of schools, departments, and colleges[37] and by community stakeholders and nonacademic scientists. These courses examine a wide range of topics, such as[38–42]

- The nature of a transdisciplinary team
- Transdisciplinary team roles
- Transdisciplinary training and research processes
- Communication skills
- Collaboration skills
- Conflict resolution

- Content knowledge and specific skills relevant to the practice and research areas

- Multilevel determinants of health and health care delivery

- Research methods

- Practice and research ethics, including community-engaged research

- Medical terminology

Oandasani and Reeves[43] suggest the following competencies for those engaged in transdisciplinary training: the ability to describe one's roles and responsibilities clearly to other professionals and community stakeholders; the ability to recognize and observe the constraints of one's role, responsibilities, and competencies while also perceiving needs in the wider framework; the ability to recognize and respect the roles, responsibilities, and competencies of other professionals; and the ability to work with other professionals to effect change and to resolve conflict in these interactions. Nash[38] suggests that transdisciplinary students also need to develop common values and cooperative behaviors that are necessary for successful transdisciplinary team functioning.

Pedagogy of Transdisciplinary Training Programs

Transdisciplinary training programs should integrate transdisciplinary coursework and experiences throughout curricula, not only in elective courses,[20] an integration that has been achieved by a few schools, such as the University of California, Berkeley, Claremont Graduate University, and Washington University. Transdisciplinary training should begin early in the educational continuum[21] and should be done accomplished through a range of instructional methods[37,39] both didactic and experiential. Technology may also expand the capacity of such programs by facilitating the use of case scenarios, vignettes, or experiential simulation laboratories to create real-world examples of patient problems.[39]

Along with problem-based learning, a common pedagogical tool used in successful transdisciplinary training programs is experiential and service learning, which puts skills into practice.[20,36,41] This learning may be conducted in community settings, facilitated by community stakeholders.[20] Lennon-Dearing, Lowry, Ross, and Dyer,[30] for example, describe a program in which students attend a hospital ethics committee meeting, tour a hospital, and interview community members together as part of their training.

Training programs should include active reflection on the transdisciplinary process, particularly reflection that accompanies real-world experiences in health care settings.[35,36] For example, the University of California, San Diego, provides transdisciplinary student training in three community clinics for vulnerable patients.[44] These community clinics afford trainees the opportunity to augment their disciplinary experiences with real-world experiences in health care settings. As part of their training program, trainees participate in a daily *learning circle*, in which everyone reflects on what he or she learned in the clinic that day. Kilgo, Aldridge, and Denton recommend that training should feature frequent reflection by disciplinary trainees because "different perspectives lead to better decision-making."[45]

Evaluation

Scholars agree that successful transdisciplinary training programs must conduct comprehensive evaluations of program processes and outcomes in order to achieve sustainability and ongoing support from administrations and funders.[29,33] This evaluation should include longitudinal measures of program graduates that map their career trajectories and the impact of the training program on their professional practice. Programs are encouraged to use both qualitative and quantitative research to demonstrate program outcomes.[20,42] Trainees' progress can also be measured through time by using a standard bibliographical approach in which manuscripts, presentations, and funding proposals prepared with or presenting transdisciplinary approaches are tracked through time. Metrics are not yet available, however, to measure improvement in a trainee's science across time.

Additional Resources

The Study Group on Interprofessional Education and Collaborative Practice of the World Health Organization is preparing an evidence-based report that will make recommendations for the education and training of transdisciplinary health care team members.[46] This report will be a helpful resource for designing and evaluating future transdisciplinary training programs.

In 1998, the US Congress created the Advisory Committee on Interdisciplinary, Community-Based Linkages (ACICBL) to help guide the secretary of the Department of Health and Human Services on policy and program development for cross-disciplinary training involving community research,[47] training that over time has become transdisciplinary in nature and scope. Authorized by the Public Health Service Act, the ACICBL includes representation from Area Health Education Centers and the disciplines and fields of geriatrics, chiropractic, podiatry, social work, psychology, and rural health.[34] Since its first report, this committee has continued to provide resources for community research and reports about the value of transdisciplinary team medical care and training, and has made recommendations that all training and grants funded by the Health Resources and Services Administration should include a transdisciplinary approach to patient care and research.

Another potential resource for transdisciplinary training is the National Public Health Training Centers Network. This program provides funding to improve the public health of vulnerable communities by cross-training students and trainees, clinicians, and community stakeholders. In 2005, this program provided training to over 5,000 students from different disciplines and community health workers.[20] This program may serve as a resource for transdisciplinary programs that wish to fund student training. Likewise, Area Health Education Centers across the country, funded through Title VII, educate students from different health disciplines and provide opportunities for them to work with underserved populations.[21] An Area Health Education Center might also be a collaborative partner for a program interested in providing transdisciplinary training.

Although not primarily focused on public health, two international websites offer some thoughts on transdisciplinary education. The website of the Centre International de Recherches et Études Transdisciplinaires (CIRET), based in France (basarab.nicolescu.perso.sfr.fr/ciret/index_en.php), has addressed issues of transdisciplinary education. The March 2005 issue of the *Bulletin Interactif du CIRET*, for example, which can be found on the CIRET website, addresses the responsibility of universities to foster transdisciplinary education. The website of the Network for Transdisciplinary Research (TD-net) of the Swiss Academies of Arts and Sciences (transdisciplinarity.ch/e/index .php) describes a Master of Arts in Transdisciplinary Studies conferred by the Zurich University of the Arts.

Summary

Successful transdisciplinary research occurs when disciplinary scholars are able to create new intellectual spaces that allow them to visualize all the determinants of complex social problems such as health disparities. To successfully train the next generation of transdisciplinary scholars, institutions must make it possible for trainees to learn the skills needed to operate in these newly created spaces between disciplines and almost certainly outside their own primary disciplines. This requires not only that they be exposed to scholarship from a range of disciplines but also that they learn to use that scholarship to devise interventions to address complex social problems.

Transdisciplinary training that combines exposure to a range of disciplinary knowledge and methods with effective instruction in processes for transforming such knowledge and methods into solutions to complex social problems through transdisciplinary teamwork is the gold standard. In this chapter we have suggested a number of successful methods through which institutions and organizations have begun to achieve this end.

Key Terms

Area Health Education Centers	Centers funded through Title VII that train students representing a variety of health disciplines and provide them with opportunities to work with underserved populations.
biopsychologist	A behavioral scientist who focuses on both psychology and biology.
Leadership Education in Neurodevelopmental Disabilities and Related Disorders (LEND)	A program funded by the Maternal and Child Health Bureau that is an example of providing transdisciplinary training on the multilevel determinants of health to students in professional programs.
National Public Health Training Centers Network	Programs that improve the public health of vulnerable communities by providing funding for the transdisciplinary training of students, clinicians, and community stakeholders.
Transdisciplinary Research on Energetics and Cancer (TREC)	A National Cancer Institute–funded initiative aimed at reducing cancer linked with obesity. Currently, it funds four centers around the country and also a coordinating center.

Review Questions

1. Why is a transdisciplinary approach a good way to study the phenomenon of health disparities?
2. What are four attributes of successful transdisciplinary teams?
3. What are some barriers to implementing a transdisciplinary education or training program?
4. What can universities do to facilitate successful transdisciplinary learning?
5. What are five topics that might be included in a transdisciplinary education or training program?
6. What teaching methods lead to successful transdisciplinary learning?

References

1. Nicolescu B. Manifesto of Transdisciplinarity. Albany: State University of New York Press; 2002.

2. Jantsch E. Towards interdisciplinarity and transdisciplinarity in education and innovation. In: Apostel L, Berger G, Michaud, G, eds. Interdisciplinarity: Problems of Teaching and Research in Universities. Paris: Organisation for Economic Co-operation and Development (OECD) and Center for Educational Research and Innovation; 1972:97–121.

3. Hoffman-Riem H, Biber-Klemm S, Grossenbacher-Mansuy W, Hadorn GH, Joye D, Pohl C, et al. Idea for the handbook. In: Hadorn GH, Hoffman-Riem H, Biber-Klemm S, Grossenbacher-Mansuy W, Joye D, Pohl C, et al., eds. Handbook of Transdisciplinary Research. London: Springer; 2008:3–18.

4. Committee on Facilitating Interdisciplinary Research, National Academy of Sciences, National Academy of Engineering, Institute of Medicine. Facilitating Interdisciplinary Research. Washington, DC: National Academies Press, 2004.

5. Gehlert S, Sohmer D, Sacks T, Mininger C, McClintock M, Olopade O. Targeting health disparities: a model linking upstream determinants to downstream interventions. Health Affairs. 2008;27(2):339–349.

6. Gehlert S, Mininger C, Cipriano-Steffens CM. Placing biology in breast cancer research. In: Burton LM, Kemp S, Leung M, Matthews SAD, Takeuchi D, eds. Communities, Neighborhoods, and Health: Expanding the Boundaries of Place. New York: Springer; 2011:57–72.

7. Warnecke RB, Oh A, Breen N, Gehlert S, Paskett E, Tucker KL, et al. Approaching health disparities from a population perspective: the National Institutes of Health Centers for Population Health and Health Disparities. American Journal of Public Health. 2008;98(9):1608–1615.

8. Warnecke R, Gehlert S, Barrett R, Darnell J, Ferrans C, Cho YI, et al. Linking multilevel approaches to issues in health policy. Journal of the National Cancer Institute (in press).

9. Gehlert S, Murray A, Sohmer D, McClintock M, Conzen S, Olopade O. The importance of transdisciplinary collaborations for understanding and resolving health disparities. Social Work in Public Health. 2010;25(3):408–422.

10. Gehlert S, Mininger C, Sohmer D, Berg K. (Not so) gently down the stream: choosing targets to ameliorate health disparities. Health & Social Work. 2008;33(3):163–167.

11. Gehlert S, Rebbeck T, Lurie N, Warnecke R, Paskett E, Goodwin J, et al., for the Centers for Population Health and Health Disparities. Cells to Society: Overcoming Health Disparities. Bethesda, MD: National Cancer Institute, US Department of Health and Human Services; 2007.

12. Gehlert S, Colditz G. Cancer disparities: unmet challenges in the elimination of disparities. Cancer Epidemiology, Biomarkers & Prevention. 2011;20(9):1809–1814.

13. Office of Portfolio Analysis and Strategic Initiatives. Overview of the NIH Roadmap. Rockville, MD: Office of Portfolio Analysis and Strategic Initiatives,

National Institutes of Health: 2009. Available at: commonfund.nih.gov/about
.aspx [accessed May 22, 2011].

14. Organisation for Economic Co-operation and Development. The Knowledge-Based
Economy. Paris: OECD; 1996. Available at: www.oecd.org/sti
/scienceandtechnologypolicy/1913021.pdf.

15. Gebbie K, Rosenstock L, Hernandez LM; Institute of Medicine, Committee on
Educating Public Health Professionals for the 21st Century, eds. Who Will Keep
the Public Healthy?: Educating Public Health Professionals for the 21st Century.
Washington, DC: National Academies Press, 2003.

16. Neuhauser L, Richardson D, Mackenzie S, Minkler M. Advancing
transdisciplinary and translational research practice: issues and models of
doctoral education in public health. Journal of Research Practice. 2007;3(2):1–24.

17. Claremont Graduate University. Why Transdisciplinary Studies. Available at:
www.cgu.edu/pages/8628.asp [accessed May 22, 2011].

18. Claremont Graduate University. Transdisciplinary Studies: Frequently Asked
Questions. Available at: www.cgu.edu/pdffiles/CreativeServicePDFs
/TransdisciplinaryBro09.pdf [accessed May 22, 2011].

19. Claremont Graduate University, School of Arts and Humanities. Transdisciplinary
Funding. Available at: www.cgu.edu/pages/8176.asp [accessed May 22, 2011].

20. Advisory Committee on Interdisciplinary, Community-Based Linkages. Best
Practices for Improving Access to Quality Care for the Medically Underserved: An
Interdisciplinary Approach. Sixth Annual Report to the Secretary of the US
Department of Health and Human Services and to the Congress. Washington,
DC: US Department of Health and Human Services; 2006.

21. Nandiwada DR, Dang-Vu C. Transdisciplinary health care education: training
team players. Journal of Health Care for the Poor and Underserved.
2010;21(1):26–34.

22. University of Pittsburgh, LEND. About. Available at: www.uclid.org [accessed
May 22, 2011].

23. University of Washington, UW LEND. Welcome to the UW LEND Program.
Available at: depts.washington.edu/lend [accessed May 22, 2011].

24. University of California, Irvine, Undergraduate Research Opportunities Program.
About ID-SURE. Available at: www.urop.uci.edu/id-sure.html [accessed May 22,
2011].

25. Misra S, Stokols D, Hall K, Feng A. Transdisciplinary training in health research:
distinctive features and future directions. In: Kirst M, Schaefer-McDaniel N,
Hwang S, O'Campo P, eds. Converging Disciplines: A Transdisciplinary Research
Approach to Urban Health Problems. New York: Springer; 2011:133–147.

26. Stokols D. Training the next generation of transdisciplinarians. Paper presented
at: NSF-University of Idaho Conference on Enhancing Communication in Cross
Disciplinary Research; September 2010; Coeur d'Alene.

27. University of Toronto, Institute of Medical Science. MSC8000Y—Transdisciplinary
Studies in Infectious Disease (using Hepatitis C as a model). Available at:
www.ims.utoronto.ca/courses/description/msc8000y.htm [accessed May 22,
2011].

28. Clark P. Institutionalizing interdisciplinary health professions programs in higher education: the implications of one story and two laws. Journal of Interprofessional Care. 2004;18(3):251–261.

29. Cooper H, Carlisle C, Gibbs T, Watkins C. Developing an evidence base for interdisciplinary learning: a systematic review. Journal of Advanced Nursing. 2001;35(2):228–237.

30. Lennon-Dearing R, Lowry LW, Ross CW, Dyer AR. An interprofessional course in bioethics: training for real-world dilemmas. Journal of Interprofessional Care. 2009;23(6):574–585.

31. Pellmar T, Eisenberg L. Bridging Disciplines in the Brain, Behavioral, and Clinical Sciences. Washington, DC: National Academies Press; 2000.

32. Sicotte C, D'Amour D, Moreault M-P. Interdisciplinary collaboration within Quebec community health care centres. Social Science & Medicine. 2002;55(6):991–1003.

33. Advisory Committee on Interdisciplinary, Community-Based Linkages. An Examination of the Healthcare Workforce Issues in Rural America. Eighth Annual Report to the Secretary of the US Department of Health and Human Services and to the Congress. Washington, DC: US Department of Health and Human Services; 2008.

34. Advisory Committee on Interdisciplinary, Community-Based Linkages. Review and Recommendations. First Annual Report to the Secretary of the US Department of Health and Human Services and to the Congress. Washington, DC: US Department of Health and Human Services; 2001.

35. Bronstein LR. A model for interdisciplinary collaboration. Social Work. 2003;48(3):297–306.

36. Clark PG. Values in health care professional socialization: implications for geriatric education in interdisciplinary teamwork. Gerontologist. 1997;37(4):441–451.

37. Allen DD, Penn MA, Nora LM. Interdisciplinary healthcare education: fact or fiction? American Journal of Pharmaceutical Education. 2006;70(2):39.

38. Nash JM. Transdisciplinary training: key components and prerequisites for success. American Journal of Preventive Medicine. 2008;35(2 suppl):S133–S140.

39. Baldwin DC, Jr, Baldwin MA. Interdisciplinary education and health team training: a model for learning and service. 1979. Journal of Interprofessional Care. 2007;21(suppl 1):52–69.

40. Frenk J, Chen L, Bhutta ZA, Cohen J, Crisp N, Evans T, et al. Health professionals for a new century: transforming education to strengthen health systems in an interdependent world. The Lancet. 2010;376(9756):1923–1958.

41. Hall P, Weaver L. Interdisciplinary education and teamwork: a long and winding road. Medical Education. 2001;35(9):867–875.

42. McPherson K, Headrick L, Moss F. Working and learning together: good quality care depends on it, but how can we achieve it? Quality in Health Care. 2001;10(suppl 2):ii46–53.

43. Oandasani I, Reeves S. Key elements for interprofessional education. Part 1: The learner, the educator and the learning context. Journal of Interprofessional Care. 2005;19(suppl 1):21–38.

44. Beck E. The UCSD student-run free clinic project: transdisciplinary health professional education. Journal of Health Care for the Poor and Underserved. 2005;16(2):207–219.

45. Kilgo J, Aldridge J, Denton B. Transdisciplinary teaming: a vital component of inclusive services. Focus on Inclusive Education. 2003;1(1):1–5.

46. Yan J, Gilbert JH, Hoffman SJ. World Health Organization Study Group on Interprofessional Education and Collaborative Practice. Journal of Interprofessional Care. 2007;21(6):588–589.

47. US Department of Health and Human Services, Advisory Committee on Interdisciplinary, Community-Based Linkages. About the Committee. Available at: www.hrsa.gov/advisorycommittees/bhpradvisory/acicbl/About/index.html [accessed May 22, 2011].

Chapter 3

Competencies in Transdisciplinary Public Health Education

Lauren D. Arnold   Anne Sebert Kuhlmann
J. Aaron Hipp   Elizabeth Budd

Learning Objectives

- Define competencies, and explain their role in public health education.
- Provide examples of competencies for transdisciplinary public health.
- Outline the steps involved in developing and implementing competencies for a transdisciplinary public health program.
- Give examples of questions to use for evaluating competencies in a public health curriculum and assessing whether students have developed transdisciplinary public health skills.

•••

The previous two chapters have laid out a definition of transdisciplinary public health; described the practical and scientific benefits of the transdisciplinary approach to research and practice; discussed how to implement transdisciplinary collaborations in the public health context, especially within teams; examined how to educate a new generation of students to function as transdisciplinary scholars to address complex problems, using the best of disciplinary knowledge and methods; and finally, explored how transdisciplinary work is developing in a range of transdisciplinary education and training programs.

This chapter maps a path from the development of core public health competencies to developing transdisciplinary competencies into curriculum for public health students. The chapter outlines specific transdisciplinary competencies potentially important to a student's training, professional development, and perhaps most important, career placement. Suggestions are given for incorporating such transdisciplinary competencies into public health coursework, with processes that faculty and programs can use for the development and implementation of these competencies. The skills important to the development of a competent transdisciplinary public health professional are explored in depth.

Competencies for Transdisciplinary Public Health

Competencies have become an important guiding principle across the spectrum of graduate education in recent years. Today, lists of competencies are commonly found on syllabi, academic program websites, professional organization websites, and in the workplace. Specifically, academic leaders and professional organizations such as the Institute of Medicine (IOM) and the Association of Schools of Public Health (ASPH) now endorse the use of competencies to guide curriculum development for graduate public health education and professional training.[1-3]

In thinking about competencies from both the student and faculty perspective, and given the focus of this book on transdisciplinary education in public health, a number of questions arise:

- What exactly are competencies, and more specifically transdisciplinary competencies?
- Why are transdisciplinary competencies important to a public health graduate student's training, professional development, and, most important, career placement?
- How should transdisciplinary competencies be integrated into coursework, and why should students be aware that this is occurring and actively involved in this process?
- What skill sets are important to the development of a competent transdisciplinary public health professional?

This chapter explores these questions, with a specific focus on transdisciplinary competencies as they affect graduate education in public health.

The concept of *competency-based education* was formally introduced in the 1970s[4,5] and describes an instructional system in which the learning process moves beyond acquisition of information to focus on application of foundational knowledge and skills.[6] *Competencies* are defined as skills, knowledge, and behaviors that are considered to be performance standards in a given field (see, for example, NC Department of Health and Human Services[7]). They describe aptitudes a person should develop to be considered proficient in both the classroom and the field or workplace and are one way to convey expectations of basic abilities in a profession or academic program. For example, MPH program graduates should be able to not only define categories of study designs and biases in data collection and analysis but also to use these concepts when critically reading and evaluating the public health literature. Ultimately, this practical skill is critical to identifying strong sources of evidence to inform public health practice, such as choice of a smoking intervention for urban youth or a breast cancer screening program for recent immigrants. Competency-based education, especially when it is founded in *action-oriented* competencies, drives student instruction and learning, contributing to communication and cohesion across all levels of academic programs.[1] Over the past few decades this pedagogical approach has been used across the spectrum of health professions training, including nursing,[8] medicine,[9-11] dentistry,[12] physical therapy,[4] and public health.[1,13,14]

Because competencies reflect abilities expected by a given profession, competency development is ideally driven by feedback from the workforce and by professional needs.[15] In this way the composition and structure of a public health student's education is directly influenced not only by *what* information she or he should know but also by *how* she or he should be able to apply that information in the workplace, as viewed by practicing professionals in the field. Accordingly, competencies can drive the educational process to employ a hands-on approach in the classroom that engages students and emphasizes activities such as role-playing, working with case studies and simulations, and engaging in group projects to address current challenges in the field. In graduate school it can be easy for MPH students to lose sight of the bigger picture as they become immersed in the details of what they are learning; for instance, when memorizing formulas in biostatistics and epidemiology courses or remembering the subtleties of theoretical frameworks in a behavioral science course. However, actively keeping program and course competencies in mind and striving to achieve them throughout classroom and practicum training will make learning more engaging, meaningful, and realistic; in turn, this can help MPH students remember why they choose public health as a career path.

As discussed in chapter 1, public health is inherently interdisciplinary: the field draws on and integrates a wide range of disciplines to address health concerns and issues on the population level. However, as the authors of chapter 1 have further described, the complexity of public health problems often requires a transdisciplinary approach that transcends disciplinary boundaries and involves the creation of new frameworks and strategies to enable translating research results to feasible, real-world solutions. This latter concept is often difficult to grasp for the MPH student, and it may not even be emphasized in training, especially when students are working through foundational courses. Therefore the transdisciplinary perspective and approach to public health needs to be underscored through the development and integration of specific transdisciplinary competencies into the MPH curriculum.

Why Should Students Care about Competencies?

In a general sense, competencies serve as both the backbone on which to develop courses and a means of ensuring that MPH graduates will be proficient in essential, core skills when they enter the workforce. Mastering competencies is important to students' ability to pass the national certification exam in public health, to become well-rounded public health professionals, and to work in interdisciplinary teams. The earlier in training that the student recognizes the role of competencies, the earlier she or he begins to understand how *book learning* translates to *real-life practice*. Striving to demonstrate competence across the spectrum of public health enables students to build and refine skills and take a role in directing their own educational and professional development. Students can then directly and confidently convey to potential employers the skill sets they have gained and the proficiencies they will bring to a public health position.

Many modern public health positions require a transdisciplinary set of competencies that reach beyond the traditional core areas of public health. It is certainly true that students trained in public health must have a core foundation in the basic principles of public health and an understanding of how these core areas relate both to one another and to disciplines outside public health, such as medicine, sociology, anthropology, and economics. However, as Stokols et al. previously described in chapter 1 of this book, public health practitioners also need to be able to work in transdisciplinary teams to conceptualize and develop new approaches to public health problems that reach beyond traditional disciplinary lines in order to identify feasible solutions to public health problems of interest. The complexity of the chronic conditions that are so often the focus of public health endeavors, such as obesity, HIV/AIDs, cancer, and Alzheimer's disease, require not only the population-level focus that comes from public health but often benefit as well from a transdisciplinary focus and competency skill set.

Core Public Health Competencies

In response to calls from the Institute of Medicine and other professional organizations in the late 1990s, the Association of Schools of Public Health began to explore developing a set of competencies for all graduates of accredited schools of public health.[1] Up to that time each school had its own requirements and expectations for MPH students, and there were no formal, standardized criteria for learning outcomes and skill development across MPH programs.[16] As a first step, ASPH formed a committee that included employer and community representatives to identify existing needs in the field. Making the students active players, ASPH also assessed students' expectations for their graduate education. From this effort it was determined that future MPH graduates should build skills not only in the five core disciplines of public health (biostatistics, epidemiology, environmental health science, health policy and management, and social and behavioral sciences) but also in cross-cutting thematic areas.[1,17] The result was a set of 119 competencies across twelve domains—the five core disciplines along with seven thematic areas that span the breadth of public health concentrations and activities: public health biology, diversity, leadership, communication and informatics, professionalism, systems thinking, and program planning.[1] These competencies, examples of which are presented in table 3.1, are intended to guide MPH program development and curricula.[1] Each school or program is responsible for building on and adapting these competencies in order to develop specific competencies relevant to its own curriculum, strengths, and mission. Today, the ASPH competencies are the focus of the national certification exam in public health, available to all graduates of accredited public health graduate programs.

Although the ASPH core competencies incorporate a number of aspects beyond the five core public health disciplines and include competencies in relevant cross-cutting areas, they do not specifically emphasize the skills and abilities needed for *transdisciplinary problem solving* and a transdisciplinary approach to public health. The IOM, which promotes the use of competencies across the range of health disciplines, highlights the need for health professionals to demonstrate the ability to collaborate and communicate in interdisciplinary teams in order to provide reliable care on both individual and community levels.[3] As described earlier by Stokols et al. in chapter 1, a natural next step is moving from an interdisciplinary to a transdisciplinary model. Being aware of the transdisciplinary approach from the beginning of MPH training will encourage students to more fully develop their potential to collaborate and serve on transdisciplinary teams, working together to address public health challenges from a variety of perspectives.

Development of Transdisciplinary Competencies

As programs and faculty work to develop transdisciplinary competencies, it is crucial that those involved understand the key features that distinguish transdisciplinary competencies from traditional competencies—an emphasis on

Table 3.1. Examples of core competencies in twelve areas of public health for MPH graduates, as defined by ASPH

Core and thematic areas	Examples of competencies
Biostatistics	Interpret statistical results in public health studies. Distinguish among measurement scales, and describe how this affects selection of statistical tests.
Environmental health science	Describe programs, guidelines, and authorities that control environmental health issues. Discuss risk management and communication approaches in relation to environmental health and equity.
Epidemiology	Evaluate limitations and strengths of epidemiological studies. Compute basic epidemiological measures (e.g., incidence, prevalence, relative risk).
Health policy and management	Describe the legal and ethical bases for public health. Apply systems thinking to address organizational issues.
Social and behavioral sciences	Describe the role of community factors in the development and resolution of public health problems. Identify behavioral and social theories used in public health.
Communication and informatics	Describe how public health data are collected, processed, and disseminated. Apply theory-based communication principles across the spectrum of audiences.

Diversity and culture	Describe the role of history and structural inequality in producing health disparities.
	Apply community-based participatory research skills to improve health of diverse communities.
Leadership	Demonstrate team-building, negotiating, and conflict management skills within the context of addressing public health problems.
	Describe and engage in strategies for building collaborations and partnerships.
Public health biology	Apply biological principles to the development of disease prevention and control programs.
	Apply biologically based principles to guide public health policies.
Professionalism	Value commitment to professional service.
	Apply principles of evidence-based decision making in public health.
Program planning	Distinguish between goals, objectives, and outcomes of a public health program.
	Develop a program budget and justification.
Systems thinking	Provide examples of feedback loops in public health systems.
	Analyze the impact of global trends on public health systems.

Note: A list of all 119 ASPH competencies is available at: http://www.asph.org/publication/MPH_Core_Competency_Model/index.html.
Source: Adapted from ASPH Education Committee, *Master's Degree in Public Health Core Competency Model*, Version 2.3 (ASPH, 2006).

creating new frameworks and approaches that draw from those used in various fields; the identification of possible solutions to health challenges based on these outside-the-box approaches; and the application of research to real-world settings. In addition, the development of transdisciplinary competencies must be guided carefully, with consideration of input from faculty, students, and practicing professionals. Transdisciplinary competencies often build on and extend the existing ASPH competencies. For example, ASPH leadership competencies include team building and engaging in strategies for building collaborations (table 3.1); taking these one step further, transdisciplinary competencies might include being able to specifically distinguish features of transdisciplinary collaboration and to develop shared conceptual frameworks from discipline-specific theories (as outlined later in this chapter).

Key Distinctions Guiding Competencies

Most public health challenges are multifaceted and cannot be addressed effectively with simple, one-dimensional solutions. For example, attempting to examine and understand low colorectal cancer screening rates in underserved populations from a solely behavioral health perspective, without consideration of sociocultural, psychological, communication, health systems, or policy perspectives, will likely limit the success of problem identification and any proposed solution. Transdisciplinary problem-solving methods require applying a shared disciplinary framework to the analysis of complex public health problems and then drawing ideas from the interaction of biological, behavioral, social, and public health approaches. It may be argued that better strategies emerge when public health professionals bring together knowledge and experience from diverse perspectives to think about problems and generate solutions in new ways. As stated earlier, public health graduate programs and courses that focus on a transdisciplinary approach will certainly encompass the ASPH core competencies. Yet in order to provide a truly transdisciplinary experience, it is necessary for faculty and students in these programs to consider additional skills, or measures of competence, that will prepare graduates for a successful career in a transdisciplinary environment.

In order to be effective in their future public health practice, students must have the applied skills; that is they must be able to *explain*, *describe*, *distinguish*, *define*, and most important, *develop* and *apply* a set of criteria, theories, or skills. The development and application of transdisciplinary skills and knowledge is the focus of transdisciplinary coursework and a critical aspect of students' professional development. Transdisciplinary work requires teamwork with diverse colleagues and community partners—whether in a virtual or an office setting—and such teamwork has repeatedly been stressed by future employers as a desired competency.

Development of Competencies

Although the development of transdisciplinary competencies may appear initially to be the responsibility of MPH program faculty and staff, the involvement of students and community members—in particular students' future employers—is essential to the process. Programs or courses that desire to develop transdisciplinary competencies and incorporate them into student learning must keep this principle in mind. Drawing on a method outlined by ASPH,[17] schools and departments can approach transdisciplinary competency development as an iterative process that includes input from faculty, students, community partners, and professionals in practice. A systematic model for the development of transdisciplinary competencies, using this iterative process, is described here; this model draws on a process used by the MPH program in the Brown School at Washington University in St. Louis, a program designed with a transdisciplinary focus at its core.

Initial Problem-Solving Competency Development

As a first step to drafting transdisciplinary problem-solving competencies, faculty teams should review ASPH's set of competencies and their own program's current competencies (if such exist), in parallel with course syllabi. The ultimate goal is to narrow down, or fine-tune, the 119 competencies to those most relevant to the program or school, while adding others that reflect the transdisciplinary nature—whether existing or desired—of the curriculum. Above all, the competencies must meld with the mission of the school or program. A list of potential competencies should then be circulated among appropriate substantive faculty, who edit them in light of the program. Redundancies should be identified, and another round of edits will ensure both parsimony and sufficient coverage of the abilities viewed as essential transdisciplinary public health skills.

Although this suggests a place to begin development of general public health competencies, the pathway to development of transdisciplinary public health competencies for public health education programs is not as clear since transdisciplinary competencies for education do not routinely exist in the literature. For this reason, faculty at Washington University's Brown School developed their own set of transdisciplinary problem-solving (TPS) competencies in 2009, via an innovative process during the conceptualization and development of competencies for the entire MPH program. Box 3.1 presents seven of the transdisciplinary problem-solving competences they created and the introduction given to students along with the competencies list. These competencies suggest one model to use when adding transdisciplinary competencies to an established degree program or curriculum.

Box 3.1: Examples of transdisciplinary problem-solving competencies

Transdisciplinary problem-solving methods require applying a shared disciplinary framework to the analysis of complex public health problems, drawing from an understanding of the interaction of disciplinary approaches from the biological, behavioral, social, and public health sciences. *Upon graduation, a student with an MPH should be able to*

1. Explain why the complex, multifactorial nature of problems in public health and health disparities requires a transdisciplinary approach.

2. Describe how social, economic, behavioral, environmental, and biological conditions contribute to health outcomes using theoretical approaches drawn from diverse disciplines.

3. Distinguish the features of transdisciplinary collaboration.

4. Develop and apply processes that integrate and promote transdisciplinary perspectives, contributions and collaboration.

5. Define problems in a transdisciplinary way and develop shared conceptual frameworks from discipline-specific theories and models.

6. Apply transdisciplinary solutions to public health problems using appropriate analytical tools drawn from public health or other disciplines.

7. Demonstrate the ability to communicate transdisciplinary research evidence to key stakeholders to influence policy and practice.

Competency Vetting

An essential step in transdisciplinary competency development is competency vetting, or the refinement of the competencies, through an iterative process that solicits input from students, community partners, internship supervisors, and employers. With respect to student input, vetting requires distributing the competencies to student representatives on the academic program's curriculum committee (or an equivalent body) and to other student organizations. Some programs or schools may strive to ensure that these student participants represent the various concentrations a program offers. The involvement of students in the evaluation of transdisciplinary competencies is somewhat complicated by their lack of experience with public health curricula. For example, students are more likely than other participants to identify omissions of key competencies they believe are currently stressed in classes and assessments, and this suggests that only the students who have taken several courses should participate in the discussion. However, it is also the case that students may not fully appreciate the depth of the transdisciplinary focus until their academic program is complete. Regardless of how students are selected to participate, various methods can be used for effectively obtaining feedback on competencies, including surveys, open forums, focus groups, and directed interviews.

Vetting with community partners and potential employers is also a critical step.[18] Conversations with these individuals should begin with an orientation to the transdisciplinary approach (to ensure that interpretation of that approach is somewhat consistent across participants), accompanied by an open-ended discussion about the importance of transdisciplinary problem solving to overcoming public health problems. Evidence suggests that community partners seek students with the ability to work with others in defining and tackling complex public health challenges. Employers of public health practitioners seek trained master's degree students with skills in problem solving as well as the ability to work in teams; draw on multiple disciplines; apply skills learned from multiple disciplines; and respectfully lead program development and implementation from multi-, inter-, and transdisciplinary perspectives. These are important skills that should be reflected in the final transdisciplinary competencies.

Mapping Competencies to Course Development

The final step in developing an effective transdisciplinary curriculum is to determine how the transdisciplinary competencies will be developed across the continuum of the curriculum, with the goal of building competent public health practitioners. One approach is to lay this out visually, using a matrix that relates the transdisciplinary competencies to courses in which they are presented. For example, table 3.2 displays transdisciplinary competencies as rows and courses in the curriculum as columns. Ideally, each competency can be addressed in more than one course, as that will contribute to the reinforcement of skill and knowledge development and to the ability to apply skills in more than one aspect of public health. During the initial matrix development and prior to each semester, instructors should review their syllabi and learning objectives to identify which of the transdisciplinary competencies are sufficiently covered by the coursework and to consider syllabus changes that would better integrate some of these skills. Faculty who developed the competencies can work in the opposite direction, taking the written competencies and denoting which course(s) should be developing them within the curriculum. Inconsistencies should be vetted by an independent group, and ultimately, the matrix should be introduced to students for feedback. The process of reviewing transdisciplinary

Table 3.2. Example of a matrix for assessing inclusion of TPS competencies in an MPH curriculum

TPS competencies	MPH courses			
	Cross-cutting themes in public health	Research methods	Program planning, implementation, and evaluation	Environmental health
1. Explain why the complex, multifactorial nature of problems in public health and health disparities requires a transdisciplinary approach.	X	X		X
2. Describe how social, behavioral, environmental, and biological conditions contribute to health outcomes, using theoretical approaches drawn from diverse disciplines.	X			X
3. Distinguish the features of transdisciplinary collaboration.	X			
4. Develop and apply processes that integrate and promote transdisciplinary perspectives, contributions, and collaboration.	X	X	X	
5. Define problems in a transdisciplinary way, and develop shared conceptual frameworks from discipline-specific theories and models.	X	X		
6. Apply transdisciplinary solutions to public health problem using appropriate analytical tools drawn from public health or other disciplines.	X	X	X	
7. Demonstrate the ability to communicate transdisciplinary research evidence to key stakeholders to influence policy and practice.	X			

competencies in parallel with individual courses, as well as with the MPH program overall, should be a continuous one, with modifications made to syllabi and overall program requirements as needed. This process should require constant evaluation of the competencies, specifically focusing on how well they are working to achieve the mission, goals, and objectives of the program and, in particular from the student's perspective, to help students obtain a set of useful and marketable skills. The process of evaluating transdisciplinary problem-solving skills is a large topic and is addressed in chapter 4.

Once the transdisciplinary competencies are finalized, the remaining challenge is to integrate them into the curriculum. Although some classes may be inherently transdisciplinary, others, such as core foundation courses, may by necessity follow a more traditional approach to coursework within the context of a particular discipline. Still other areas for integration are the practicum and culminating experience (for example, paper, presentation, exam, or capstone seminar), required components of all MPH programs. The next section provides suggestions for the implementation of transdisciplinary competencies in a transdisciplinary course, a core MPH course, and a culminating experience.

Implementation of Transdisciplinary Competencies in the MPH Curriculum

In designing and facilitating the MPH curriculum, faculty should focus on course elements (for example, assignments, group work, discussions, and evaluations) that guide students toward strong competence in applying transdisciplinary problem solving to public health.

Assignments

Although the transdisciplinary competencies should clearly outline specific knowledge and skills that demonstrate an understanding of both transdisciplinary problem solving and how to apply these skills to public health, assignments in the courses are the crucial elements that teach students how to apply transdisciplinary skill sets. Each assignment in a course, whether a mock grant proposal, policy brief, or reading, should be designed to help students develop specific transdisciplinary competencies. Figure 3.1 illustrates a way for faculty and students to assess how TPS course competencies map to specific course assignments throughout a semester. Mapping these relationships at the start of the semester is a useful way to see where, in theory, competencies will be addressed. One way to verify that assignments actually provide opportunities to build the competencies is to review the competency list and check off each one that applies to an assignment as the semester progresses. Ideally, this should be an ongoing process, so that if desired competencies are not met with

		Assignments			
	Transdisciplinary competencies	Readings & discussion	Paper #1	Group project	Group presentation
Knowledge	Define a public health issue using a transdisciplinary lens	✓			
	Explain the distinguishing features of a transdisciplinary approach	✓			
	Describe the importance of collaborating with diverse communities and constituencies				
Skills	Communicate effectively with transdisciplinary partners	✓			
	Modify and develop strategies that consider transdisciplinary collaboration	✓			
	Demonstrate team-building, negotiation, and conflict management skills				
	Develop strategies to motivate others for collaborative problem solving, decision making, and evaluation				
	Analyze determinants of health and disease using an ecological framework	✓			

Figure 3.1. Mapping transdisciplinary competencies to specific course assignments
Source: From Debra Haire-Joshu's course "Transdisciplinary Problem Solving: Chronic Disease, Policy, and Prevention for Public Health" (unpublished material), Washington University in St. Louis; 2011.

a specific assignment as planned, the criteria for other course assignments can be modified to address those competencies.

It is important for students and faculty to consider assignments with transdisciplinary elements in broad terms, beyond the traditional take-home tasks such as papers or problem sets that students complete individually. Assignments can be completed in class or can involve group work, they may have formal grading criteria or may solicit students' thoughts, and they may occur only once or regularly throughout the course. Integrating a variety of assignments into a course helps students to learn, practice, and apply a variety of transdisciplinary knowledge and skills. For example, at-home readings followed by in-class discussions can occur regularly throughout the course. To integrate a transdisciplinary approach, readings that incorporate a mix of sources and styles, such as peer-reviewed articles, news stories, and agency websites (for the Food and Drug Administration or Centers for Disease Control and Prevention, for example), can introduce students to the wide range of perspectives about a particular issue that they should be aware of and consider when working from a transdisciplinary perspective. Regardless of source, readings can serve to define a transdisciplinary approach to public health problem solving, provide various viewpoints (such as those of interest groups) on public health issues, or discuss newly instituted policies that influence public health. Professors should aim to select readings that highlight knowledge competencies and should prepare guidance for students in doing the readings, so that they pay attention to crucial information. Similarly, throughout the semester, encouraging—or even requiring—students to contribute readings relevant to transdisciplinary problem solving will serve to reinforce the transdisciplinary competencies through active learning.

Discussions

Class discussions provide students with an opportunity to practice thinking and communicating through a transdisciplinary lens. To highlight this mindset, for example, on the first day of class students can be asked to name disciplines that could potentially contribute to solving public health problems that are a focus of the class (for example, childhood obesity, adolescent tobacco use, or cancer screening among middle-aged adults). The disciplines can be recorded so the class as a whole can review the list it has generated (figure 3.2 shows an example, a PowerPoint slide listing disciplines that students suggested were related to a course). Students can then work together to elaborate on how the disciplines listed relate to a specific public health problem of interest and how

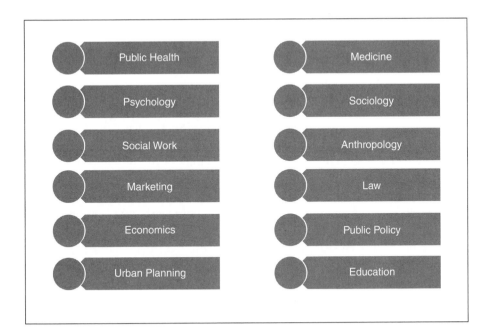

Figure 3.2. Disciplines students identified as likely to be relevant to solving a particular public health challenge
Source: From Debra Haire-Joshu's course "Transdisciplinary Problem Solving: Chronic Disease, Policy, and Prevention for Public Health" (unpublished material), Washington University in St. Louis; 2011.

Box 3.2: Questions for students to ask themselves to actively integrate transdisciplinary competencies into their coursework

1. What makes the approach mentioned in the article or reading transdisciplinary?
2. Why is it important to include diverse perspectives in the design stage of the solution offered?
3. What are the priorities of the disciplines represented in the reading?
4. Do these priorities complement or compete with public health priorities?
5. Which disciplines that were not represented in the reading might contribute to a solution?
6. What might a social worker, clinical psychologist, nurse, or city planner think was missing from the intervention mentioned in the reading?
7. Which theories or approaches from disciplines other than public health might inform this problem?

---

they can contribute to the solution; that is, students can actively pursue some transdisciplinary problem-solving competencies. Such a list can also be used as a backdrop during each class discussion to remind the students of the many disciplines that potentially contribute to solutions of the public health issues at hand. Even if such an exercise is not formally done on the first day of a course, students can proactively do it on their own and use the result as a framework for guiding their learning and thought processes throughout the semester.

Another approach is to use discussion questions, such as those presented in box 3.2, that are designed to encourage students to consider a transdisciplinary approach when reviewing readings. Such questions can be applied to readings throughout the breadth of public health coursework to continuously emphasize the transdisciplinary nature of complex problems—and potential for transdisciplinary work—across the spectrum of public health.

Group Work

In a transdisciplinary approach to public health education, it is critical to make assignments that require the students to work together. Transdisciplinary problem solving outside the classroom involves gathering and analyzing the various, and sometimes conflicting, perspectives of colleagues, politicians, community members, and organizations. Group projects enable students to work with others with diverse backgrounds and experience to practice such skill-based competencies as negotiation, collaboration, and incorporation of diverse perspectives into a solution. For example, requiring students to work in small groups to draft a survey about tobacco use in adolescents may pair students with backgrounds in social work, statistics, biology, and psychology. Each student can bring his or her training to the table by suggesting different vantage points from which to conceptualize the issue and direction of the survey. Ultimately, the final survey should reflect these different perspectives and put them to use so they work together and not against each other.

Evaluations

Providing honest, constructive feedback and evaluation of colleagues is a key professional skill for working in a transdisciplinary environment and for assessing the important skill of teamwork. Evaluating fellow students as part of group work in courses gives students an opportunity to practice this critical skill. Thus course grading criteria should include both self-evaluation and peer evaluation, reflecting the equal importance of competence in working independently and with others. Requiring students to evaluate group members' contributions to a project provides accountability and practice with conflict management, as well as another opportunity to reflect individually on the ways in which a transdisciplinary approach was used. Table 3.3 provides

Table 3.3. Questions to assess transdisciplinary aspects of group work

Component	Evaluation questions
Transdisciplinary approach	What fields were represented by the group? What strength(s) did each field offer to the assignment?
Contribution	How was discussion enriched by different perspectives?
Respect	Did group members encourage others to contribute to their ideas?
Flexibility	Were group members flexible when disagreements occurred, particularly when they arose through a conflict in approaches owing to different disciplines or backgrounds?

Source: From Debra Haire-Joshu's course "Transdisciplinary Problem Solving: Chronic Disease, Policy, and Prevention for Public Health" (unpublished material), Washington University in St. Louis; 2011.

examples of questions students can consider, whether through formal or informal evaluation, when assessing success of the project and group members' contributions.

Integrating Transdisciplinary Competencies into Nontransdisciplinary Coursework

It would defeat the intent of transdisciplinary problem solving if transdisciplinary competencies were not incorporated throughout the curricula, including foundational public health coursework. As described earlier, it is important for faculty, students, and community partners to work together to identify transdisciplinary competencies and find ways to develop them into skill sets.

For example, consider transdisciplinary competencies 1 and 2 in box 3.1. In an environmental health foundation course, a key learning objective is the pathway from source of environmental toxin to health effect. These pathways are often complex and multifactorial. Understanding and solving them always requires a transdisciplinary approach. Exposure to mercury from coal-based power plants provides an example. First, *what is the industrial process in energy production that emits mercury?* This is best understood by environmental and industrial engineers. The majority of mercury is emitted to the air via smokestacks. *Where does it travel and settle?* Chemical engineers can assist with weight analysis, and meteorologists can assist with prevailing wind patterns in the community. A large proportion of mercury settles into waterways and aquatic food chains, which can best be modeled and sampled by ecologists and biologists. Sociologists, nutritionists, and epidemiologists can then help to determine the populations most exposed to local fish. *How is mercury absorbed once ingested and what organs in the human body may serve as natural sinks for mercury? What health effects could mercury have on humans, and is there a threshold exposure?*

This example illustrates the multifactorial challenge that is typical of many public health problems and that requires transdisciplinary approaches to understanding and mitigation.

Integrating Transdisciplinary Competencies into the MPH Culminating Experience

The transdisciplinary competencies also relate to the culminating experience required of all public health graduate students. The Council on Education for Public Health (CEPH) suggests that this educational component may be a paper, presentation, or capstone seminar. To encourage a transdisciplinary approach to the culminating experience, each student should be asked to define and apply transdisciplinary problem solving to a public health challenge above and beyond the required coursework and the practicum experience. Students may build on their internship work as well as coursework in designing their culminating experience, but they must also demonstrate that their work extends beyond what was developed during the fieldwork or during class time. A presentation, for example, is an opportunity for students to demonstrate their grasp and use of transdisciplinary problem solving in a real-world setting. Students can then be assessed on their ability to think and work across disciplines and on their demonstration of knowledge of the traditional core disciplines of public health.

Development of a Transdisciplinary Public Health Professional

Although this chapter has focused on concrete academic skills that may be required from a practical standpoint for a public health professional, it is also clear that working as a transdisciplinary professional solving public health problems as part of a team of professionals may require a unique set of perspectives and other skills. What are these unique skills necessary for working effectively in such an environment?

As previously discussed, students must first develop a strong base in the five foundational areas of public health—biostatistics, environmental health science, epidemiology, health policy and management, and social and behavioral sciences. That is, in order for public health professionals to apply skills in a transdisciplinary way, or know how to meld together disciplinary skills, it is important for them first to have a solid grounding in competencies in each of these core disciplinary areas. Without this foundation, public health professionals rarely begin to understand and reason through the multifactorial challenges of important public health problems. After all, the key point is that transdisciplinary methods provide insights beyond disciplinary insights. That means that disciplinary methods can still be applied, but transdisciplinary methods can provide additional concepts and methods. (For example, traditional environmental health methods provide insights into the problem of mercury exposure from coal-based power plants, but transdisciplinary methods provide broader insights.)

Competence in the core areas of public health is only the beginning, however. A second goal must be to build skills in transdisciplinary problem solving that go beyond these five core areas. These skills include the ability to understand and explain the complex nature of problems; to employ theoretical perspectives from a range of disciplines; to develop a shared conceptual framework of a problem based on a variety of disciplinary perspectives; and to apply appropriate analytical tools to the problem, regardless of the tools' disciplinary origin.[19] Building these competencies will require students to take courses that present a holistic perspective on a particular topic; to reach out and engage with experts, students, and information from a variety of disciplines; and to be comfortable entertaining new analytical tools even if they may be unfamiliar.

Public health students and professionals should also recognize that only a few people on a team in a transdisciplinary work environment may have a formal education in public health; indeed, they might be the only team member with this background. They will bring a population-level perspective, with a focus on disease prevention and health promotion, to the team, and this perspective may differ somewhat from that of other disciplines, particularly those whose work is more individually focused, such as medicine, nursing, social work, or counseling. Public health students and professionals should be prepared to articulate a public health perspective on the issue at hand to students and professionals from other disciplines, and this viewpoint can contribute to understanding and addressing that issue. For example, if a student is part of a task force charged with improving the health of Hispanics in the Atlanta metropolitan area, she may find that the initial inclination of the task force members is to focus on increasing access to health care services—a clinical and somewhat individually focused perspective. If she advocates for consideration of the population-level perspective of public health, that might steer the task force toward considering broader aspects of the issue, such as the disproportionate burden of pedestrian injuries and fatalities found among Hispanics,[20] and that might shift the focus of the task force toward also considering policy change and funding to build more sidewalks.

Students need to know that effective transdisciplinary public health requires that professionals be self-aware, respectful of others, and flexible in their thinking. Public health professionals need to be aware that professionals from other disciplines may use different terminology than the public health professionals would to describe particular concepts—or that similar terminology may be applied differently. For example, an epidemiologist might use the term *cohort* to refer to a study that follows a defined population over time in order to compare outcomes among those exposed to suspected risk factors and those not exposed,[21] while a social worker who uses the same term might be referring to a longitudinal study of a specific population in which a new subsample of the population is selected to participate in each round of data collection.[22] Awareness that people may use terminology differently depending on their disciplinary training can save time and frustration in meetings and can facilitate working relationships among professionals across disciplines.

Public health professionals working in a transdisciplinary environment must be flexible in their thinking. This means being willing to entertain and explore ideas that may challenge one's existing public health knowledge. It also means being respectful of others and their perspectives—listening to their ideas patiently, thinking about how those ideas may fit with or challenge one's existing ideas, and asking questions to clarify any misunderstandings.

Finally, as future professionals, public health students have the responsibility to seek out colleagues with different backgrounds and collaborations with these colleagues. Students should be learning to think from a systems perspective about the various stakeholders and disciplines that may be working on an issue and seek out collaborations to work together as appropriate. Engaging in transdisciplinary public health does not mean that every project has to involve representatives from as many disciplines as possible; it does mean, however, thinking about the disciplines that may have important contributions or insights for a particular project and seeking out those collaborations. Although it may feel more comfortable and seem easier to work with professionals who have similar training and background, public health professionals (and thus public health graduate students) must be willing to seek out collaborators from a variety of disciplines. For example, Mark J. Manary, who is a professor of pediatrics at Washington University in St. Louis and the University of Malawi and whose professional goal is to "fix malnutrition for kids in Africa," stresses the need to work with biotechnology firms, the food industry, and the agricultural industry—not just medical and public health professionals—to address issues of malnutrition globally.[23] Even though many professionals in medicine and public health may be uncomfortable establishing these types of collaborations, they are critical for addressing malnutrition from a transdisciplinary problem-solving perspective.

Transdisciplinary public health professionals need to be able to communicate effectively to diverse audiences and, in doing so, be able to distinguish between information that might be general knowledge and information that might be discipline specific. This too requires seeking out colleagues with other backgrounds and forming partnerships with them as appropriate and having a willingness to read publications, attend lectures and presentations, and find experts in other disciplines. For example, a public health professional working on a team interested in the potential of community mobilization as a strategy to prevent HIV/AIDS among a high-risk population should not be limited to the public health and medical literature in assessing the evidence base for such a strategy. Knowledge about community mobilization produced by psychology, sociology, political science, and international development must also be sought and considered. This may involve searching unfamiliar databases, talking to individuals in both academic and community settings, and seeking learning opportunities such as a conference or course that traditionally might fall outside the realm of public health. Transdisciplinary public health professionals must also be willing to present their work and findings to professionals from a range of disciplines in various settings. Any discipline-specific

Box 3.3: Examples of questions for reflecting on and assessing progress toward mastering transdisciplinary public health skills

1. Do you have a strong understanding of each of the core areas of public health—biostatistics, environmental health science, epidemiology, health management and policy, and social and behavioral sciences?
   - If not, in which areas do you feel weaker?
   - How do you plan to strengthen your skills in each of these areas?

2. Have you ever explained the complex nature of a particular topic to someone who is unfamiliar with the topic?
   - If yes, what parts of your explanation can you improve?
   - If not, with whom can you practice this skill?

3. Can you explain what the public health (population-level) perspective is for a particular topic?
   - How does this perspective differ from an individual-level perspective on the topic?

4. How do you react when you hear a professor or student from a different discipline discuss a topic you have covered in another class?
   - Do you consider how their perspective challenges what you already know?
   - Do you pay attention to terminology and theories mentioned to identify similarities and differences?
   - Or, do you dismiss what they are saying because it does not match your existing knowledge?

5. What other disciplines may be relevant to the particular topic of interest to you?
   - Where will you find the existing knowledge on the topic from these disciplines?
   - Who might be appropriate colleagues or organizations representing these disciplines to collaborate with on this topic?

information may require additional explanation for a broader audience. Box 3.3 provides a list of questions for students to ask themselves as a self-assessment of their progress toward becoming a public health professional skilled at working in a transdisciplinary environment.

Summary

This chapter provides a path from the development of core public health competencies to the ways transdisciplinary competencies can be developed and implemented, with processes that faculty and programs can use. Suggestions are also given for ways in which such transdisciplinary competencies can be implemented into public health coursework. The skills important to the development of a competent transdisciplinary public health professional are explored here, with a specific focus on what students need for professional development and, perhaps most important, career placement.

In recent years, professional organizations such as the Institute of Medicine and the Association of Schools of Public Health have placed a great deal of emphasis on the importance of transdisciplinary and cross-cutting skill sets but have provided limited guidance for integrating them into curriculum development. Transdisciplinary competencies are a way to articulate the transdisciplinary skill sets for guiding the development of transdisciplinary education. These competencies can assist faculty in development of courses, students in the understanding of skills they need to be effective and useful in their careers, and employers in assessing whether transdisciplinary education programs are effective at delivering competent public health professionals.

Key Terms

competencies	Skills, knowledge, and behaviors considered to be performance standards in a given field.
competency-based education	A learning process that moves beyond acquisition of facts and information to focus on application of knowledge and skills.
competency vetting	The refinement of competencies through an iterative process that seeks input from all stakeholders, such as students, community partners, internship supervisors, and employers
culminating experience	A paper, presentation, or capstone seminar required of MPH students at CEPH-accredited schools and programs.

Review Questions

1. What are competencies, and how do competencies guide an individual's educational and professional development?

2. What distinguishes transdisciplinary competencies from foundational and cross-cutting thematic MPH competencies?

3. Why is it important to include public health faculty, students, professionals, and employers in the development of transdisciplinary competencies, and what role does each group play in this process?

4. What are the basic ways of integrating transdisciplinary competencies into the graduate public health curriculum?

5. How can MPH students reflect on and assess their progress toward mastering transdisciplinary public health skills as they advance through their graduate training?

References

1. Calhoun JG, Ramiah K, Weist EM, Shortell SM. Development of a core competency model for the master of public health degree. American Journal of Public Health. 2008;98(9):1598–1607.

2. Council on Education for Public Health. Accreditation Criteria: Schools of Public Health. Washington, DC: Council on Education for Public Health; 2005.

3. Committee on the Health Professions Education Summit; Board on Health Care Services; Ann C. Greiner, Elisa Knebel, eds. Health Professions Education: A Bridge to Quality. Washington, DC: National Academies Press, 2003.

4. May BJ. Competency based education: general concepts. Journal of Allied Health. 1979;8(3):166–171.

5. Rosinski EF. A generic definition of a competency-based education. American Journal of Pharmaceutical Education. 1975;39(5):557–559.

6. Westera W. Competences in education: a confusion of tongues. Journal of Curriculum Studies. 2001;33(1):75–88.

7. NC Department of Health and Human Services. Banding Guide Definitions. 2008. Available at: www.ncdhhs.gov/humanresources/banding/hrguide_definitions .html [accessed November 19, 2012].

8. del Bueno DJ. Competency based education. Nurse Educator. 1978;3(3):10–14.

9. Albanese M, Mejicano G, Gruppen L. Perspective: competency-based medical education: a defense against the four horsemen of the medical education apocalypse. Academic Medicine. 2008;83(12):1132–1139.

10. Bell HS, Kozakowski SM, Winter RO. Competency-based education in family practice. Family Medicine. 1997;29(10):701–704.

11. Leung WC. Competency based medical training: review. British Medical Journal. 2002;325(7366):693–696.

12. Yip HK, Smales RJ, Newsome PR, Chu FC, Chow TW. Competency-based education in a clinical course in conservative dentistry. British Dental Journal. 2001;191(9):517–522.
13. Dandoy S. Educating the public health workforce. American Journal of Public Health. 2001;91(3):467–468.
14. Wright K, Rowitz L, Merkle A, Reid WM, Robinson G, Herzog B, et al. Competency development in public health leadership. American Journal of Public Health. 2000;90(8):1202–1207.
15. Council on Education for Public Health. Competencies and Learning Objectives. Washington, DC: Council on Education for Public Health; 2006.
16. Clark NM, Weist E. Mastering the new public health. American Journal of Public Health. 2000;90(8):1208–1211.
17. Association of Schools of Public Health. Master's Degree in Public Health Core Competency Development Project, Version 2.3. Washington, DC: Association of Schools of Public Health; 2006.
18. Moser JM. Core academic competencies for master of public health students: one health department practitioner's perspective. American Journal of Public Health. 2008;98(9):1559–1561.
19. Brown School of Social Work. MPH Competencies. St. Louis, MO: Washington University in St. Louis; 2011.
20. Beck LF, Paulozzi LJ, Davidson SC. Pedestrian fatalities, Atlanta Metropolitan Statistical Area and United States, 2000–2004. Journal of Safety Research. 2007;38(6):613–616.
21. Gordis L. Epidemiology. 2nd ed. Philadelphia: W.B. Saunders; 2000.
22. Rubin A, Babbie ER. Research Methods for Social Work. 7th ed. Belmont, CA: Thomson/Brooks/Cole; 2010.
23. Mark Manary. [Faculty bio.] Department of Pediatrics, Washington University School of Medicine. Available at: peds.wustl.edu/faculty/Manary_Mark_J.

Chapter 4

Measuring Success

An Evaluation Framework for Transdisciplinary Public Health

Douglas A. Luke
Sarah Moreland-Russell
Stephanie Herbers

Learning Objectives

- Describe an evaluation framework for planning and implementing evaluations of transdisciplinary training programs in public health.
- Develop a framework for the evaluation of transdisciplinary initiatives.
- Explore methods and measures for evaluations of transdisciplinary training and education programs.
- Describe assessment methods that provide objective indices for assessing transdisciplinary training programs.

•••

As noted in previous chapters, there is a growing recognition that finding solutions to many of the most pressing and complex public health problems and scientific questions will require new interdisciplinary (ID) and transdisciplinary (TD) approaches. As a mode of discovery and education, the practice of transdisciplinarity in public health has delivered much already and promises more—a deeper understanding of the interactions of social, behavioral, and genetic health factors and how they affect health outcomes, new technologies, more effective and innovative practices and policies, and in turn, improved health outcomes.[1-5]

The institutionalization of TD public health (both within and across institutions) is essential for creating a new generation of public health scholars and practitioners who are well equipped to address the world's most pressing public health challenges.[6-8] TD public health programs nurture future scientists by providing collaborative opportunities, exposure to disciplines other than their own, mentorship from faculty, and training in TD methods and theories.[9] These features enrich scholars' *depth* and *breadth* of knowledge, and allow them to transcend traditional discipline-based boundaries.[4] Such innovative education and training gives students and professionals the opportunity to reorganize their thinking and practice around TD public health and is essential for continuing to advance practices and policies and promote long-term and long-lasting solutions to complex problems in human health.

However, the promise of TD public health needs to be proven. Evaluation of public health TD initiatives is critical for tracking implementation and assessing the effects of these programs on students, faculty, and academic institutions over time. Although the benefits of TD public health have been frequently suggested, actual assessment of TD programs has been infrequent.[6] As a result, it is difficult to compare different training programs, let alone evaluate their quality or impact. Given the substantial federal and private resources that have been allocated to establish and maintain TD initiatives, it is essential that concerted efforts be made to evaluate their near-, mid-, and longer-term collaborative processes and outcomes.[10-13] The purpose of this chapter is to present an evaluation framework for planning and implementing evaluations of transdisciplinary training programs in public health.

In the next section we highlight previous evaluations of TD initiatives. While there have been a variety of previous studies, few frameworks have allowed for evaluation of a TD initiative across an institution. Thus the remaining sections of this chapter will present an evaluation framework that provides objective indices for assessing TD training programs and institutional TD integration in an academic setting, an example of how such an initiative is currently being implemented, and recommendations for future evaluations.

Overview of TD Initiative Evaluation

According to Irwin Feller, the reality of transdisciplinary evaluation is shaped by "multiples": multiple actors who make multiple decisions in multiple organizational settings that have multiple context-dependent measures of quality.[14] Such heterogeneity highlights the fact that measuring the essential attributes of TD programs, let alone monitoring processes or describing the outcomes, is a complicated task.[6,15] A small number of evaluations on inter- and trans-disciplinary programs have been published, and they provide valuable guidance for new evaluation designs. However, there is little consistency across these studies—they vary in scope, from small-scale studies of centers and specific training programs to large-scale studies of national initiatives.[16] The methodology and conceptual frameworks used in these investigations differ as well.

Most evaluation studies of inter- and transdisciplinary public health or health-related programs have focused on curriculum development and assessment. These studies provide good examples of how to use process and outcome indicators for evaluating training elements and outcomes.[6,17–20] However, these studies have not examined longer-term career outcomes, effects of TD training on academic faculty and staff, or higher-level effects on organizational structures and processes.

A critical element of TD evaluation is the assessment of those factors that are hypothesized to be most related to important TD training outcomes, including positive knowledge, attitudes, and beliefs about TD science.[5,7,9,13,16,21] For example, a number of studies suggest that TD collaboration during and after training is a key indicator of TD training success. Indicators of TD collaboration include development of and attendance in inter-, multi-, and transdisciplinary courses, level of interaction and scholarly exchanges with faculty members and fellow students, number of internship experiences providing opportunities for students to collaborate with scholars from diverse fields, and number of completed dissertations that include TD methodology and committees comprising TD faculty.[2,6,7,9] The capacity of these TD programs to enhance individual competencies (for example, effective teamwork or communication skills) is also highlighted as a measure of training effectiveness.[7] Again, while these studies suggest specific tools for evaluating and promoting TD education and collaboration, the actual evaluation focuses specifically on the quality, novelty, and scope of student and faculty work and does not consider the factors and institutional qualities that go beyond promoting TD collaboration and supporting TD integration.[7,15]

We can also learn about useful TD evaluation approaches by considering larger-scale TD research initiatives. Stokols et al. offer a conceptual and programmatic framework for evaluating the collaborative processes and research and organizational outcomes of transdisciplinary science in a research center initiative.[13] Specifically, they employ a variety of qualitative and quantitative methods to evaluate TD scientific collaboration within and between Transdisciplinary Tobacco Use Research Centers (TTURCs). The presentation of this multicenter evaluation offers a comprehensive framework for tracking the scholarly, institutional, and societal outcomes of large-scale research initiatives; however, training and curriculum development are not explored.

As suggested by this review, many of the existing evaluation studies of TD training in public health focus on the curriculum and classroom and on the direct effects of TD training on students and trainees. A central tenet of the evaluation model we will propose in this chapter is that effective and sustainable TD training is driven by a number of factors that exist outside the classroom. Students certainly may learn about TD research from their practicums, from their experiences working with public health research projects, from attending guest lectures and brown-bag lunches, and so on. Also, any number of faculty and administrative processes and characteristics may support successful TD training. For example, hiring faculty with demonstrated interest and skills in TD science would presumably be positively associated with good TD training outcomes. Essentially, evaluators must take a broad, ecological view of the entire academic organization when evaluating processes and outcomes of major TD training initiatives. Thus the evaluation framework presented here will be the first ecological model of TD evaluation that takes into account curriculum, student, faculty and staff, and organizational levels of analysis. The evaluation of TD initiatives is still a relatively new enterprise, so our hope is that this framework can stimulate further discussion and development of TD evaluation methods and products.

An Ecological Evaluation Framework

Effective TD training programs affect and are affected by almost all parts of an academic institution. For instance, TD programs can contribute toward the formative phase of a scientist's intellectual development, advance the scholarly work of faculty and staff, introduce new curriculum strategies, and result in multi-institutional funding. To develop our evaluation framework, we engaged in a logic-model building process,[22] basing our work on the TD evaluation literature, with input from the leadership of the Washington University transdisciplinary public health program.

Our ecological TD evaluation framework, presented in figure 4.1, highlights the components of a TD initiative within an academic setting and its expected outcomes. The framework is not an exhaustive list of all of the activities and outcomes of a TD program but rather outlines the core components needed for a successful initiative.[23] The framework is organized across four levels: (1) institution, (2) faculty and staff, (3) students, and (4) curriculum. We will now walk you through each level of this model.

Institution

Several stakeholders are integral to a TD initiative: those in a position to make or influence decisions about the initiative, those involved in the operations of the initiative, and those served by the initiative.[24] The influence of these

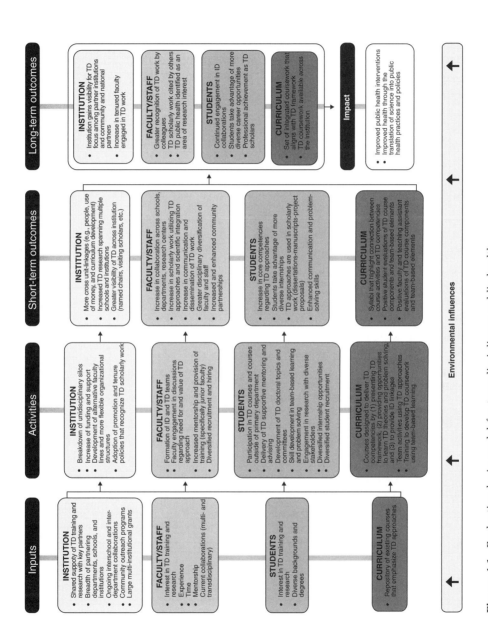

Figure 4.1. Evaluation logic model for transdisciplinary public health

stakeholders on the success of a TD initiative must be included in any evaluation in order to identify facilitators and barriers to achieving the initiative's goals and to determine opportunities for intervention to ensure future success. For example, the larger academic institution in which the TD initiative is housed can have a significant influence on the implementation of TD programs.[7,23,25] The institution often determines the policies that promote or discourage collaboration across departments, schools, and other institutions. By supporting TD programs with funding for the development of new curricula and policies (such as tenure policies) that promote TD scholarly work, the institution can influence cross-unit linkages, collaboration on TD research across schools and other institutions, and the visibility of TD work within the institution and in the larger community it serves.

Faculty and Staff

Faculty and staff play a significant role in the decisions regarding the development of TD training programs and their implementation. While institutional support influences the work of faculty, staff, and students, there must first be faculty and staff who are committed to TD training and research if any program or larger initiative is to be successful. Faculty and staff are ultimately responsible for forming TD teams, collaborating on scholarly work, developing curricula and training programs, hiring other faculty and staff, and recruiting the students who will be trained in TD values and approaches. Thus it is essential to engage faculty and staff in discussions on the value of TD approaches, training and mentorship in TD implementation, and recognition of TD work within and outside the institution.[2,9,23,26]

Students

Students are often the primary stakeholders served by TD training in an academic setting. Successful TD programs will recruit students from diverse backgrounds, engage them in TD courses within and outside their primary departments, provide opportunities for skill development in team-based learning and problem solving, and provide them with mentorship that is supportive of TD approaches in research and practice. Through their participation in such efforts, students are expected to integrate concepts and findings from multiple fields throughout their work; illustrate enhanced communication, leadership, and problem-solving skills; take advantage of more diverse training and career opportunities; and show greater success in team-based settings where individuals from a variety of disciplines must collaborate.[6,9,23,27]

Curriculum

Beyond the primary stakeholders of an academic TD initiative, another main area of important focus is curriculum development and implementation.

Curriculum guides the work of faculty, staff, and students and often serves as the core around which TD initiatives are organized. The goal for a TD curriculum is the development of a set of integrated courses designed to provide training in TD competencies by (1) presenting a framework for conceptualizing TD research and practice, (2) providing sessions that focus on TD theories and problem solving, and 3) promoting opportunities for linkages across disciplines within and outside the academic setting. A successful TD curriculum will include faculty, staff, and students from across the institution, involve partners from outside the institution as instructors and mentors, promote team-based learning, and result in participants who have more positive attitudes toward TD approaches and who can successfully employ the approaches in their work.

In addition to outcomes expected for each of these four levels, this framework highlights anticipated impacts of a TD initiative. These are based loosely on the impacts identified by Stokols et al.[13] and include improved public health interventions and improved health through the translation of science into public health practice and policy. The framework also highlights the importance of environmental influences that can affect TD initiatives, including federal funding in support of TD work, the existence of interuniversity collaborations, the availability of supportive faculty, and so forth.

Strategies for Implementing a TD Initiative Evaluation

The evaluation of TD initiatives in academic institutions has the potential not only to inform the implementation of initiatives in individual institutions but also to contribute to the current state of knowledge in the evolving field of TD training and practice. Thus adequate resources and support dedicated to evaluation are strongly encouraged. This effort includes identifying faculty and staff responsible for overseeing the evaluation, dedicating financial support and other resources to the evaluation, and making a commitment to sharing results with stakeholders within and outside the institution. The "Framework for Program Evaluation in Public Health Practice," disseminated by the Centers for Disease Control and Prevention (CDC), is a useful guide for planning and implementing an evaluation.[24] This framework outlines steps, or strategies, that serve as starting points for tailoring evaluations for public health. The steps are common practices for any program evaluation and can be useful for planning the evaluation of your own TD initiative. In this section, we will walk you through these strategies.

First, the CDC's guidelines recommend engaging stakeholders and bringing them together to describe the program.[24] Stakeholders should include those responsible for implementing your TD training program as well as those that have influence on its implementation, as outlined in our framework (figure 4.1).

Engaging a variety of stakeholders can ensure that the evaluation will address important elements of your TD initiative and gain buy-in early on in the process. Using a logic model will help you describe your program and what is to be evaluated.[22,28] As illustrated by our framework, logic models are pictures of how your program works. They can describe the necessary resources, activities to be implemented, and expected effects of your efforts.[22,24,28] Facilitating a logic modeling process with your stakeholders can identify gaps between your program's actions and its desired effects and also identify the areas most important for evaluation.[22] In accordance with our framework, we recommend engaging stakeholders in the development of a logic model that is tailored for your TD training program and any broader TD initiative in your institution.

Once you have a logic model, it is important to focus your evaluation to ensure that it is assessing issues of greatest concern to stakeholders while efficiently using stakeholders' time and other resources.[24] To help with focusing your evaluation, consider the stage of the initiative (for example, development, initial implementation, or expansion); how data will be used (for example, in identifying opportunities for improvement and justifying funding and other support); and what you and your stakeholders want to know. Identifying your primary evaluation questions can also help with focusing your evaluation by identifying the aspects of the program that will be addressed.[24,29] Using your logic model as a guide, brainstorm with stakeholders to get a comprehensive list of evaluation questions to be asked. Then narrow the list down by prioritizing the questions based on the overall program goals, the program stage, the data available for answering the questions, and the financial support available for the evaluation.[30]

After prioritizing the evaluation questions, you can determine what kinds of data and data collection methods will be most useful for evaluating your TD program. For the evaluation of the doctoral training program in social ecology at the University of California, Irvine, Mitrany and Stokols suggested two areas of focus: processes and products.[6] Process measures include the assessment of coursework, mentorship, and communication and their influence on TD attitudes and behaviors of students. Product measures focus on the assessment of the TD qualities of tangible products (such as papers and dissertations) produced through student and faculty work. These two areas are useful for identifying the TD program qualities and outcomes to be measured. To expand this approach to the larger initiative level, we recommend incorporating measures that also assess the influence on program success of broader organizational factors (such as support of the institution, integration across departments, and involvement of faculty and staff) and the outcomes and benefits achieved by multiple stakeholders (including students, faculty and staff, and the institution).

To ensure that your evaluation conveys a comprehensive picture of your TD program, we recommend using multiple quantitative and qualitative data measures and sources. You can use existing data or collect new data. When choosing methods, keep under consideration who will be responsible for data collection and analysis, the resources available for evaluation, and the potential burden on participants. Table 4.1 presents examples of potential data measures and sources for the evaluation of your TD efforts for each domain area outlined in our framework. It lists many sources that are currently available at your institution (such as attendance, promotion, and tenure dossiers) as well as measures you would need to collect via new sources (such as interviews with faculty and staff) or adaptations of existing sources (such as course evaluations). Works cited in this table offer further information on specific tools and descriptions of how measures and sources might be used. To date, tools for assessing students' TD learning are most prevalent,[9] as cited in table 4.2. Fewer validated instruments are available for other domains in the framework, though a variety of potential data sources are available to inform evaluation of TD initiatives, as illustrated in table 4.1.

Once you have completed these steps, you will want to compile your decisions into an evaluation plan. This is a document that stakeholders can reference to understand what you are evaluating, how you are evaluating it, and when. In addition to developing your logic model and evaluation questions and determining appropriate data measures and sources, it is also important to identify who will be responsible for carrying out the evaluation and a timeline for the primary activities.[31] Analysis protocols and dissemination plans are also helpful and should be considered early on as part of your evaluation planning process. The quality of evaluation data cannot be improved once data have been collected, thus it is important to outline at the beginning how data will be collected, analyzed, and communicated.[32] There are many resources available for guiding the collection, analysis, and interpretation of evaluation data,[33-37] thus we will not go into detail here.

Evaluation of TD programs should be an iterative process in which evaluation findings are regularly reviewed and communicated. As you gather and interpret the evidence, ensuring use of the evaluation findings by sharing results and lessons learned is important.[24] This includes working with other stakeholders to give and receive feedback and to identify recommendations for moving forward. The evaluation of TD initiatives is a relatively new area of focus for public health programs, thus sharing results with stakeholders within your institution as well as those outside it is vital to the further development of TD training programs and broader initiatives.

In the next section, we present a case study that provides a real-world example of how a TD initiative is being implemented in an academic setting,

Table 4.1. Transdisciplinary program evaluation measures and sources

Framework domain	Measures	Data sources
Institution[7,25]	• Tenure policies that reward TD work • Organizational policies that support cross-unit appointments • Funding for TD initiatives within the institution • Research projects with collaborators across the institution	• Organizational policies • Faculty appointments and affiliations • Annual budget report • Grants tracking database
Faculty and staff[2,12,38]	• Collaborative activity • TD attitudes • Readiness to be a TD mentor • Participation in TD-related professional development • TD presence in scholarly work and other products	• Faculty and staff surveys or interviews • Partner relations tracking • Grants tracking database • Publication and citation tracking • Curriculum vitae • Promotion and tenure dossiers • Product assessments
Students[2,6,7,9]	• Participation in TD courses • TD attitudes • Collaborative activity • TD presence in products • Career paths	• Student attendance • Student surveys or interviews • Team assessments • Curriculum vitae • Product assessments • Alumni tracking database
Curriculum[9]	• Coverage of TD content in curriculum • Integration of courses for TD training • Student satisfaction with and assessment of course content • Faculty satisfaction	• Course syllabi • Course catalogues • Course evaluations

Table 4.2. Assessment tools for evaluation of TD students

Tool	Description
Behavior change collaborative activities index[9]	Eight-item scale that has students acknowledge any TD collaborative behaviors (e.g., participating in groups with researchers from other fields, designing a new collaborative study, or taking classes outside their major)
Interdisciplinary perspective index[9]	Six-item scale that measures TD orientations and values; evaluates students' attitudes about using MD approaches and methods
Team project participation scale[9]	Five-item scale that gauges students' evaluations of team projects
Laboratory impressions scale[9]	Five-item scale that assesses the collaborative qualities of students' research settings
Interdisciplinary scientific appreciation index[9]	Four-item scale that measures the degree to which students valued and enjoyed ID or TD collaboration
Product evaluation[6,9]	Ten-point scale that assesses the extent to which there is successful integration of concepts, methods, and findings from different fields in a scholarly product

how it aligns with the components of the framework, and what initial lessons have been learned that will influence future implementation and evaluation.

Case Study: Applying the Framework to an Initiative

The TD evaluation framework presented earlier in this chapter is meant to be generally useful for a wide variety of TD public health training initiatives. Thus its domains and indicators are somewhat generic and would normally be more precisely defined for a specific TD initiative. To provide a more grounded example of how this framework might be used for a real initiative, we apply the TD framework to the current TD public health training initiative being implemented at the Brown School at Washington University in St. Louis. Many of the components of this program (for example, the TD problem-solving classes) are described in more detail in other chapters of this book. Although a formal evaluation of the Brown School initiative has not been implemented, it is still useful to examine progress toward the goals of the initiative, using the important elements of our evaluation framework.

The Brown School TD public health initiative had its genesis in late 2008, when a group of public health faculty and school administrators started planning a new MPH program at Washington University. Much of the time and energy of this group was devoted to curriculum development, faculty hiring, program marketing, and other administrative activities required to get a new graduate program off the ground. However, very early on the MPH leadership group decided to incorporate a new vision of TD public health training into the program. This TD approach would not be limited to the classroom but would touch all aspects of public health at the Brown School, from competencies to faculty hiring, mentoring, and promotion. The long-range plan was to extend this TD vision of public health across the university.

At the time of the writing of this chapter, the first cohort of MPH students has just graduated, in May 2011. The MPH program only recently received CEPH accreditation, and the public health program is only now at its full faculty complement. So it is still early in the TD initiative to examine outcomes to assess the success of the initiative. However, it is instructive to use the framework to assess progress toward goals and to determine what types of evaluation activities should be implemented in order to chart progress over time.

Table 4.3 presents an informal assessment of the Brown School TD initiative, using the indicators of short- and long-term outcomes from the TD evaluation framework (figure 4.1). A variety of formal and informal data sources are used in this table. Although the formal evaluation of this initiative has not been done, a variety of monitoring systems (such as class evaluations, student feedback focus groups, and practicum feedback) have been started to track the success of the MPH program, and these provide some good early data points on the TD initiative as well.

As table 4.3 suggests, the TD initiative is already seeing some early successes. MPH curriculum and course activities are strongly influenced by the TD vision, and evaluation criteria are shaped by TD competencies. Faculty and students are particularly excited about the transdisciplinary problem-solving classes. Students from other programs are asking to participate in the TD courses and student activities. Faculty hiring is already being shaped by the TD focus, and the Brown School is starting to see faculty with more diverse disciplinary backgrounds interested in joining its faculty. Perhaps most encouraging for the long-term prospects of the TD initiative is the support at the university-level for TD programs. In the past year Washington University has provided funding support for the development of new interdisciplinary courses and has also established a new funding program to develop new inter- and transdisciplinary research collaborations.

Informal assessment of the first years of the TD initiative also reveals a number of challenges. Although there is much student enthusiasm for TD public health, there is also a fair amount of confusion. We are learning that faculty need to do a better job of communicating the TD vision and plan to students, other faculty, and local community partners. Also, although faculty have started discussing more broadly how TD public health relates to their

Table 4.3. Mapping the evaluation framework onto the Washington University TD initiative

TD outcomes	Status	Notes
Curriculum		
1. Syllabi that highlight connection between course activities and TD competencies	All TPS [transdisciplinary problem solving] course syllabi highlight connection to TD competencies.	Working to ensure that all regular (non-TPS) MPH course syllabi highlight connections to TD competencies.
2. Positive student evaluations of TD course components	Sixty-six percent of students report positive experience with TPS courses; only 8% report negative experience.	Student satisfaction appears to be increasing over time as new TPS courses are developed.
3. Positive faculty and TA evaluations of TD course components	Informal discussion and faculty retreat conversations indicate support and enthusiasm.	
4. Set of integrated coursework that aligns with TD framework	Alignment of MPH courses with TD approach is a critical part of the MPH accreditation documents.	
5. TD coursework available across the institution	Many of the MPH TD courses are available to students in other graduate programs.	Have not examined yet the existence of TD courses in other schools.
Students		
1. Increase in core competencies regarding TD approaches	Set of [10] core TD competencies established in 2009.	TD competencies used in course activities, evaluations, and MPH culminating exams.
2. Students take advantage of more diverse internships		No formal tracking system in place yet.
3. TD approaches are used in scholarly work	In early evaluations and focus groups, students report excitement but also confusion about TD approaches in public health.	No formal tracking system in place yet.
4. Enhanced communication and problem-solving skills	Coursework developed to provide rich communication and team problem-solving experiences.	

(*Continued*)

Table 4.3. (*Continued*)

TD outcomes	Status	Notes
5. Continued engagement in TD collaboration		Not enough time yet to assess.
6. Students take advantage of more diverse career opportunities		Not enough time yet to assess.
7. Professional achievement as TD scholars		Not enough time yet to assess.
Faculty and staff		
1. Increase in collaboration across institution	Over past two years, development of a small number of new research collaborations taking a TD focus, such as the Washington University Network of Dissemination & Implementation Researchers (WU-NDIR).	
2. Increase in scholarly work using TD approaches	Faculty are currently somewhat unclear on how to categorize their TD work.	Need to establish clear definitions before assessing progress.
3. Increase in dissemination of TD work	Faculty report wanting to take advantage of new TD dissemination opportunities, such as those provided by the Policy Forum (see below).	Need to establish clear definitions before assessing progress.
4. Greater disciplinary diversification of faculty and staff	Recent faculty searches have aimed at broader set of disciplines; strong faculty candidates (including some new hires) have responded to job advertisements because of TD focus.	
5. Increased community partnerships	Faculty are only beginning to have discussions with community partners about TD approach.	

Table 4.3. (*Continued*)

TD outcomes	Status	Notes
6. Greater recognition of TD work by colleagues	Faculty are considering changes to promotion and tenure guidelines that would recognize impact of TD work.	
7. TD scholarly work cited by others	Faculty are currently somewhat unclear on how to categorize their TD work.	
8. TD public health identified as an area of research interest	Public health faculty have clearly established TD as a broad area of interest.	This book is one clear sign of established interest.
Institution		
1. More cross-unit linkages	New and planned university institutes designed to promote inter- and transdisciplinary collaborations (e.g., Institute of Public Health; Policy Forum)	No formal plan to implement cross-unit hiring yet.
2. Increased TD research spanning multiple schools and units	University has established new funding opportunity to promote new inter- and transdisciplinary research collaborations among faculty (URSA—University Research Strategic Alliance).	
3. Greater visibility of TD across institution	University has established new Cross-School Interdisciplinary Teaching Grants, and [4] new TD courses will be developed in 2012.	
4. Institution gains visibility for TD focus among partner institutions		Not enough time yet to assess.
5. Increase in tenured faculty engaged in TD work		Not enough time yet to assess.

own work, it is clear there is a lot of work to do on the specifics; for example, universities and departments must decide how TD work will be evaluated and valued in promotion and tenure decisions.

The biggest challenge in using this TD evaluation framework at Washington University may lie in establishing the data collection mechanisms needed for assessing the longer-term outcomes. For example, it is relatively easy to get feedback from current public health students while they are resident in the program. However, as we stated earlier, we expect that effective TD training will influence the entire career arc of public health professionals. So we need to establish a contact and feedback system that engages students in the years after they leave the MPH program, so we can learn what jobs they take, how they engage diverse stakeholders and collaborators, and how they incorporate TD approaches into their professional lives.

Summary

This chapter presented a general framework for evaluating TD initiatives in public health training and education settings. Although there has been much progress in defining transdisciplinarity in public health and in identifying its core principles (see chapter 1), there are few examples of fully evaluated TD initiatives and a lack of guidance on how to design and implement an appropriate evaluation. The primary innovation in the framework we present is the adoption of an ecological model that recognizes that TD activities and outcomes are organized across multiple levels—namely the curriculum, students, faculty and staff, and institution. In particular, although many of the most important TD activities are focused on the classroom and how public health students are trained, both the evaluation model presented here and the experience of implementing the TD initiative at Washington University underscore that faculty and staff and institutional factors are also important. Just as TD approaches hold the potential for transforming public health, a transformed public health educational institution is required to deliver and sustain this new way of training the next generation of public health scientists and practitioners.

Key Terms

assessment tools	Tools aimed at understanding and measuring student learning.
evaluation	A systematic method for collecting, analyzing, and using information to answer questions about projects, policies, and programs.
logic model	A tool used to evaluate the effectiveness of programs and the logical linkages among program

	resources, activities, outputs, audiences, and outcomes related to a specific problem or situation.
measure	The extent, quantity, amount, or degree of what is being analyzed, determined by a calculation.

Review Questions

1. What are the details of an evaluation framework for evaluating transdisciplinary training programs in public health? What are the core components of the evaluation framework?

2. The logic model is described as a useful framework for the evaluation of transdisciplinary initiatives. What is a logic model, and how is it best adapted to the evaluation of a TD imitative in public health?

3. Within each domain of the framework for evaluation, what is at least one measure for the evaluation of transdisciplinary training and education programs, and one data source for that evaluation? What are the strengths and weaknesses of the measures and data sources?

4. What are three methods for assessing TD training programs, and how do they provide (or not provide) objective indices? What are some alternative measures?

References

1. Kessel F, Rosenfield PL. Toward transdisciplinary research: historical and contemporary perspectives. American Journal of Preventive Medicine. 2008;35(2 suppl 1):S225–S234.

2. Nash JM. Transdisciplinary training: key components and prerequisites for success. American Journal of Preventive Medicine. 2008;35(2 suppl 1):S133–S140.

3. Paul BD, ed. Health, Culture, and Community: Case Studies of Public Reactions to Health Programs. New York: Russell Sage Foundation; 1955.

4. Committee on Facilitating Interdisciplinary Research, National Academy of Sciences, National Academy of Engineering, Institute of Medicine. Facilitating Interdisciplinary Research. Washington, DC: National Academies Press; 2004.

5. Taub A. Transdisciplinary approaches to building the capacity of the public health workforce. Ethnicity & Disease. 2003;13(2 suppl 2):S45–S47.

6. Mitrany M, Stokols D. Gauging the transdisciplinary qualities and outcomes of doctoral training programs. Journal of Planning Education and Research. 2005;24(4):437–449.

7. Nash JM, Collins BN, Loughlin SE, Solbrig M, Harvey R, Krishnan-Sarin S, et al. Training the transdisciplinary scientist: a general framework applied to tobacco use behavior. Nicotine & Tobacco Research. 2003;5(suppl 1):S41–S53.

8. Lattuca LR. Creating Interdisciplinarity: Interdisciplinary Research and Teaching among College and University Faculty. Nashville, TN: Vanderbilt University Press; 2001.

9. Misra S, Harvey RH, Stokols D, Pine KH, Fuqua J, Shokair SM, et al. Evaluating an interdisciplinary undergraduate training program in health promotion research. American Journal of Preventive Medicine. 2009;36(4):358–365.

10. Rhoten D, Parker A. Risks and rewards of an interdisciplinary research path. Science 2004;306(5704):2046.

11. Klein JT. Evaluation of interdisciplinary and transdisciplinary research: a literature review. American Journal of Preventive Medicine. 2008;35(2 suppl 1):S116–S123.

12. Mâsse LC, Moser RP, Stokols D, Taylor BK, Marcus SE, Morgan GD, et al. Measuring collaboration and transdisciplinary integration in team science. American Journal of Preventive Medicine. 2008;35(2 suppl 1):S151–S160.

13. Stokols D, Fuqua J, Gress J, Harvey R, Phillips K, Baezconde-Garbanati L, et al. Evaluating transdisciplinary science. Nicotine & Tobacco Research. 2003; 5(suppl 1):S21–S39.

14. Mansilla B. Assessing expert interdisciplinary work at the frontier: an empirical exploration. Research Evaluation. 2006;15:17–29.

15. Stubblefield C, Houston C, Haire-Joshu D. Interactive use of models of health-related behavior to promote interdisciplinary collaboration. Journal of Allied Health. 1994;23(4):237–243.

16. Thompson-Klein J. Afterword: the emergent literature on interdisciplinary and transdisciplinary research evaluation. Research Evaluation. 2006;15:75–80.

17. Bradbeer J. Barriers to interdisciplinarity: disciplinary discourses and student learning. Journal of Geography in Higher Education. 1999;23(3):381–396.

18. Clarke JH, Agne, RM. Interdisciplinary High School Teaching. Needham Heights, MA: Allyn & Bacon; 1997.

19. Pezzoli K, Howe D. Planning pedagogy and globalization. Journal of Planning Education and Research. 2001;20(3):365–375.

20. Wineberg S, Grossman P, eds. Interdisciplinary Curriculum: Challenges to Implementation. New York: Teachers College Press; 2000.

21. Rosenfield PL. The potential of transdisciplinary research for sustaining and extending linkages between the health and social sciences. Social Science & Medicine. 1992;35(11):1343–1357.

22. W.K. Kellogg Foundation. Logic Model Development Guide. Battle Creek, MI: W.K. Kellogg Foundation; 2004.

23. Misra S, Stokols D, Hall KL, Feng A. Transdisciplinary training in health research: distinctive features and future directions. In: Kirst M, Schaefer-McDaniel N, Hwang S, O'Campo P, eds. Converging Disciplines: A Transdisciplinary Research Approach to Urban Health Problems. New York: Springer Science+Business Media; 2011:133–147.

24. Centers for Disease Control and Prevention. Framework for program evaluation in public health practice. MMWR. 1999;48(RR-11):1–40.

25. Nyden P. Academic incentives for faculty participation in community-based participatory research. Journal of General Internal Medicine. 2003;18(7):576–585.

26. Kessel F, Rosenfield P, Anderson N. Interdisciplinary Research: Case Studies from Health and Social Science. New York: Oxford University Press; 2008.

27. Chang S, Hursting S, Perkins S, Dores G, Weed D. Adapting postdoctoral training in interdisciplinary science in the 21st century: the Cancer Prevention Fellowship Program at the National Cancer Institute. Academic Medicine. 2005;80(3):261–265.

28. McLaughlin J, Jordan G. Using logic models. In: Wholey J, Hatry H, Newcomer K, eds. Handbook of Practical Program Evaluation. 2nd ed. San Francisco: Jossey-Bass; 2004:6–32.

29. W.K. Kellogg Foundation. Evaluation Handbook. Battle Creek, MI: W.K. Kellogg Foundation; 2004.

30. Grembowski D. The Practice of Health Program Evaluation. Thousand Oaks: Sage; 2001

31. Taylor-Powell E, Steele S, Douglah M. Planning a Program Evaluation. Madison: University of Wisconsin-Extension; 1996.

32. Mattessich P. The Manager's Guide to Program Evaluation. Saint Paul, MN: Fieldstone Alliance; 2003.

33. Wholey J, Hatry H, Newcomer K, eds. Handbook of Practical Program Evaluation. 2nd ed. San Francisco: Jossey-Bass; 2004.

34. Steckler A, Linnan L, eds. Process Evaluation for Public Health Interventions and Research. San Francisco: Jossey-Bass; 2002.

35. Stufflebeam D, Shinkfield A. Evaluation Theory, Models, and Applications. San Francisco: Jossey-Bass; 2007.

36. Rubin H, Rubin I. Qualitative Interviewing: The Art of Hearing Data. Thousand Oaks, CA: Sage Publications; 1995.

37. Krueger R, Casey M. Focus Groups: A Practical Guide for Applied Research. 3rd ed. Thousand Oaks, CA: Sage Publications; 2000.

38. Stokols D, Harvey R, Gress J, Fuqua J, Phillips K. In vivo studies of transdisciplinary scientific collaboration: lessons learned and implications for active living research. American Journal of Preventive Medicine. 2005; 28(2 suppl 2):202–213.

Part 2

Cross-Cutting Themes in Transdisciplinary Research

Chapter 5

Transdisciplinary Approaches
Sorting Out the Socioeconomic Determinants of Poverty and Health

Timothy D. McBride   Abigail R. Barker
Lisa M. Pollack   Leah M. Kemper

Learning Objectives

- Explain how transdisciplinary approaches can help us to understand the relationships between poverty, income, and health.
- Understand conceptual and transdisciplinary models of the relationships between income and health.
- Understand analytical approaches used to disentangle the effects of income, poverty, and wealth on health (and effects in the reverse direction as well).
- Understand how to use transdisciplinary models to analyze social policies.
- Explain how to translate and disseminate findings from transdisciplinary models to policymakers.

•••

The United States, along with the rest of the world, is experiencing drastic increases in income inequality that are raising serious concerns about inequality and social justice across society, not the least of which are concerns about the health status of individuals. Researchers have long recognized the need to use transdisciplinary perspectives to address the problems of income inequality, poverty, and social justice and the associated complex health and social problems. As the understanding of these complex health and social problems has evolved over time, researchers and practitioners have increasingly pushed for ideas that transcend the boundaries of traditional disciplinary fields, for more complex empirical methods, and for a more complex transdisciplinary approach, such as the approach described by Stokols et al. in chapter 1.

For three decades after World War II, the incomes of all families generally grew together, but this growth ceased after the 1970s.[1] Since the 1970s, the top 1 percent of families has seen nearly a 300 percent increase in their after-tax, inflation-adjusted incomes, whereas the middle class has experienced an increase of less than 40 percent over that same period. Put another way, owing to the income growth for the top 1 percent of families in the last three decades, the *increase* in their annual income (over $1 trillion), exceeds the *entire* annual income of the bottom 40 percent of households in the United States.[1] "Not since the Roaring Twenties has the share of income going to the very top reached such high levels," Alan Krueger, chair of President Obama's Council of Economic Advisers, concluded in a speech interpreting these trends.[2]

A consequence of these momentous shifts in income is that the middle class is shrinking in the United States, from 50 percent of households in 1970 to 42 percent of households in 2010. Income inequality in our society has been increasing in the last three decades, whereas in the years before 1970, the United States had made major progress in reducing income inequality.

This chapter explores a range of transdisciplinary approaches to public health problems, with a specific focus on the insights these models provide about social and economic determinants (in particular, poverty and income) of health. The first section discusses theoretical approaches, starting with familiar approaches from public health, as grounding for the discussion. Moving on from there, the chapter presents two less-familiar models that are inherently transdisciplinary—the health capital model and the livable lives model. The second section moves from theoretical approaches to empirical approaches and describes the development in recent decades of a wide range of complex empirical approaches. Developed by teams drawing on methods from a range of disciplines (that is, using the science of team science, as described in chapter 1), these new methods are being used in attempts to address health disparities. They capture the transdisciplinary nature of complex economic, health, and social systems but also apply across households, the health care system, and over the life course.

The final section of this chapter presents an example showing how these models have been used recently to provide an analytical framework for understanding what may be the most important piece of social legislation passed in the last few decades—the Affordable Care Act of 2010—which potentially will mitigate the income inequality changes described previously. This section concludes by discussing how the results of this work can be disseminated to the public, to public health practitioners, and to policymakers.

Models of Health Behavior

Public health researchers have employed multiple models to explain health behavior, from the *health belief model* to the *social ecological model*.[3] Many of these models offer a transdisciplinary approach, drawing on the multiple disciplines of public health but also extending to concepts beyond public health in such areas as medicine, psychology, economics, and the environment. For example, the social ecological model describes how to implement health promotion interventions and what to expect from them, looking at the ways in which multiple levels of factors (individual, interpersonal, community, organizational, and societal)[4] influence lifestyle, behavior choices, and health.[5]

This inherently transdisciplinary model (depicted in figure 5.1), starts with individual-level behaviors, much as the health belief model does, and thus important variables influencing behavior will be the individual's family situation (demographics, race, ethnicity, income, poverty, marital status), as well as the individual's interactions with his or her physical and sociocultural surroundings (that is, environments).[6] This model can integrate constructs from models that focus on psychological, social, and organizational levels of influence and can provide a comprehensive and transdisciplinary framework for

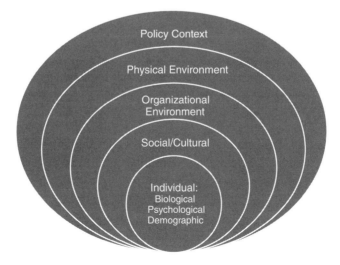

Figure 5.1. A social ecological model of health behavior

incorporating multiple theories, consideration of environments, and policy.[4] The central tenant of ecological models is that they consider both individual-level and environmental or policy-level interventions to achieve changes in health behaviors, because research has shown that healthy behaviors are maximized when environments and policies support these choices.[7] Ecological models are well respected as they are applied to health behavior, as evidenced by the frequency with which authoritative organizations report using these models to guide public health programs (consider, for example, the Institute of Medicine's Healthy People 2010 reports on health behaviors and the World Health Organization's strategy for diet, physical activity, and obesity[4]).

A Transdisciplinary Health Economics Approach: The Health Capital Model

As noted earlier, health behavior approaches have tended to draw on models such as the health belief model or social ecological model to understand how economic determinants affect health status, and how these variables interact with other environmental factors. In recent decades, however, as economists and others from other disciplines have increasingly become involved in the analysis of health behavior, a range of new models have been introduced to the discipline of public health. The application of economic models to health behavior in a major way dates to Kenneth Arrow's seminal article in 1963 and the birth of the subdiscipline of *health economics*.[8,9] After Arrow developed and tailored his insights to health markets, health economists have more recently developed a new set of models, sometimes described as a *health capital* approach, and have used this approach to understand the relationship of a range of variables to health (see, for example, Grossman[10]). This class of models, while originating from the economics literature on human capital theory and investment, represents a significant departure from that literature because it incorporates multiple insights from other disciplines, as discussed below.

In the health capital model the demand for medical care is a *derived demand*, meaning that it is derived from individuals' demand for health—both for its own sake and for its ability to generate income that can purchase other desired goods (which is the traditional human capital approach that economist Gary Becker observed). In the *human capital* approach, the accumulation of education is viewed as a means to expand skills, income, wealth, and well-being over time.[11] Similarly, in the health capital model, each person is endowed with a stock of *health capital*, and that stock of health can be increased by spending time producing health with purchased goods. Medical care is one of these goods; health might also be improved by purchasing other goods, such as nourishment, vitamins, and exercise, to produce investment in health. These purchases will be affected by an individual's knowledge of health—for which overall educational level may be taken as a proxy—as well as the presence of preexisting or chronic conditions. A person's health will decline (depreciate) if he does nothing to improve it. Therefore a person is motivated to invest in health to reduce the time spent being ill, as health stock depreciates.

In the health capital model, each person makes choices to maximize utility, in this case overall well-being, and in the process determines the optimal level of investment in health. The opportunity costs of investing are the dollar amount spent on medical care and the amount of time spent in investing in health, less the amount by which a person's health stock depreciates. It is assumed that health depreciation rates accelerate with age; that is, that people's health deteriorates more rapidly as they age. It is also assumed that the rate of depreciation is affected by other external factors, such as pollution and hazardous employment (that is, environmental health conditions), so that it is more costly for older persons living in polluted areas to attain any given level of health. The optimal level of health a person chooses determines the amount of medical care he or she demands in a specified time period. The main ideas of the model are summarized in the diagrams in Figure 5.2.

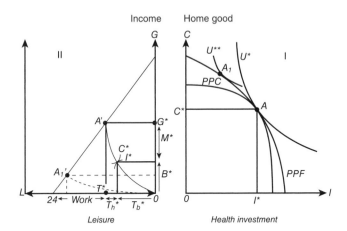

Figure 5.2. Investment and consumption in the health capital model
Source: A. Goodman, M. Stano, and J. M. Tilford, "Household Production of Health Investment: Analysis and Applications," *Southern Economic Journal,* 1999;65(4):791–806.
Note: Diagram I axes: L = leisure; G = total consumption of goods; PPF = production possibilities frontier; Tb = time spent on bread; diagram II axes: B = consumption of bread; C = consumption; I = investment; M = consumption of medical care; Th = time spent on health; U = utility.

The main ideas of this approach are as follows:

1. Health is a form of human capital; it lasts for more than one period and depreciates, but it does not depreciate instantly.

2. The demand for health has two important aspects: (a) a pure investment aspect (health is desired because it also increases the healthy days available for work and thus increases income; figure 5.2, diagram I), and (b) a pure consumption aspect (health is desired because it makes people feel better; figure 5.2, diagram II).

3. The consumer does not purchase investments in health passively in the marketplace but instead *produces* them, spending time on health-improving efforts in addition to purchasing medical care inputs (figure 5.2).

4. Health status is determined by a number of economic factors, including the opportunity cost of time and the value of health to the individual (its investment aspect). The economic factors in health have both direct and indirect price effects, which are immediate as well as dynamic.

5. The demand for medical care is a derived demand. In other words, it is not medical care per se that consumers want but rather health itself; so they demand inputs to produce it.

Because the individual is both a producer and a consumer of health, and time spent being ill generates an opportunity cost (as economists describe it, because there is less time available for work, which ultimately translates into lower income and wealth and therefore potentially higher poverty), individuals' differing opportunity costs are likely to have both direct and indirect effects. It is important to determine whether these effects offset each other or are additive.

Like all theoretical models, the health capital model is useful only if it can be used to generate testable hypotheses and an understanding about how the world works. The health capital model leads to a range of important testable conclusions about the relationships among the direct costs of investments in health (such as the costs of obtaining medical care and the time costs of producing health), the indirect costs (such as depreciation), the indirect benefits (such as greater future earnings), and the total amount of health chosen by individuals. Of particular focus in this chapter is the relationship among economic status, social determinants, and health status. In particular:

○ Higher wages lead individuals to want to invest more in their health and medical care because of the long-term payoff in terms of income; however, higher-income persons who must invest time to improve health are less likely than lower-income persons to do so because they face a higher opportunity cost of time. Thus these factors offset each other to some extent.

In contrast, for lower-income persons, the effects will be the opposite because their long-term payoff is less and opportunity cost of time is less. Thus the model provides an explanation for lower health status among lower-income persons, albeit an explanation that is relatively novel.

○ Health is a *consumption good*, and individuals with higher incomes may be able to invest in health because they have more income available to them— that is, they can invest in health clubs, healthy foods, and time spent producing health, investments that may not be available to lower-income persons, who are less likely to have the necessary time or resources.

○ As in the typical demand model for medical care, health is produced like other commodities. Health is a product of medical care, and more income leads to more production of medical care, so higher incomes lead to a higher production of health.

Conversely, low-income persons will demand less medical care, and invest less in *healthy goods*, and these are two additional explanations for the correlation between income and health status.

○ A major insight provided by the health capital model is derived from the assumption that education can increase the marginal productivity of inputs to health capital, thus increasing the stock of health. This assumption says that a more educated person will be more effective at targeting strategies and behaviors to improve health.

Therefore, empirical results that find a positive coefficient here provide one explanation for the widely observed correlation between health status and education: perhaps it is a supply-side response from increased efficiency in the production of health. The model does not, however, capture the demand-side responses that could arise from a stronger "taste" for healthy goods, nor does it isolate the effects of education on wages. Obviously, education is a major component of the wage and income differences mentioned in the first two bullets.

○ The health capital model is a dynamic, life-course model.[12] Thus decisions at one point in time affect decisions at another point in time. Persons with lower incomes can be affected by chronic disease, chronic poverty, and lack of wealth over time.

Including all the various interconnected decisions made by people over time in a rather complicated transdisciplinary health capital model that includes such variables as education, health, demographics, and family status helps us to understand the social determinants of health and their relationship to economic status in particular. Thus, as the health capital model is a model of the social determinants of health that describes health status over the life course, especially for low- and moderate-income persons, it is inherently a transdisciplinary model.[12] Furthermore, the fact that this model was created on an investment model from classical economics with modifying assumptions from the fields of public health, education, and psychology reinforces its trans-disciplinary label.

Many of the conclusions of the health capital model, and the reasoning behind them, are not obvious outside that model's framework (for example, the opportunity costs of time, the investment and consumption aspects of health, and the countervailing ways these factors work in determining impacts of health investment). For this reason, the health capital model offers a distinct and significant contribution to our understanding of health as the outcome of decisions made by the individual and at the same time offers insights that can affect policy.

For instance, it is a standard assumption in economics for the *marginal utility of income* to be positive; that is, an additional dollar of income increases a person's well-being, and moreover, each additional dollar adds less utility than the previous dollar (one result is that an extra dollar of wages benefits a person in poverty more than that same dollar benefits a wealthy person). This raises important public health implications when applied to the production of health for individuals or across individuals. Applying this model to health, a given investment in health production generates a greater value in terms of its utility for health status (or well-being) when applied to people with lower incomes than the same investment applied to higher-income persons does, all else being equal. The wealthy person has been described in some literature as being on the *flat of the curve* because further investments in medical care will generate little utility or value. This suggests that from society's point of view, a small amount of investment in low-income persons can have a particularly large effect on the well-being of society.

However, the model can also lead to significant paradoxes that are impor-tant for public health. From the perspective of the low-income individual, it may not be rational to spend time investing in health because he can gain more well-being (or utility) from more hours worked than he can from any potential return on health investments. This is so because the *return on investment* from time spent on improving health (measured by wages) is quite low for low-income persons. In contrast, high-income persons have a high return on investments in health. This in turn suggests that it may be appropriate to make policy interventions to address these perverse incentives, because working while neglecting investment in health may have long-run consequences (for example, obesity or chronic conditions), and this may be a partial explanation for higher rates of chronic disease among lower-income persons. A cross-disciplinary team of researchers would be well suited to

Table 5.1. Summary of effects of health capital model variables on health status

Variable	Direction of effect on health status	Causal reason or explanation from health capital model
Higher income	Positive	High investment effect: health investments have a high payoff. High income and wages increase affordability of health improvement and medical care.
	Negative	High opportunity cost of time, owing to high wages.
Lower income	Negative	Low investment effect: health investments have a low payoff. Low income and wages make health improvement less affordable, and medical care may not be affordable either.
	Positive	Low opportunity cost of time, owing to low wages.
Higher level of education	Positive	Operates through an efficiency effect: individual makes improved health decisions.
Lower level of education	Negative	Operates through an inefficiency effect: individual makes poorer health decisions.

identifying the exact mechanisms through which such perverse incentives might be reversed.

In summary, the health capital model is a transdisciplinary approach that provides insights about the effects of income and poverty on health status (table 5.1). As Stokols et al. laid out in chapter 1, transdisciplinary models present novel ideas or approaches that synthesize or extend discipline-specific perspectives. While it is certainly not novel to suggest that income affects health, the health capital model brings novel explanations for why that might be happening, including a life-course perspective, opportunity costs, and the role of education as an *efficiency effect*.

A New Transdisciplinary Approach: The Livable Lives Model

In recent years, low- and moderate-income families in the United States have faced major challenges in many areas of their lives. As noted earlier, the United States has experienced growing income and wealth inequality since the early 1970s, with nearly all the economic gains over the last thirty-five years concentrated in the upper fifth of the income and wealth distributions. Most workers have been falling behind financially. For example, the median earnings of men working full-time fell from $47,000 in 1973 to $45,000 in 2007 (adjusted for inflation). In addition, one out of every three jobs in the

United States is currently classified as low wage, paying less than $11.50 an hour. The deep recession that hit in late 2007 particularly affected low-wage workers, who faced sustained unemployment, significant economic risk and vulnerability, high consumer debt, rising social strains on families and communities, and significant gaps in the social safety net (especially in the health services sector).

Notwithstanding significant advances and expenditures in the field of medicine, the United States lags behind the rest of the world with respect to health status. A recent Commonwealth Fund study found that the quality of the American health care system ranks low in comparison to the systems of other industrialized countries.[13] Many low-income populations struggle to live healthy and productive lives due to disparities in access to and delivery of medical care. Individuals with low incomes or low educational levels and people of color often face exceptional challenges in maintaining good health and are less likely than others to have quality medical care.

Prior to the passage of the Affordable Care Act of 2010, the social safety net had frayed for many low-income persons as income inequality continued to increase.[2] Recent public policy changes such as income tax cuts have exacerbated inequality, as have highly regressive subsidies for health insurance, housing, and assets (via tax policies regarding home ownership, retirement savings, and other social purposes). Middle- and lower-income families benefit little or not at all from these massive asset-building subsidies because such families are less likely to hold jobs that offer benefits and are less likely to own homes—especially high-priced homes with large mortgages.

Thus the changes in well-being since the early 1970s have not been evenly spread across individuals, sociodemographic groups, geography, or a number of other determinants. While the troubling trends in inequality among ethnic groups have received much attention, less attention has been paid to the disparities across geographical regions (for example, economic growth has been more rapid on the coasts than in the middle of the country and in urban areas than in rural areas).

Livable Lives Defined

According to Sherraden et al., a society should be able to provide *livable lives* for its citizens; "that is, lives with a reasonable degree of social, health, and economic security; [they should] have the resources available to take care of their basic needs (shelter, nutrition, health, education) and satisfaction in life, and raise and educate their children successfully."[14]

Public health policy—and private sector action—has a major role to play in fostering these fundamental goals of basic well-being, social and economic stability, and active, engaged citizenship. Moreover, the focus of the livable lives model is transdisciplinary because it extends beyond the basic consumption orientation of traditional public health policy and social welfare policy, focusing attention on the positive conditions that should be achieved for public health and social and economic development.

The livable lives model requires a transdisciplinary theoretical formulation that may be essentially linear (quite common in the social sciences) or dynamic (requiring sophisticated dynamic models of the type addressed later in this chapter). While there is plenty of room for both inductive and deductive approaches in the model and for incorporation of multiple disciplinary contributions, applied social science is essentially deductive, and the essential test of this model is fundamentally an empirical test.

Conceptualizations from a variety of academic disciplines and applied professions can contribute to a transdisciplinary approach to the understanding and investigation of the challenge of making livable lives possible. In particular:

- Public health professionals can focus on prevention of disease across populations by exploring linkages among social, economic, demographic, and environmental determinants of health.

- Sociologists can focus on class, race, and other segmentations as structural issues in society, and some sociologists view individuals from a dynamic, life-course perspective. They may also contribute through analysis of the impact of social networking.

- Social work professionals can look fundamentally at the person-in-environment in order to highlight disparities in social and economic conditions across different groups and promulgate policies and programs that can reduce disparities.

- Psychologists can pay particular attention to individual attitudes and behaviors, and social psychologists can focus on the individual in his or her social context, an emphasis similar to the focus on person-in-environment in social work theory and practice. The idea of *human flourishing*, espoused by social philosophers, also articulates a vision of human growth and attainment of human potential.

- Economists can focus first on income and level of consumption (assumed to represent well-being, or *welfare*). Recently, economic scholars have looked more closely at assets and net worth as having direct effects on well-being, independent of the effects of income. Economists sometimes empirically link economic status and the ability of individuals to achieve general well-being. For example, the health capital model put forward by health economists is an attempt to use dynamic models to link economic status, education, and other social factors to long-term improvements in health.

- Medical researchers often concentrate on the impacts of biology, genetics, and medical care delivery on the ability of individuals to improve their health status.

- Political scientists can offer theories of citizenship and civic engagement.

- Business scholars can provide important views of production, marketing, and consumption in households.

- Law scholars can offer essential legal frameworks, particularly relevant for consumer protections and taking research knowledge into effective public policy.

- Art and architecture professionals are increasingly engaged with low-income communities, drawing on theoretical approaches to creativity and insight in art, and spatial relationships and functionality in architecture.

- Researchers in engineering are already partnering in various ways, particularly on the social aspects of public acceptance of engineering innovations.

The Livable Lives Model and the Life-Course Perspective

The livable lives model requires an understanding of how individuals and families progress across the life course. This includes understanding how individuals deal with life crises and shocks and how they recover from these events. Stated most positively, are individuals able to reach their potential, achieve their dreams, and live out their lives to the fullest extent? What conditions are necessary to make this possible? In particular, when individuals are faced with negative health shocks, how do these setbacks affect their ability to achieve their life goals?

Although there are no limits to the disciplines or topics that might fall into this model, it seems likely that major areas of focus would include the following:

1. *Financial*, including income, savings, asset holdings, and financial capability.

2. *Physical and mental health*, including nutrition, public health, and health care.

3. *Employment*, including stability, working conditions, transitions, and benefits.

4. *Housing*, including both rental housing and home ownership.

5. *Child development and education*, including preschool, primary and secondary school, and postsecondary enrollment and degree attainment.

6. *Community well-being*, especially social engagement honoring diversity.

7. *Political access and representation*, particularly civic engagement and voting.

8. *Environmental sustainability* in the form of responsible consumption (until recently few connections were made between the environment and social and economic issues, but in the twenty-first century this is likely to change fundamentally).

The term *livable lives* also suggests a positive and activist orientation, which rests on three key assumptions for individuals: (1) livable lives are within reach, (2) conditions sometimes have to be created to make this possible, and (3) both public policy and private sector action are required to achieve this goal.

Because it is inherently transdisciplinary, the livable lives approach encompasses much more than traditional policy approaches such as the *living wage* or *family wage*. It embraces a full range of social conditions and policy supports that can make life with a low or moderate income stable, secure, satisfying, and successful in raising children.

Analytical Tools for Addressing Poverty and Health

As Stokols and his colleagues state in chapter 1, traditional multidisciplinary research is typically understood as the "sequential or additive *combination* of ideas or methods drawn from two or more disciplines or fields to address a problem," whereas interdisciplinary research involves the "*integration* of perspectives, concepts, theories, and methods from two or more disciplines or fields to address a problem." For tackling complex public health or social problems, even the theories described in the previous section have not been adequate. Therefore analysts from a range of fields, such as biostatistics, economics, epidemiology, and psychology, have sought transdisciplinary empirical methods to tackle complex public health issues, using, in the words of Stokols et al., an "integrative process whereby scholars and practitioners from both academic disciplines and nonacademic fields work jointly to develop and use novel conceptual and methodological approaches that synthesize and extend discipline-specific perspectives, theories, methods, and translational strategies to yield innovative solutions to particular scientific and societal problems."

To tackle complex systems made up of heterogeneous elements that interact with one another, often with properties that are not explained by an understanding of the individual elements, and that persist over time and adapt to changing circumstances, public health analysts are using results from systems science studies to shape practice and policy.[15] This family of empirical models, often described as simulation models, network models, agent-based models, or system dynamics models, typically integrate a variety of methodological approaches from a range of disciplines and call for sophisticated methods of application.[16] Though familiar in some disciplines, such as economics or engineering, these models are not as widely known or featured in public health education and training. However, it is often the case that the usefulness of these models is significantly enhanced by the formation of teams of scientists from multiple disciplines and fields, and that these teams may seek advice from (or add) practitioners, policymakers, and community members. This transdisciplinary empirical work requires the integration of a variety of disciplinary methods and approaches and has often led to what Stokols et al. describe in chapter 1 as "the *creation* of fundamentally new conceptual frameworks, hypotheses, and research strategies that synthesize diverse approaches and ultimately extend beyond them to *transcend* preexisting disciplinary boundaries" (see also Krueger,[2] Grossman[10]).

The remainder of this section describes in-depth simulation, an approach that has been used as a tool for modeling or describing the complex social, behavioral, and economic relationships that govern health and social behaviors. In the final section, we present an example of using such models.

Systems Science and Simulation Models

Health and poverty are inexorably linked, and the family of systems science models (including, as mentioned, agent-based models, simulation models, and system dynamics models) offers the modern empirical approach to acknowledging this complex relationship. Questions regarding health status—measured in several ways, depending on the interests of researchers—and health care utilization rates are tangled together with questions about the sources of poverty and ways to combat it. Simulation models explore the effects of health policies on outcomes and costs in the short or long term, using a range of economic variables.[17] Comprising a set of equations drawn from real-world analysis and combined into a structural framework that can be used to model real or hypothetical systems, simulation models have been applied extensively to a range of public health and health economics questions, often where there is a paucity of analytical evidence.[18] In fact, it is clear that poor health status is both a cause and an effect of living in poverty, meaning that in statistical terms a serious endogeneity problem exists. The approach of systems science is to combine the results of previous research, often across different disciplines, into one model that allows all the variables to play a role simultaneously as they interact with each other in complex ways, an approach similar in principle to that of the health capital model. Systems science models begin with a large sample population, often drawn from nationally representative surveys (such as the Current Population Survey) that contain a wide range of actual demographic, income, and health data on individuals, usually at one point in time. Then, guided by peer-reviewed literature, researchers apply a set of behavioral rules to govern the choices and behaviors of individuals and organizations at one point in time as well as over time. The simulation evolves over time, tracking changes in the individuals' status or the community's status or the interaction of the organizations with the individual (a major focus of system dynamics models), and the model is run over the life course to obtain results.

To apply systems science methodology to the complexities of health, poverty, and social dynamics, it is necessary to tap into disciplines such as psychology, behavioral economics, demography, and organizational behavior. The rules followed by patients or consumers may, for example, have a *present bias*. This acknowledges the lack of purely rational decision making when it comes to making decisions over time: people tend to prefer gratification now. There may be an element of critical mass in certain types of behavior as well. For example, if a certain percentage of the population smokes cigarettes, this may increase the chance that a particular individual will start smoking also. This is important in capturing neighborhood, peer group, cohort, or other social network effects, which are known to be significant in both health and poverty research. Demographic relationships, in particular birthrates by demographic group, need to be explicitly factored into the model as well. Additionally, physicians are an essential part of the model, and their actions and decisions will be influenced within the context of the organization for which they work. Incentives or other policy schemes meant to alter physicians' behavior would be transmitted through the hierarchy of an organization to change the rules for these actors in the simulation.

This type of analysis can be integrated with methods well established in the health literature, such as survival and event history analysis. In such a framework, the variable of interest is the probability of survival or the number of periods until a particular event takes place. For example, in a study of cancer survivors, researchers are interested in the expected number of months the patient remains cancer free. Standard analysis involves plotting survival rates across different subpopulations and testing for statistical differences. From a policy perspective, researchers would like to identify ways to increase survival—and this is what systems science and simulations can do, as a complete data set is generated for every hypothetical policy change.

Transdisciplinary Models in Policy Work: Solutions for Fragmented Systems

The fragmented US health and social welfare systems fail to use a comprehensive transdisciplinary approach to address the needs of low-income uninsured or underinsured individuals. Numerous programs have been created to provide health insurance, health care services, and income maintenance to the low-income population in the United States. However, these programs are often narrowly focused on a particular problem, and thus they address narrowly a particular problem in a person's life, without acknowledging related problems and applying a transdisciplinary perspective.

Within the health care system, the Medicare and Medicaid insurance systems—and within these systems Medicare Parts A, B, C, and D—are fragmented and complex, as are the fifty-one different state Medicaid and state Children's Health Insurance Program (CHIP) systems, which are often loosely linked to income programs such as Supplemental Security Income (SSI) and Temporary Assistance for Needy Families (TANF) programs, as well as other non-income-based programs such as housing assistance. Each of these programs fills a critical need for low-income persons, but they can work at cross-purposes at times for their respective populations. For example, each program has a separate needs test, and sometimes these accumulate so that each additional dollar of income is subject to what is essentially a tax rate that is quite high. This can create perverse incentives for individuals to avoid seeking health capital to improve their well-being, as described by the socioecological and health capital models presented earlier.

A transdisciplinary understanding of health and public health leads to the suggestion that the health and social welfare systems be integrated, so that critical services will be provided that enable low-income individuals to improve health. Findings from models such as the health capital model, the livable lives models, and complex simulation models lead researchers to conclude that there are numerous factors affecting the lives and health of people that must be addressed to have a greater impact on the health of the individual and individual demand for health care services. Furthermore, these models show that the process is dynamic and takes place over a person's life course.

Innovative Transdisciplinary Policy Interventions

The Affordable Care Act of 2010 (ACA)—perhaps the most significant piece of social legislation passed in decades—is an example of a comprehensive and complex piece of health and social legislation that offers a wide range of opportunities to improve the delivery of assistance for health care and social services to low-income individuals. It also provides new funding and initiatives aimed at improving health and preventing disease that begin to address some of the issues raised in this chapter. For instance, with the passage of the ACA, low- and moderate-income individuals will be able to address a wide range of concerns, including

- Access to affordable health insurance for all citizens below the poverty line, starting in 2014 through state-based health insurance exchanges (although this will be limited in any states that reject federal funds for Medicaid expansion)

- Subsidies for individuals with incomes above 133 percent of the poverty line to purchase affordable health insurance through state-based health exchanges

- Reforms in health insurance markets so that no individuals will be denied coverage based on prior health conditions

- The ability for individuals to navigate easily between programs (such as going from Medicaid to private insurance), reducing the stigmas or problems that have plagued low-wage workers and their employers

- Public health measures designed to create incentives to keep individuals healthy, including reductions in the prices for preventive care, incentives for community and clinical prevention activities, funds for public health infrastructure activities, funds for prevention research and training, and the creation of the National Prevention, Health Promotion, and Public Health Council

It is clear that the ACA takes a different approach to health promotion and improvement than has been typical, and that it comes from a tradition represented by the models described in the first two sections of this chapter, such as the theoretical models (socioecological, health capital, or livable lives models) and the empirical models (simulation approaches) that recognize the complexity of the problems of health care access, cost, and quality. Thus, whether the ACA will improve the lives of low- and moderate-income persons or not depends on how it affects not just the health dimensions but the many other dimensions of their lives: income, education, food, housing, and other necessities. The ACA recognizes that the problems of low- and moderate-income persons are not static but dynamic and that they have a lifelong dimension. For example, treatment of chronic diseases such as obesity, diabetes, and heart disease can be much more effective if it is undertaken early in life and offers a range of interventions, including preventive care, recognized by many aspects of Title IV of the ACA.

The development of the ACA created major challenges for the policy community on a level not approached by any major piece of legislation preceding it. By 2010, due to constant and ongoing methodological improvements and computational power, analysts were able to provide policymakers with quick turnaround analyses of the effects of the ACA. Largely, these results were based on detailed microsimulation models.[19] Two of the most prominent models developed during the health reform effort were the Congressional Budget Office's model[20] (a complex simulation model that took over two years to develop, in anticipation of the health reform debate), and the Urban Institute's health insurance reform simulation model (HIRSM).

As the health reform debate unfolded over 2009 and 2010, the estimates generated by the Congressional Budget Office's microsimulation model became the crucial arbiter in the debate in ways that were unprecedented in public policy. In fact, the legislation could not be passed until the CBO completed its analysis of each change in the legislation as it worked through the process, and the analysis was publicly announced and delivered to the Congress.[21] Other organizations and analysts, such as the Urban Institute, Robert Wood Johnson Foundation, and others, also produced parallel and independent analyses of the health legislation, using simulation models and produced in real time.[22]

In a systematic review of the flurry of simulation models, Glied found that simulations of health reform proposals in recent years have helped policymakers clarify potential unanticipated consequences of policies, and they have illustrated the likely magnitudes of policy-induced changes with reasonable certainty.[19] Baseline estimates of key empirical variables are drawn from sample surveys and empirical literature, and they measure imprecisely, with sampling error and statistical error. However, Glied found that the estimates resulting from the simulation models, compared with realized outcomes of actual implemented policies, suggests these models are "moderately successful" in forecasting, with the estimates falling within about a 30 percent range of the realizations, and she concludes that the models are useful with this range of error, for the reasons discussed here.

Disseminating Results of Transdisciplinary Analysis

If researchers have important transdisciplinary findings, isn't it a key step to disseminate these findings to policymakers and practitioners? And what are the challenges in doing so, with transdisciplinary work, especially when dealing with complex public health and social problem problems?

There is widespread agreement that health services research should be more accessible and useful to policymakers and other key stakeholders at the national, state, and local levels.[23] The health research community has issued reports offering detailed recommendations to research and funding audiences for promoting greater research dissemination and use.[23] A 2000 conference employed a discussion format to offer detailed recommendations to research and funding audiences for promoting greater research dissemination by researchers to policymakers and greater research use.[24] Both of these approaches identified a set of issues and potential solutions for expanding policymakers' access to and use of health services research through improved products and dissemination. More recently, the Coalition for Health Services Research noted that "health services research when appropriately funded, coordinated and disseminated plays a critical role in addressing problems related to the nation's health care system" (p.1).[25] In addition, federal funders are seeking ways to strengthen the links between researchers and important target audiences by identifying the information needs of end users and developing mechanisms for promoting effective research dissemination.[24] Research has identified several strategies critical for effective dissemination and expanded use of public health and health services research.

1. *Engage end users when framing research.* Researchers should anticipate users' needs by developing long-term agendas that consider emerging health issues. Researchers should engage users in framing research agendas. One way to do this is by establishing a research-to-policy network comprising researchers and users. Another is by developing *synthesis* products that summarize what is known on a topic, in an accessible, readable format, in order to identify additional research needed. Research conducted with a transdisciplinary approach particularly benefits from such a summary because it establishes a common ground for researchers who are coming together from different intellectual backgrounds and who may have different types of knowledge. Researchers should monitor policy developments so that previously released research findings are communicated when they are relevant to current policy debates.

2. *Researchers should tailor the design of products to meet the needs of diverse end users.* Different products are needed for different stakeholder groups. Thus research delivered to policy audiences must be packaged to fit certain needs and also to appeal to the audience in general. Policymakers prefer short, to-the-point, user-friendly products, such as policy briefs or summary fact sheets that contain key information relevant to policy discussions. Moreover, policy briefs containing main descriptive findings can be disseminated while the researcher is preparing a journal article containing detailed statistical analysis on the same subject. Policy briefs or other dissemination products should have well-written titles that reflect vital "takeaways" from the research, should include strategic visuals (such as simple and clear graphs and charts), and should be structured to include key findings easily noticed by the reader. The briefs should also include detailed information on local areas (for example,

states, counties, or congressional districts) that appeal to policymakers (since "all politics is local"). While it is important to stress the limitations of the analysis on the brief or fact sheet itself, information about the statistical methods should be available mainly via references or internet links.

Other end users may have different needs, which the dissemination product must be tailored to meet. One advantage of a transdisciplinary team is that the message may be customized for different audiences by relying on different members of the research team to interpret the results, perhaps framing these results in the vocabulary of their own research specialty as appropriate, in order to facilitate communication across disciplines.

3. *Make research products easily accessible to end users.* Users may need to provide research results to policymakers immediately (in minutes, not hours or days). Research utilization by users is predicated on users having ready access to research findings, and multiple communication channels are needed to reach various audiences, including policymakers, associations, advocacy groups, and media. Changes in modern communication strategies have led to a preference for e-mail announcements with links to new research findings; e-mail dissemination allows timely access to information and active routing of documents directly to interested parties. In addition, well-designed, professional, and accessible websites draw users to relevant research findings.

4. *Expand contact and working relationships with end users.* When research is used to inform policy, users must trust that the information they receive is reliable and credible, and they will often rely on personal contacts with researchers they trust. Thus the most effective means of disseminating research to policy users is through direct, sustained interpersonal contact. Researchers earn the trust of policymakers when they present accurate and evidence-based information, acknowledge data or information limitations, provide an objective and nonpartisan viewpoint, work diligently to be recognized experts in their fields, respond to staff requests in a timely fashion, and provide policy relevant information specific to staff needs. Researchers should provide timely and objective analysis, even if it conflicts with established policy views. Although researcher-policymaker relationships develop best through interpersonal interaction, trust also can develop through electronic communication or shared written documents. High turnover in policy staff careers necessitates that researchers regularly renew efforts to establish and nurture relationships with new staff. The obvious point of contact for researchers is with policy staff associated with the researcher's own state, though staff who support members of committees with jurisdiction over the issues may offer a possible connection. Advocacy groups may also serve as intermediaries to provide research findings to policymakers. However, this creates a different dimension to the relationship for researchers and may call

into question the credibility of the researcher's work. Researchers can protect themselves from this questioning by providing unambiguous results (not subject to interpretation) to the groups. Transdisciplinary research teams insulate themselves further from this problem by their very nature, because their work is automatically perceived as having a consensus view.

5. *Invest in developing greater capacity for effective dissemination.* Effective dissemination efforts require dedicated resources to support specialized knowledge and skills, in addition to the resources needed for the research activity. The imperative to produce timely, useful, and accessible information creates competitive pressure for many researchers. Researchers should have a plan and budget for effective dissemination that identifies resources consistent with meeting the needs of the relevant policymakers, trade organizations, and practitioners. A possible menu of resource options includes writers (such as science writers or journalists), public relations specialists, a publications budget that includes website development and management, support for telephone and electronic communications, travel to sustain relationships, and staff time for dissemination. Scientifically sound research is the core ingredient of effective dissemination, but policy communication skills are particularly important for the development and dissemination of products valuable to policy audiences.

Summary

The profound increases in income inequality affecting the United States have important social justice and public health implications that have become a major focus of the literature on the social determinants of public health. Transdisciplinary modeling approaches lend the greatest insight into the effects of income and poverty, and this chapter has explored some recent innovative models that are providing insights from both theoretical and empirical perspectives but that are not widely known to the public health field. On the theoretical side, the chapter presented the health capital model and the livable lives model, and on the empirical side the chapter discussed the family of models often called simulation and system dynamics models, with a specific focus on microsimulation models. Microsimulation models, which are inherently very broad and transdisciplinary, have been used recently to model the effects of the most far-reaching piece of social legislation passed in the last half-century in the United States, the Affordable Care Act, which may reverse the trend of rising income inequality that has been occurring in the last three decades and which will have profound effects on health inequality as well, for the reasons enumerated in this chapter.

Key Terms

health capital model	A model that describes the demand for health from a theoretical and life-course perspective.
life-course perspective	An approach that examines how a sequence of socially defined events and roles that the individual enacts over time may influence future decisions and events such as marriage and divorce, fertility, and health.
simulation	The imitation of the operation of a real-world process or system over time, using a model developed to represent the key characteristics or behaviors of individuals or communities or organizations.

Review Questions

1. Why are transdisciplinary approaches especially useful for understanding the relationships between poverty, income, and health?

2. What are the leading models for exploring the relationships between income and health? What are the strengths and weaknesses of these models?

3. What analytical approaches are commonly used to disentangle the effects of income, poverty, and wealth on health? What difficult statistical issues are faced in this analysis?

4. What common public health policy problems are well suited to researchers' use of the income and health conceptual models?

5. Why is it important to translate and disseminate transdisciplinary results to policymakers, and what challenges are faced in this process?

References

1. US Census Bureau. The Changing Shape of the Nation's Income Distribution: 1947–1998. Washington, DC: US Census Bureau; June 2000.
2. Krueger A. The rise and consequences of inequality in the United States. Speech delivered to the Center for American Progress, January 12, 2012.
3. McLeroy KR, Bibeau D, Steckler A, Glanz K. An ecological perspective on health promotion programs. Health Education Quarterly. 1988;15(4):351–377.
4. Glanz K, Rimer B, Viswanath K. Health Behavior and Health Education Theory, Research, and Practice. 4th ed. San Francisco: Jossey-Bass; 2008.

5. Israel B, Checkoway B, Schulz A, Zimmerman M. Health education and community empowerment: conceptualizing and measuring perceptions of individual, organizational and community control. Health Education Quarterly. 1994;21(2):149–170.

6. Stokols D. Establishing and maintaining healthy environments. American Psychologist. 1992;47(1):6–22.

7. Ottawa Charter for Health Promotion. Ottawa: Canadian Public Health Association; 1986.

8. Arrow, KJ. Uncertainty and the welfare economics of medical care. American Economic Review. 1963;53(5):941–973.

9. Fuchs VR. The Future of Health Policy. Boston: Harvard University Press; 1998.

10. Grossman M. On the concept of health capital and the demand for health. Journal of Political Economy. 1972;82(2):223–249.

11. Auster R, Leveson I, Sarachek, D. The production of health: an exploratory study. Journal of Human Resources. 1969;4:411–436.

12. Grossman M. On optimal length of life. Journal of Health Economics. 1998;17(4):499–509.

13. Davis K, Schoen C, Stremikis K. Mirror, Mirror on the Wall: How the Performance of the US Health Care System Compares Internationally, 2010 Update. Washington, DC: Commonwealth Fund; June 2010.

14. Sherraden M, McBride T, Rank M. Livable lives: a concept note. Working paper, Center for Social Development, Washington University in St. Louis; 2009.

15. Luke DA, Stamatakis KA. Systems science methods in public health: dynamics, networks, and agents. Annual Review of Public Health. 2011;33:357–376.

16. Gilbert N, Troitzsch KG. Simulation for the Social Scientist. New York: Open University Press; 2005.

17. Merz J. Microsimulation—a survey of methods and applications for analyzing economic and social policy. MPRA Paper 7232, University Library of Munich, Germany; 1994.

18. Orcutt GH, Caldwell S, Wertheimer RF. Policy Exploration through Microanalytic Simulation. Washington, DC: Urban Institute; 1976:1–12.

19. Glied S, Tilipman N. Simulation modeling of health care policy. Annual Review of Public Health. 2010;31:439–455.

20. Congressional Budget Office. CBO's Health Insurance Simulation Model: A Technical Description. Washington, DC: Congressional Budget Office; 2007.

21. Congressional Budget Office. Analysis of the Major Health Care Legislation Enacted in March 2010. Washington, DC: Congressional Budget Office; 2010.

22. The Urban Institute. The Urban Institute's Health Microsimulation Capabilities. Washington, DC: Urban Institute; July 2010.

23. George Mason University, Center for Health Policy Research & Ethics, RUPRI Center for Rural Health Policy Analysis; US Agency for Healthcare Research and Quality; US Office of Rural Health Policy. Linking Rural Health Services Research with Health Policy: Conference Report. Fairfax, VA: George Mason University, Center for Health Policy Research & Ethics; 2000.

24. Mueller KJ, Coburn AF, Wakefield MK, McBride TD, Slifkin RT, MacKinney AC, for the RUPRI Rural Health Panel. Bridging Rural Health Research and Policy: Dissemination Strategies. August 2007. Available at: www.rupri.org/Forms /Health_Panel_Aug07.pdf.

25. AcademyHealth. Placement, Coordination, and Funding of Health Services Research within the Federal Government. AcademyHealth report. Washington, DC: AcademyHealth; 2005.

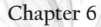

Chapter 6

Transdisciplinary Public Policy
The Roles of Law and Public Health in Creating Public Policy

Sidney D. Watson

Learning Objectives

- Understand how to implement transdisciplinary research through the use of law and public policy.
- Explore the ways in which law and public policy are at the core of transdisciplinary public health research and practice.
- Develop methods for more effectively using transdisciplinary teams to use public policy and law.
- Explore methods for putting science into practice in ways that are community focused and intervention oriented.
- Understand how public health law is implemented through constitutional and other judicial decisions, statutes and ordinances, regulations, public policy, and institutional rules.

●●●

As has been outlined in the previous chapters, transdisciplinary methods for public health research involve using broadly constituted teams of researchers

The author thanks Scott Burris for reading and commenting on this chapter, and Jamille Fields, Saint Louis University, for research and editing assistance.

working across disciplines to create real-world solutions to public health problems.[1] Public health (and other) collaborative research tends to be interdisciplinary and multidisciplinary, involving a single discipline working with one or two or other disciplines on an issue of mutual interest. Such research uses the tools of the principal investigator's discipline complemented by coinvestigators with additional skills from other disciplines.[1] Thus it was cancer specialists and epidemiologists working in such interdisciplinary teams who identified the correlation between secondhand tobacco smoke and lung cancer, establishing a previously unknown pathway for lung cancer.

Transdisciplinary research goes further, seeking not just to identify causes but also to create innovative solutions that are beyond the scope of any one discipline. In transdisciplinary research participants seek to adapt their own discipline's theories and research to the needs of the other disciplines represented in the research group and to view problems through a variety of disciplinary lenses. The practice ramifications of a transdisciplinary approach are that it pushes disciplines from silos, side by side with their respective traditions, so they can intermingle with and inform each other. As disciplines learn from each other and boundaries erode, the hope is that problems are defined in novel ways and solutions become more creative. This pushing across disciplines tends to grow the research team and change the research dynamics. For example, a transdisciplinary cancer research team might include, in addition to a physician and epidemiologist, an economist, psychologist, environmental engineer, and lawyer. Together, the research team members might model and compare alternative policy interventions for reducing secondhand smoke, including economic incentives to reduce smoking, methods to alter smoking behaviors, and environmental changes. This kind of team approach draws across disciplines, helping researchers to learn from each other and, in doing so, to define the problem and solution in innovative ways.

Transdisciplinary research is concerned with getting science into practice, so it tends to be community focused and intervention oriented.[1,2] Among the primary tools for implementing transdisciplinary research are law and public policy. Therefore this chapter focuses on two areas. First, it discusses why law and public policy are at the core of transdisciplinary public health research and practice. Second, it describes how public health professionals can work more effectively as part of transdisciplinary teams using public policy and law.

Why Policy and Law Are Important to Public Health

"Public policy can be one of the most effective approaches to protecting and improving the health of the population."[3] This statement made by an Institute of Medicine committee reflects the fact that public policy and law have long played a key role in improving community health.[4] For example, once physician and public health pioneer John Snow had evidence that the source of the 1855 London cholera outbreak was water from the now-infamous Broad Street pump, he needed legal authority from the locality's board of guardians to remove the pump handle in order to stop people from drinking that water and stop the epidemic.[5] And one of the first laws passed by the first US Congress was a provision to fund quarantine inspections of all ships entering US ports.[6]

Most public health policies are implemented through law.[3,7,8] Laws authorize public health functions like vaccination and quarantine, criminalize risky behaviors like speeding and driving while intoxicated, and discourage other forms of risky behavior through a variety of tools including warnings on tobacco and alcohol and sin taxes. In addition, as public health policies are implemented, these policies stretch into all the disciplines encompassed by public health, suggesting an inherently broad transdisciplinary focus. One can argue here that the implementation of public health policy through law is in itself the interpretation of the goals of the public health disciplines in legal language, and then the implementation of these laws in practice, often or usually requiring a transdisciplinary focus.

While the term *public policy* is often invoked to mean the positions, principles, and priorities that inform high-level decision making in all branches of government, the term is also used to refer collectively to statutes, regulations and rules, executive agency strategic plans, executive agency guidance documents, executive orders, and judicial decisions and precedents.[3] Although public health practitioners sometimes use the term *law* to refer narrowly to statutes created by the legislature, legal scholars define *law* more broadly to also include regulations, constitutional law, judicial decisions, and the norms to which public and private actors conform their behavior and that are treated as authoritative (table 6.1).[5]

Law—like public policy—is more than just the rules written down in statutes and court decisions: it also encompasses the institutional arrangements and day-to-day practices through which law influences behavior and attitudes.[9-12] Constitutional law provides the organizational structure for government. It provides the ground rules through which policies are debated, codified, implemented, and interpreted. Law also gives legitimacy to social norms, by, for example, prohibiting certain forms of discrimination and protecting free speech.[13] In the private realm, contract law shapes our concepts of how the economy should function and civil society should be ordered. Family law shapes our ideas of how to form our most intimate relationships.[12]

Much of the law and policy that influences public health operates in the private realm. US health care is primarily provided by private actors, and most of the law that regulates health care delivery and financing influences the private activity of hospitals, doctors, pharmaceutical companies, and insurers. As such, public policy enacted through law is often what makes public health

Table 6.1. Defining law and public policy

Constitutional and other judicial decisions	These are current court interpretations of the US Constitution and state constitutions and of federal and state statutes, regulations, and common law. These decisions are based on decisions made by previous courts (precedents).
Statutes and ordinances	These are generally produced by the legislative branch of government, including Congress, state legislatures or assemblies, city councils, school boards, and the like. Laws passed by Congress or a state assembly are called statutes. Laws passed by local units of government are called ordinances.
Regulations	These are rules, procedures, and administrative codes promulgated by the executive branch of government, such as federal or state agencies, to achieve a specific objective or discharge specific duties. These are applicable only within the jurisdiction or purpose for which they are made.
Public policy	This term refers to the broad arena of positions, principles, and priorities that inform high-level decision making in all branches of government, but it is often used to refer collectively to laws, regulations and rules, executive agency strategic plans, executive agency guidance documents, executive orders, judicial decisions, and precedents. Some public policies do not have the force of law (that is, they are not enforceable in a court of law or by a public agency), but they may have an impact similar to that of law in the actions they produce.
Institutional rules	These are policies and guidelines adopted by private actors that govern how these actors operate internally and externally. Some institutional rules may be required or encouraged by statute, regulation, court decision, or public policy. Others may be the result of private ordering among the parties, without guidance from government.

Source: Adapted from Institute of Medicine, Committee on Public Health Strategies to Improve Health, *For the Public's Health: Revitalizing Law and Policy to Meet New Challenges* (Washington, DC.: National Academies Press; 2011).

goals manifest in the private health sector. Similarly, public health laws that seek to alter risky activity typically operate in the personal and private sphere of individual behavior, whether they are seat belt laws or prohibitions on unprotected sex, suggesting a broad scope of influence.

Using law and policy to further public health goals requires attending to the difference between law as it is written in statutes, regulations, and court decisions and law as it happens in practice, the divide between "law on the books and law in the streets."[1,14,15] Laws once enacted must be implemented. Sometimes, however, implementation is stifled because of lack of funding. For example, the federal health care reform law of 2010, the Affordable Care Act (ACA), provides for important investments in growing the public health workforce through new scholarships, loans, and loan forgiveness for public health professionals.[16] However, these programs are dependent upon Congress appropriating the funds necessary to create these programs. Without these appropriations, these important programs will be initiatives on the books but will never come into practice.

At other times, laws on the books do not make it into practice because public officials do not administer and enforce those laws. In the 1952 *Brown v. Board of Education* decision, the US Supreme Court declared school segregation to be unconstitutional and ordered schools to integrate with "all deliberate speed," but for over twenty years Southern officials dragged their feet, avoiding implementing the Court's ruling.[17,18] Domestic violence is an area where, for years, statutes making it a criminal offense to batter a spouse routinely went unenforced because local law enforcement officials either took no notice of the law or were not persuaded of the need to enforce it.[19]

Finally, law on the streets can be different from law on the books because the public's perception of the law can be quite different from what is actually required by the statute, court decision, or agency policy.[3] For example, state legislatures and Congress have passed laws prohibiting workplace genetic discrimination, and empirical studies show that such discrimination is rare, but members of the general public nevertheless believe such discrimination occurs frequently.[20] In the early days of the AIDs epidemic, at-risk individuals were so afraid that they would be stigmatized by a positive test that laws providing for anonymous testing had little impact.[3,5]

Roles for Law and Public Policy in Public Health

Law and public policy play three roles in public health: (1) *infrastructural* public health laws authorize the government to use its power for public health purposes, (2) *interventional* laws are designed to achieve a specific health objective by modifying a health risk factor, and (3) a whole range of incidental public health laws enacted primarily for some nonhealth purpose have intended and unintended health effects.[3,5,12] The scope of these roles brings a range of disciplines into the discussion of the implementation of law and public policy for public health; that is, it creates the need for a transdisciplinary discussion of public health issues.

First, as indicated, public health infrastructural laws create the governmental powers that administer public health by authorizing, organizing, and empowering governmental public health agencies.[3] They also typically set boundaries on public health interventions, balancing individual interests in privacy and property against community concerns about the general welfare.[5] At the turn of the twentieth century, such enabling laws were used to create boards of public health, establish clean water supplies, require the vaccination of children, and allow the inspection of workplaces for safe conditions. Infrastructural laws also establish the foundation for epidemiology, mandating collection of vital statistics data and requiring reporting of communicable diseases.[5] Controversy about the appropriate scope of infrastructural public health law has been at the heart of the public policy debate about the public health response to bioterrorism.[21]

Second, interventional public health laws alter a risk factor in order to produce a desired health outcome.[3] Some risk factors result from personal behavior, such as unsafe driving habits, unsafe sexual habits, and other hazardous behaviors. Mandatory seat belt laws aim to change automobile drivers' and passengers' habits; statutes providing for anonymous HIV testing are meant to encourage individuals to be tested. Some public health laws are aimed at institutional actors who may be creating particular risk factors. For example, the Clean Air Act discourages companies from polluting. Tort liability for lead paint is meant to discourage the creation of a social and environmental hazard.[5] Zoning laws prohibit certain types of development in certain neighborhoods.

Public policy has a transdisciplinary toolbox of interventional legal tools that can be used to modify risks factors with the aim of improving population health (table 6.2).[2,5,22] These include tax and spending initiatives, often drawn from economics and health services research; requirements to supply information through labeling and disclosure; policies that alter the built or the natural environment; and three forms of regulation: direct, indirect, and deregulation.[5] Public health law is not merely about enacting laws that require the public to do certain things (such as wearing seat belts) or prohibit them from doing other things (such as polluting the environment). Laws can create a wide array of financial, informational, and behavioral incentives for healthier communities, and this often brings in the disciplines of health behavior and also economics.

Interventional public health laws have been at the center of some of the most important public health successes of recent years. The combined use of cigarette taxes, package warning labels, advertising restrictions, bans on smoking in public places, and tort litigation has altered social norms and significantly reduced tobacco use and tobacco-related deaths.[23-25] Strong evidence, drawn from biostatistics, economics, and health behavior studies, links the decline in the rate of motor vehicle injuries per mile driven to an array of interventional public health laws including highway and new car safety standards, reduced speed limits, stricter enforcement and harsher penalties for

Table 6.2. Examples of interventional public health laws

Types of interventional law	Examples
Taxes, incentives, and federal spending authority	Cigarette and other sin taxes Tax deductions for green technology Federal highway funding to states Medicaid's federal match to states
Requirements to provide information	Food and drug labeling Disclosure of health information
Policies that alter the built environment	Zoning regulations Toxic waste regulations
Policies that alter the natural environment	Clean water regulations Clean air regulations Environmental justice litigation
Direct regulation	Seat belt and helmet laws Iodized salt provision Pasteurized milk provision Licensure of hospitals
Indirect regulation	Tort litigation over lead paint injuries Tort litigation over tobacco injuries
Deregulation	Decriminalization of HIV risk behaviors Distribution of sterile injection equipment

Source: Adapted from Institute of Medicine, Committee on Public Health Strategies to Improve Health, *For the Public's Health: Revitalizing Law and Policy to Meet New Challenges* (Washington, DC: National Academies Press; 2011).

drunk driving, and mandated use of seat belts and child restraints.[5,26] Workplace safety laws have reduced the incidence of occupational injuries.[27] Legal restrictions on lead paint have reduced blood lead levels among children.[26] Fluoridated water has reduced dental cavities in children.[26]

The third and final role played by law in public health is seen in the array of laws enacted primarily for some nonhealth purpose but having unintended health effects.[3,28,29] For example, federal agriculture subsidies were enacted to fulfill agricultural, economic, and trade objectives, but we now know that corn subsidies may contribute to unhealthy American diets and lead to obesity, diabetes, and cardiovascular disease.[30,31] Criminal laws aimed at curbing illegal drug use may increase the risk of drug users contracting HIV.[32] Corporate and tax laws that determine the tax status of hospitals and other health care organizations have an indirect impact on health to the extent they either encourage or fail to encourage the provision of certain services and care for those without insurance.[12]

These incidental public health laws affect public health by influencing the nature and scope of the economic and the social environment, and understanding these impacts requires a transdisciplinary focus (see chapter 1). Even though these laws may not have been intended to address public health, transdisciplinary research has shown that incidental public health laws likely have an even greater impact than interventional public health laws on community health.[28,33] In her book *Populations, Public Health, and the Law*, Wendy Parmet provides four excellent examples of such law.[12] First, because of the strong correlation between higher educational level and better health status, laws requiring that children attend school may actually do more to improve a population's cardiovascular health than policies that target medical or public health interventions to those at high risk of heart disease.[12,34,35] Second, by encouraging or discouraging walking, zoning laws almost certainly have a greater impact on obesity than laws requiring insurers to pay for weight reduction surgery.[12] Third, laws that modestly alter the sexual practices of a large population, for example, by regulating the portrayal of sex in the media, may prevent more cases of HIV than would laws that directly target a few individuals who knowingly infect their sexual partners.[5,12] Fourth, given the increasing evidence that income levels and the extent of inequality are important social determinants of health, it increasingly appears that laws that have a broad effect on the distribution of wealth have a more substantial impact on the health of large populations than so-called core public health laws do.[30]

Public health academics, practitioners, and agencies have promoted the use of public health enabling laws and interventional laws. More recently, they have prompted policymakers to think about the health implications of incidental public health laws. As those in public health engage in public policy and law to solve problems, they are acting with not only a public health perspective but also a transdisciplinary perspective. The next section discusses how public health practitioners can help to break down the disciplinary silos that can separate them from others who engage in public policy.

A Public Health Perspective on Public Policy and Law

Public health organizations and practitioners have a long tradition of engagement with public policy and law advocacy. During the 1855 London cholera outbreak, John Snow needed legal authority from the board of guardians of St. James Parish to remove the pump handle, so he personally appealed to the board. His action not only led to disabling the pump but also prompted a public debate that led to two legal directives, the Public Health Act of 1858 and the Sanitary Act of 1866.[3,5] Public health pioneers pushed for interventional laws like sanitation regulations and mandatory immunization provisions.[12] In recent years, public health has been as the forefront of law reform efforts ranging from bioterrorism and flu preparedness to health insurance reform.

While nineteenth-century legal scholars thought of law as *natural law*, something that could be discerned from the natural order of things, since the progressive era, legal scholars and practicing lawyers have recognized that law is a means for ordering society that draws from many disciplines. Political science and philosophy inform constitutional law. Theories based in psychology and sociology fuel the ongoing debate about whether criminal law discourages criminal behavior better through the threat of punishment or through penalties that rehabilitate. Economic theory has been one of the most powerful influences on late-twentieth century law, influencing torts and contracts as well as health insurance law. Public health brings a unique perspective to law that can help move a policy discussion toward a transdisciplinary, not merely interdisciplinary, perspective.

The public health point of view infuses policy and law discussions with a specific set of values and measurement tools. Public health's focus on community and population health, for example, offers a counterbalance to more individualistic perspectives. Moreover, public health emphasizes the *public good* aspects of health, which, at least theoretically, can be measured by objective health statistics.[5] This means that public health brings to transdisciplinary teams both a tangible focus and measureable goals that can focus the search for public policy and legal interventions. It is important, though, for public health practitioners and researchers to appreciate how this public health perspective expands and challenges the perspectives that other disciplines bring to public policy and law.

Public health has a deep communitarian ethic.[5] It has a nuanced appreciation of the interconnected nature of health, well-being, individuals, and communities.[5] Public health recognizes that the health of others has an impact on the community as a whole.

Public health also recognizes that the health of individuals depends at least in part on social and environmental factors beyond their control, requiring a transdisciplinary focus.[5] As public health professionals have studied population health, social epidemiologists have recognized that social conditions (the so-called social determinants of health) help to determine the health of an individual. This suggests that those interested in shaping public health policy cannot understand the causes of an individual's health status by looking only at factors intrinsic or unique to that individual, be they genes, lifestyle choices, or behaviors. Policymakers also need to focus on the individual's social environment to better understand how that environment affects the individual's risk factors and health. This *cells to society* approach to understanding public health problems is an important transdisciplinary focus that is being increasingly captured in public policy.

Public health practitioners should not assume that other disciplines or policymakers are familiar with the groundbreaking work of epidemiologist Geoffrey Rose. In 2001, Rose's comparison of blood pressure readings for middle-aged men in two populations—Kenyan nomads and London civil servants—demonstrated how a population health perspective leads to more effective policy strategies to improve health, as compared to the individual-oriented strategies typically proposed by law and medicine.[31] Rose showed how looking at the incidence of heart disease and high blood pressure just among middle-aged male civil servants in London might lead epidemiologists and others to conclude that the disease was caused by these workers' behavior or genes, factors that are commonly treated as individual risk factors or the result of personal choices. However, when Rose compared the overall rate of heart disease among these middle-aged male London civil servants with the rate among middle-aged male Kenyan nomads, he found that even those Londoners considered to have "normal" blood pressure had elevated rates compared to the Kenyans' rates. By comparing different populations, Rose was able to begin the process of identifying factors affecting British society and the environment at large that contributed to heart disease, factors that would be missed if one looked only at the clinical status of individuals or at British health alone. Rose's work implies that subtle social and environmental factors, rather than individual genes or behavior, can affect an entire population and be the primary factors in hypertension.[31]

On one level, Rose's research merely confirms what many people and policymakers sense intuitively—where we live and work can make us sick. What Rose and other researchers in the burgeoning field of social epidemiology contribute to transdisciplinary research is the ability to measure the impact of social conditions on health and wellness, thus creating empirical proof based on statistics and probabilities. Public health researchers' population-based studies have demonstrated the connections between smoking and cancer, and seat belt use and auto fatalities. These epidemiological studies have had a powerful impact on legal interventions designed to reduce harmful social and environmental conditions and thereby to improve individual and population health.

Rose's research also illustrates how public health's population focus points to legal and policy strategies different from those favored by disciplines with a more individual-oriented focus. Typically, public health policy interventions focus on the people with the most severe health problems; for example, those with the highest blood pressure. It labels them at risk and seeks to remedy their condition through some combination of treatment and lifestyle intervention.[12] However, a remedy aimed only at the sickest in Rose's British group might miss the majority of preventable cases of hypertension. A strategy aimed at the subtle, societal level factors that affect the population as a whole and account for the higher overall rates of hypertension in the British group as compared to the Kenyan group might prevent more cases, even though its impact on any one individual is likely to be less noticeable.[31]

Public health researchers call this the *prevention paradox*: interventions that operate even slightly upon larger populations can, at times, reduce the overall incidence of disease more significantly than those that act more robustly on only high-risk individuals or other narrowly defined groups.[36] For example, getting people to use seat belts has a greater impact on driving fatalities than policies aimed at removing drunk drivers from the road.[12] Public health, through its transdisciplinary focus on population health and its tools of epidemiology and biostatics, offers unique insights into both the problems that contribute to poor community health and innovative, potentially far-reaching solutions. Public health research is helping policymakers understand that health is not merely about biology but is the result of complex interactions of environmental, social, and behavioral factors. Public health is also helping policymakers move beyond individual-focused policies to broader population-based approaches.

Understanding community health through a broad ecological lens has also pushed the boundaries of public health beyond its traditional core areas of epidemiology, biostatics, environmental health science, health policy and management, and social and behavioral sciences and into transdisciplinary work that includes informatics, genomics, communication, cultural competence, community-based participatory research, policy and law, and global health and ethics.[1] Law offers the vehicle for applying this broad view of public health to public policy making.

However, public health practitioners need to remember that public health also has its own perceptions about the role of government and law that can differ from those of other fields and disciplines. Because public health is concerned about improving health and has its roots in efforts, like John Snow's, to create legal edicts in aid of community health, it is not reticent to use governmental authority.[37] In contrast, many other disciplines see a more limited role for government. Economists, for example, are concerned about maximizing markets and typically propose governmental action only when they see an identifiable market failure.[37] Physicians have historically been concerned that governmental authority will interfere with the doctor-patient relationship and have, until recently, strongly opposed government efforts to expand health insurance. Public health theory also differs from the political theory that underlies much of US constitutional law in that the latter tends to emphasize the rights of individuals and seeks to limit the spheres of governmental authority.[5]

Public health's communitarian ethic and reliance on governmental action sometimes stands in stark contrast to the individualistic values that underlie much of US law. The philosophical theory that informs the Bill of Rights is one that respects the importance of individual autonomy and seeks to protect it from governmental action that restricts individual choice, free speech, or personal expression. At times, the values of law and public health—one individual based and the other community based—have clashed bitterly. In the early days of the AIDS epidemic, civil rights lawyers and public health officials took opposite sides in a heated policy debate about the relative merits of required testing, mandated reporting, and other coercive governmental action intended to control the spread of the infection.[38] Transdisciplinary research and practice offers a venue for bringing these views into collaboration in order to identify public health policies that both protect the community and respect individual choice. Recent efforts to control the spread of contagious diseases such as SARS (severe acute respiratory syndrome) reflect just such a new, more transdisciplinary approach.

Public health's communitarian objectives can also create tensions with those espousing economic objectives and market-based solutions.[3] This occurred during the Industrial Revolution, when workplace health and safety was often pitted against large industrial interests. It remains true today as large corporations seek profits by shaping consumers' desire for sugar-sweetened foods and beverages, tobacco, and alcohol, which can have negative individual and population health impacts.[3] As public health professionals learn to make better use of economic analysis, they will be able to participate in these policy debates on a transdisciplinary basis that addresses both economic concerns and public health objectives.

As the field of public health increasingly attends to the broadest social and environmental determinants of health, it enters a public policy debate where the controversy between communitarian and individual values can be especially contentious. The pathways by which social conditions that are most distant from individual behavior influence population health behavior are the most complicated to explain—conditions like economic inequality, urbanization, mobility, cultural values, and attitudes related to discrimination and intolerance on the basis of race, sex, and other difference. The connections in these cases are especially complex from cause to effect and occur over particularly long time frames.[3] Underlying values about community and notions of individual choice and responsibility tend to become default positions in the absence of good science to help inform opposing individuals' or groups' worldviews.[39,40]

This means that public health researchers and practitioners will often need to translate their assumptions about the proper role of government into language and policy constructs that will resonate with an American public (and with other researchers) that tends to default to individualistic and private sector approaches. Recent work in the emerging transdisciplinary field of public health law research is establishing the population health impacts of a wide array of laws, both those intended to improve public health and those that have unintended impacts.[28] While the operation of law cannot often be studied in experimental designs, the expanded use of observational studies, rapid assessments, qualitative methods, and modeling is being deployed to understand better how laws affect community health.[28] This kind of evidence-based research can help to move the policy discussion to a new transdisciplinary level—one that takes us beyond the old disputes that divide the policy options into binary choices.

Summary

Transdisciplinary work in public health and law has the potential to bring new collaborations to public policy. However, this transdisciplinary work will require that lawyers have a richer understanding of public health and that public health practitioners have a more robust appreciation of what law is and the myriad ways it influences personal and public health.

Key Terms

constitutional and other judicial decisions	Current court interpretations of the US Constitution and state constitutions and also federal and state statutes, regulations, and common law. Legal decisions are based on decisions made by earlier courts (precedents).
institutional rules	Policies and guidance adopted by private actors that govern how they operate internally and externally. Some institutional rules may be required or encouraged by statute, regulation, court decision, or public policy. Others may be the result of private ordering among the parties, without guidance from government.
public policy	Broadly speaking, the positions, principles, and priorities that inform high-level decision making in all branches of government. This term is also often used to refer collectively to laws, regulations and rules, executive agency strategic plans, executive agency guidance documents, executive orders, judicial decisions, and precedents.

regulations — Rules, procedures, and administrative codes promulgated by the executive branch of government, such as federal or state agencies, to achieve a specific objective or discharge specific duties. Applicable only within the jurisdiction or purpose for which they are made.

statutes and ordinances — Generally produced by the legislative branch of government, including Congress, state legislatures or assemblies, city councils, school boards, and so forth. Laws passed by Congress or a state assembly are called statutes. Laws passed by local units of government are called ordinances.

Review Questions

1. Why is a transdisciplinary approach that includes a legal perspective so important for analyzing public policy?

2. What are the core methods for using transdisciplinary teams effectively to develop and use public policy analysis, advocacy, and research?

3. Why is it important to develop a community-focused and intervention-oriented transdisciplinary approach to public policy?

4. How is public health law implemented, and what transdisciplinary perspectives are useful for understanding these methods?

References

1. Gebbie K, Rosenstock L, Hernandez LM; Institute of Medicine, Committee on Educating Public Health Professionals for the 21st Century, eds. Who Will Keep the Public Healthy?: Educating Public Health Professionals for the 21st Century. Washington, DC: National Academies Press, 2003.

2. Gostin L. Public Health Law and Ethics: A Reader. Revised and updated ed. Berkeley: University of California Press; 2010.

3. Institute of Medicine, Committee on Public Health Strategies to Improve Health. For the Public's Health: Revitalizing Law and Policy to Meet New Challenges. Washington, DC: National Academies Press; 2011.

4. Institute of Medicine, Committee for the Study of the Future of Public Health. The Future of Public Health. Washington, DC: National Academy Press; 1988.

5. Moulton A, Goodman R, Parmet W. Perspective: law and great public health achievements. In: Goodman R, Hoffman R, Lopez W, Matthews G, Rothstein M,

Foster K, eds. Law in Public Health Practice. 2nd ed. New York: Oxford University Press; 2007:3–21.

6. Jacobson P, Hoffman R, Lopez W. Regulating public health: principles and application of administrative law. In: Goodman, R, Hoffman R, Lopez W, Matthews G, Rothstein M, Foster K, eds. Law in Public Health Practice. 2nd ed. New York: Oxford University Press; 2007:69–88.

7. Burris S. Thoughts on the law and the public's health. Journal of Law, Medicine & Ethics. 1994;22(2):141–147.

8. Gostin L. Public health law in a new century, part 1: law as a tool to advance the community's health. JAMA. 2000;283(21):2837–2841.

9. Ewick P, Silbey S. The common place of law: stories from everyday life. Chicago: University of Chicago Press; 1998.

10. Sarat A. Power, resistance and the legal consciousness of the welfare poor. Yale Journal of Law & the Humanities. 1990;2:343–379.

11. Burris S. Introduction: merging law, human rights and social epidemiology. Journal of Law, Medicine & Ethics. 2002;30(4):498–509.

12. Parmet WE. Populations, Public Health, and the Law. Washington, DC: Georgetown University Press; 2009.

13. Sarat A, Kearns TR. Beyond the great divide: forms of legal scholarship and everyday life. In: Sarat A, Kearns TR, eds. Law in Everyday Life. Ann Arbor: The University of Michigan Press; 1993:27–61.

14. Boden L. Policy evaluation: better living through research. American Journal of Industrial Medicine. 1996;29(4):346–352.

15. Cotton-Oldenburg NU. Bringing two worlds closer: a three-year review of council activities. The Link. 2001;14(1):1–4.

16. Affordable Care Act § 5310 (to be codified, scattered 42 USC) 2010.

17. Kelly A. The Fourteenth Amendment reconsidered: the segregation question. Michigan Law Review. 1956;54(8):1049–1086.

18. Brown v. Board of Education of Topeka, 347 US 483 (1954).

19. Jain N. Engendering fairness in domestic violence arrest: improving police accountability through the equal protection clause. Emory Law Journal. 2011;60:1011–1049.

20. Rothstein L. Redefining disability: legal protections for individuals with HIV, genetic predispositions to disease, or asymptomatic diseases. Journal of Health Care Law and Policy. 2000;3(2):330–351.

21. Matthews GW, Abbot EB, Hoffman RE, Cetron MS. Legal authorities for interventions in public health emergencies. In: Goodman, RA, Hoffman R, Lopez W, Matthews G, Rothstein M, Foster K, eds. Law in Public Health Practice. New York: Oxford; 2000:262–283.

22. Gostin L. Public Health Law: Power, Duty, Restraint. Revised and expanded ed. Berkeley: University of California Press; 2008.

23. Rabin R. The tobacco litigation: a tentative assessment. DePaul Law Review. 2001;51:350–351.

24. McVey D, Stapelton J. Can anti-smoking television advertising affect smoking behaviour?: controlled trial of the Health Education Authority for England's anti-smoking TV campaign. Tobacco Control. 2000;9:273–282.

25. Centers for Disease Control and Prevention. Law as a Tool for Preventing Chronic Diseases: Expanding the Spectrum of Effective Public Health Strategies. Atlanta, GA: Centers for Disease Control and Prevention; 2004.

26. Isaacs S, Schroeder S. Where the public good prevailed. American Prospect. 2001;12(10):26–30.

27. Achievements in public health, 1900–1999; improvements in workplace safety—United States, 1900–1999. MMWR. 1999;48(22):461–469.

28. Burris S, Wagenaar AC, Swanson J, Ibrahim JK, Wood J, Mello MM. Making the case for laws that improve health: a framework for public health law research. The Milbank Quarterly. 2010;88(2):169–210.

29. Gostin L, Jacobson P, Record K, Hardcastle L. Restoring health to health reform: integrating medicine and public health to advance the population's wellbeing. Pennsylvania Law Review. 2011;159:1777–1823.

30. Wilkinson R, Pickett K. The Spirit Level: Why Greater Equality Makes Societies Stronger. New York: Bloomsbury Press; 2009.

31. Rose G. Sick individuals and sick populations. International Journal of Epidemiology. 2001;30:427–432.

32. Friedman SR, Cooper HL, Tempalski B, Keem M, Friedman R, Flom PL, et al. Relationships of deterrence and law enforcement to drug-related harms among drug injectors in US metropolitan areas. AIDS. 2006;20(1):93–99.

33. Burris S, Kawachi I, Sarat A. Integrating law and social epidemiology. Journal of Law, Medicine & Ethics. 2003;30:510–521.

34. Parmet WE, Robbins A. Public health literacy for lawyers. Journal of Law, Medicine & Ethics. 2003;31(4):701–713.

35. Rudd R, Moykens B, Colton T. Health and literacy: a review of the medical and public health literature. In: Comings J, Garner B, Smith C, eds. Annual Review of Adult Learning and Literacy. Vol. 1. San Francisco: Jossey-Bass; 2000:158–199.

36. Gostin L, Burris S, Lazzarini Z. The law and the public's health: a study of infectious disease law in the United States. Columbia Law Review. 1999;99(1):59–128.

37. Starr P. Social Transformation of American Medicine. New York: Basic Books; 1982.

38. Shilts R. And the Band Played On. New York: St. Martin's Press; 2000.

39. Lakoff G. Don't Think of an Elephant!: Know Your Values and Frame the Debate. White River: Chelsea Green Publishing; 2004.

40. Lakoff G. Moral Politics: How Liberals and Conservatives Think. Chicago: University of Chicago Press; 1966.

Chapter 7

Sociocultural Perspectives Applied to Transdisciplinary Public Health

Bradley P. Stoner

Learning Objectives

- Understand the cultural perspectives on health.
- Explore how the cultural approach contributes to transdisciplinary practice and research in public health.
- Explore the systems approach for gauging population health in a global context.
- Understand how to analyze solutions to public health problems in a cultural context and especially by using medical anthropology.

• • •

Increasing attention is being paid in public health to issues of culture and the ways in which culture affects health, for better and for worse. Issues of culture loom large in transdisciplinary public health, specifically because cultural factors are often involved in determining what people do and why they do it. As the understanding of complex health and social problems has evolved over time, social scientists such as anthropologists and others working in the field of public health have long explored from a transdisciplinary perspective the important role cultural beliefs and practices can play to protect against health problems or, conversely, to increase health risks.[1,2] Increasingly, transdisciplinary approaches in public health research and practice (such as the approach described in chapter 1) include explicit attention to cultural factors, which engage anthropologists in these approaches in meaningful and important ways.[3] This chapter explores the ways in which anthropologists and other social scientists contribute to transdisciplinary practice through examining cultural perspectives on health, and integrate these cultural approaches into interventions to minimize health risks.

Problem Analysis

Understanding the interaction between culture and health requires some attention to what anthropologists mean when they use the term *culture*. A good place to start is the definition put forth in the nineteenth century by Tylor: "Culture, or civilization, taken in its broad, ethnographic sense, is that complex whole which includes knowledge, belief, art, morals, law, custom, and any other capabilities and habits acquired by man as a member of society."[4] Tylor's work set into motion the development of the modern field of anthropology, which considers culture one of its central concerns, seeing it as the ideas, beliefs, and practices of human groups who self-identify as sharing certain core characteristics. Cultural groups may be grounded by shared ethnicity, geography, behavior, age, or other fundamental features, and it is this shared sense of identity that affects how people think, act, and feel in a particular setting. Throughout the twentieth century, anthropologists struggled to come to terms with whether culture should refer primarily to the cognitive aspects of human life (such as language, symbols, and meaning) or should be applied more broadly to the range of behaviors and practices that structure human social organization and daily life.[5,6] Today, medical anthropologists invoke the term *culture* to mean the ways in which shared group beliefs and values can affect a population's risks for developing and sustaining adverse health outcomes.[7] The types of food one eats, the manner of making a living, modes of recreation and relaxation, religious and funerary practices—all of these are embedded in culture and can be examined from a perspective that specifically addresses these concerns.

Several tenets follow from this perspective on culture. Because culture is learned, it should be amenable to interventions to reinforce it if it is helpful or to change it if it is harmful. Cultural information is not transmitted genetically but rather vertically across generations (from elders to youth, and increasingly with regard to modern technology, from youth to elders) and also horizontally among peers, friends, and acquaintances. Public health workers seek to use culture to provide added impact or leverage to attain desired health outcomes, such as taking up healthy behaviors or refraining from unhealthy ones. Also, because culture is widely integrated into people's lives, interventions in one area may spill over to achieve positive effects in another. And finally, because culture is increasingly recognized as a driving factor in individual decision making, it is being prioritized for additional study by public health researchers in a variety of settings, including investigations of infectious and chronic diseases of all kinds.

One problem for researchers and practitioners who want to gain insights from culture or to use it as a tool is identifying the extent to which it is truly shared by people within a cultural group or setting. Anthropologists continue to struggle with this problem, and it is far from resolved. To what extent does culture permeate people's conception of who they are, what they believe, and the decisions they make, and to what extent are these decisions individual, personal, and at times idiosyncratic? Certainly, intracultural variation is an extremely important phenomenon, and understanding the range of behaviors within particular cultural or subcultural groups can be essential for determining the impact of culture on health. Anthropologists argue against the tendency to totalize and trivialize cultural groups by assuming that everyone within a particular group shares the same ideas and beliefs about a particular topic.[5] Nevertheless, even though intracultural variation can confound some attempts to elucidate cultural impacts on health, it should not dissuade investigators from trying piece together the elements of culture that are most important for maintaining health and wellness.

Today, culture is operationalized as much more than ethnic heritage. Anthropologists working on cultural models address common concerns of individuals who make up shared affinity groups and who are as often linked together by demographics or behavior as they are by common ancestry. For example, anthropologists might speak of the culture of aging and the health-related effects on persons facing the physical and cognitive challenges of old age, regardless of their geographical or ethnic identity.[8] Similarly, cultural approaches have been employed among adolescents, particularly with regard to sexual practices that put them at increased risk for sexually transmitted infections.[9] Sometimes affinity groups are further identified as subcultures, embedded within the larger general culture in which they reside and live their daily lives—hence culturally appropriate intervention efforts targeting injection drug users are increasingly employed.[10]

Culture and Health

Culture has been linked to transdisciplinary public health in important and meaningful ways. Certain cultural practices have been shown to increase health risks. Nations identifies increased adverse health outcomes linked to cultural practices surrounding dietary customs, child care patterns, religious practices, migration patterns, agricultural techniques, kinship relations, and traditional medical treatments.[11] Food preparation practices loom large in this discussion. Consumption of undercooked food products can lead to a variety of infectious ailments. "Drunken crabs," popular in the Far East, in which freshwater crabs and crayfish are soaked in brine, vinegar, or wine and then consumed, have been cited as a cause of *Paragonimus* lung fluke infection. Similarly, sushi prepared with contaminated fish can result in infection with *Diphyllobothrium*, or fish tapeworm. Trichinosis, caused by infection with the *Trichinella* parasite, is more commonly reported among persons who consume homemade sausages prepared according to traditional ethnic recipes.[12] With regard to child care, the use of "dog nurses" by the Turkana of Kenya has been linked to high rates of *Echinococcus* infection; according to Nelson, these dogs are trained to lick children clean after defecation and vomiting, leading to transfer of infectious larvae from dog to child.[13] Religious practices bear mentioning in this regard as well: increases in communicable diseases are routinely seen during the ritual Muslim hajj, or pilgrimage, causing religious leaders and public health officials to call for increased monitoring and vigilance among pilgrims making the journey.[14]

Of course, culture can be protective as well. Scholars have long pointed to religious injunctions and codes against consumption of particular foods—for example, the avoidance of pork among Muslims and Jews—as possible mechanisms to protect against food-borne illness. This health-related explanation for food preferences has been challenged by cultural materialists,[15] who claim that ecological constraints rather than disease avoidance are the more logical explanation for cultural patterns of food consumption. Nevertheless, the end result serves to protect the population from exposure to harmful pathogens carried by infected food products. Similarly, male circumcision, long a religious practice among Jews, Muslims, and other groups, and long without a demonstrable direct health benefit, has recently been shown in clinical trials to be protective against acquisition of human immunodeficiency virus (HIV).[16] Indeed, cultural groups who have not routinely circumcised are now expressing greater interest in adopting the practice due to its protective effects against this disease.[17]

Systems Approach to Transdisciplinary Public Health

Beginning in the 1970s, anthropologists turned their attention toward ecological understandings of health, viewing human health and illness within a larger context of adaptation to environmental stressors. It was also around this time that medical anthropology established itself as a discipline, defined as "a subfield of anthropology that draws upon social, cultural, biological, and linguistic anthropology to better understand those factors which influence health and well-being (broadly defined), the experience and distribution of illness, the prevention and treatment of sickness, healing processes, the social relations of therapy management, and the cultural importance and utilization of pluralistic medical systems."[18] As a discipline, medical anthropology is transdisciplinary because it draws on many different theoretical approaches, such as epidemiology, politics, sociology, anthropology, and medicine. Medical anthropologists, like other anthropologists, focus on cultural norms and social institutions as well as globalization, as each of these affects local worlds.

Following Alland,[19] this ecological approach emphasizes population health as the result of a complex interplay among biotic and abiotic systems, with culture mediating the harsh effects of the environment. In this view, physical stressors such as excessive heat, cold, drought, or flooding are mitigated by cultural adaptations to maintain and promote wellness; for example, mastery of fire to process food and ward off predators, use of clothing to enable survival in harsh climates, and forms of social organization that enable food sharing during times of shortage. This biocultural view of health recognizes human health as a consequence of biological and cultural factors working to together to achieve adaptive outcomes. Consequently, health cannot be fully understood without consideration of these complex processes. More recently, political economic models have shown how health is affected by larger social forces affecting individuals' ability to respond and adapt to stressful conditions. Models of *structural violence* invoke the powerful effects of colonialism, oppression, and subjugation that limit individual agency to respond to stressors.[20] Anthropologists are now working toward a "new biocultural synthesis" to accommodate these disparate approaches.[21]

From a public health perspective, the systems approach emphasizes the importance of gauging population health within a larger contextual understanding of the stresses and stressors posed by the environment in which humans live and thrive. Globalization challenges us to take an integrated approach to conceptualizing these stressors. For example, nutritional deficiencies must be understood within a broad framework that includes not only cultural influences on food preference and preparation patterns but also processes of food production and the global factors that affect food availability and distribution. These factors can include natural disasters such as drought or famine and also human activities such as war, political conflict, and economic calamity. Infectious diseases such as HIV need to be contextualized within a matrix that includes not only cultural influences on sexual norms and practices but also the politics of antiretroviral medication costs and availability. Cultural models of health directly address a systems approach to health when they take into consideration the ways in which culture is embedded in larger sociopolitical and economic spheres of influence.

Cross-Cultural Adaptations in Transdisciplinary Public Health

Humans have, over centuries, developed numerous cultural approaches to lifestyle and social organization that have clear health-related benefits. Many of these adaptations may not have developed specifically as health-promoting activities, but they have nevertheless enabled human communities to survive and thrive in the face of ongoing health threats. One important example involves the development of patterns of residence and population movement that serve to minimize the risk of malaria. An instance of such a pattern is the cultural preference for traditional stilt houses commonly seen among indigenous communities in northern Vietnam. People in these areas construct their living quarters on stilt props, which raise their dwellings several meters above the marshy riverbed below. Researchers suggest that this cultural housing pattern developed over centuries of cohabitation with malaria and, in some sense, represents a response to this endemic disease: the typical dwelling floor is above the flight ceiling of the *Anopheles* mosquito, which carries the malaria parasite.[22] Observational studies of stilt houses in West Africa seem to bear out the observation that persons living in these dwellings encounter much lower mosquito concentrations than people living at ground level.[23]

Cultural patterns of habitation and social organization in Sardinia offer another compelling example of adaptation to malaria, discussed extensively by Brown.[24] Sardinian settlements are typically located at altitudes above the normal habitation ranges of *Anopheles* mosquitoes, and area herders practice inverse transhumance, taking their herd animals down to valleys for grazing. This settlement pattern has several implications for reducing population-level risk of malaria. Permanent areas of occupation are located out of the normal mosquito habitat, and even though herders will be at some risk for exposure to malaria when tending to their animals, this is a relatively small number of people. Social organization patterns permit wealthier Sardinians to occupy mountain vacation homes in the late summer, which tend to be located at even higher altitudes (and therefore have fewer mosquitoes) than the permanent villages. While the Sardinian settlement pattern was not likely an intentional cultural intervention to reduce malaria risk when it first began, it has been reinforced over centuries, in no small part due to its positive health impact on the population at large, and represents an example of a cultural adaptation with a health benefit.

Solution Analysis

Medical anthropologists have come to view culture as a factor that can be mobilized to modify risk environments and help achieve positive health outcomes. This often means assessing the cultural contributions to risk behaviors and actively engaging communities to develop and implement culturally meaningful solutions. This approach can be especially important when trying to modify behaviors that have deep cultural roots but that are also closely tied to adverse health consequences when left unaddressed. Recognizing a need to go beyond merely achieving cultural competency,[25] anthropologists are likely to work toward community involvement in the research process and its implementation, also known as *participatory action research*. This can have great benefits when community partners work alongside public health workers to jointly devise solutions to problems at multiple levels.

Social Conditions in Health and Disease

A central tenet of medical anthropology is the distinction between *disease* (defined as biological dysfunction) and *illness* (defined as the perception of dysfunction by the individual).[26] Disease and illness commonly go hand in hand: infection with influenza virus generally makes a person feel achy, feverish, and generally "not well." However, instances of disconnect also often occur, as in the case of individuals with a bona fide disease (such as malaria or HIV infection) who do not feel ill or the case of persons who feel ill (with chronic fatigue, for instance) but for whom medical science can find no objective malady. *Sickness* is generally held to be the social recognition of disease or illness; that is, when other people perceive that an individual is unwell.[27]

The recognition that sickness is a social process is validated by the numerous social obligations and expectations surrounding individuals who adopt a "sick" role; for example, they need to obtain a doctor's note to be excused from school or work, and friends and coworkers display sympathy. From an anthropological perspective, these social influences on health and wellness can be mobilized to promote adherence to health-promoting behaviors and avoidance of behaviors that are health threatening. For example, the engagement of "popular" peers to model appropriate risk reduction behaviors has been shown to promote adherence to safer sex practices among men who have sex with men, thereby reducing the likelihood of HIV acquisition.[28] And peer influences have been shown to be important determinants of smoking avoidance and smoking cessation among teens.[29]

At the macro level, health and illness follow steep sociodemographic gradients. In developing and emerging economies, key health indicators track closely with national per capita income, whereas in developed countries income inequality accounts for much of the variance in health outcomes.[30,31] Poverty, racial and ethnic discrimination, and low educational attainment are widespread risk markers for adverse health outcomes. Globally, gender inequality is common: in many societies women have limited influence over health care decision making at the household level, with resources preferentially directed toward boys and men.[32] Understanding the dynamics of social organization is essential for developing and implementing culturally appropriate interventions to improve health outcomes and reduce health disparities.

Transdisciplinary Interventions and Impacts

Several important examples highlight the ways in which anthropologists, working in transdisciplinary teams, have integrated cultural perspectives into their intervention work. The best of these involve sharing workloads with members of affected communities and ceding key decision-making authority to community-based colleagues and outreach workers. These approaches are important for achieving success in addressing multilevel, multisystem health problems.

Culturally specific intervention messages were used by Shain et al.[33,34] to help African American and Hispanic women develop the necessary skills and behavior change to reduce their risk of sexually transmitted infections. Intervention messages were developed through standard theory-based approaches to AIDS risk reduction, augmented by ethnographic research on the study populations. The intervention was delivered through several small-group sessions that emphasized personal responsibility and commitment to changing unsafe sexual behaviors. At the six- and twelve-month follow-ups, intervention participants were significantly less likely than matched controls to have acquired gonorrhea or chlamydia, demonstrating the importance of culturally tailored messaging.

Culturally specific messaging was used to great effect in the transdisciplinary Hartford Drug Monitoring Project.[35] In order to gauge the changing use of street drugs in Hartford, Connecticut, and provide the most robust outreach services, researchers combined epidemiological and ethnographic methods to foster a research and policymaking community partnership with local health officials and representatives of the drug-using community. Using a participatory action research model, health workers identified emerging trends in drug use and presented observations and concerns to a community response team that was empowered to make decisions about appropriate public health reactions. Ethnography was employed specifically in settings where drugs were consumed, and was combined with in-context, informal interviewing and key informant interviewing of active drug users to create a vivid picture of the daily lives of affected community members. When new data emerged documenting the widespread use of "dust" by youth and young adults (which later proved to be PCP), the project staff were poised to react in short order with a dust awareness and prevention campaign. Working closely with the Hartford Hispanic Health Council, health workers designed and implemented dust prevention images and messages to reach youth and young adults on their own terms. Although funding limitations prevented a formal impact assessment, it is clear that the project engaged local community members in culturally meaningful ways, and to a degree heretofore not commonly seen in prevention interventions of this type.

Finally, it is instructive to consider the transdisciplinary work of Schoenberg et al.,[36] who used ethnographic methods to explore *lay discourses* on diabetes and their relationship to perceived levels of stress. Using formal sampling methods across multiple study sites, the researchers examined how the concept of stress figured into local understandings of how, when, and why people develop diabetes. Working with African Americans, Mexican Americans, Great Lakes Indians, and rural whites, the research team offered the informants' own narrative descriptions to richly illustrate how stress is thought to work as both a precipitating factor and a consequence of diabetes. Respondents agreed, regardless of their ethnicity or location of residence, that stress can cause or precipitate the onset of diabetes, can directly exacerbate diabetes once it occurs, and can serve to trigger diabetes complications. Stress could be a sudden event or a protracted series of events. It could be temporally proximate to the onset of diabetes or distal to its occurrence. What is interesting about this study is the extent to which stress, which loomed so large in respondents' narratives, is virtually absent from biomedical conceptualizations of diabetes, and how the primacy given to patients' concerns in this study stands in stark contrast to typical health messaging about blood sugar, medication compliance, and the like.

Summary

The future of public health is transdisciplinary, so it stands to reason that cultural perspectives on health will be increasingly incorporated into public health education, research, and practice. Anthropologists working in public health will benefit from increasing familiarity with the terms and methods of sister disciplines in public health, so that the findings of anthropological research can be readily translated and transmitted among practitioners with different training backgrounds. Anthropologists who value collaboration and teamwork have much to offer public health in the new millennium, due to the transactional and boundary-crossing nature of truly transdisciplinary collaborations.[3]

Cast against this backdrop, future priorities for anthropologists in public health should include

- *Increased opportunities for cross-disciplinary training.* This may include formal coursework in biology, statistics, psychology, and other sciences that are fundamental to the public health enterprise.
- *An increased transparency in anthropological writing.* Field reports, study methods, and interpretations should strive to be interesting, accurate, and readily understandable by health professionals with other disciplinary backgrounds.
- *An expanded focus on macrolevel determinants of health.* Anthropologists will be wise to consider the extent to which culture is shaped by, and constrained by, forces of politics, economics, and history.

- *The adoption of global perspectives on health.* Local health responses in disparate locations are often critically linked in an increasingly globalized world. Anthropologists are well positioned to consider both the similarities and the differences in health outcomes across national boundaries and class barriers.

Key Terms

culture	The ideas, beliefs, and practices of human groups who self-identify as sharing certain core characteristics. Some of these ideas, beliefs, and practices can affect a population's risks for developing and sustaining adverse health outcomes.
ecological understanding of health	The view that human health and illness is best understood within the context of adaptation to environmental stressors.
medical anthropology	A subfield of anthropology that draws upon social, cultural, biological, and linguistic anthropology to better understand those factors which influence health and well-being (broadly defined), the experience and distribution of illness, the prevention and treatment of sickness, healing processes, the social relations of therapy management, and the cultural importance and utilization of pluralistic medical systems.

Review Questions

1. What are the characteristics of the cultural perspective on health, and how do different disciplines contribute to this perspective?

2. How does the cultural perspective contribute to transdisciplinary approaches to solving public health problems?

3. What is the systems approach to gauging population health within a global context? What are some important examples of public health problems that are well suited to a transdisciplinary approach?

4. How do medical anthropology methods help researchers to develop culturally meaningful solutions to public health problems?

References

1. Dunn F, Janes C. Introduction: medical anthropology and epidemiology. In: Janes C, Stall R, Gifford S, eds. Anthropology and Epidemiology: Interdisciplinary Approaches to the Study of Health and Disease. Dordrecht: Reidel; 1986:3–34.

2. Trostle J. Epidemiology and Culture. New York: Cambridge University Press; 2005.

3. Hahn R, Inhorn M. Introduction. In: Hahn R, Inhorn M, eds. Anthropology and Public Health: Bridging Differences in Culture and Society. 2nd ed. New York: Oxford University Press; 2009:1–31.

4. Tylor E. Primitive Culture. New York: Harper & Row; 1958 [1871].

5. Miller B. Cultural Anthropology. 6th ed. New York: Prentice Hall; 2010.

6. Nielsen F. Culture. In: AnthroBase Online Dictionary of Anthropology; 2011. Available at: www.anthrobase.com/Txt/N/Nielsen_F_S_06.htm [accessed July 25, 2011].

7. McElroy A, Townsend P. Medical Anthropology in Ecological Perspective. 5th ed. Boulder, CO: Westview Press; 2008.

8. Sokolovsky J. The Cultural Context of Aging: Worldwide Perspectives. 3rd ed. Westport, CT: Praeger; 2008.

9. Halpern CT. Reframing research on adolescent sexuality: healthy sexual development as part of the life course. Perspectives on Sexual and Reproductive Health. 2010;42(1):6–7.

10. Small W, Shoveller J, Moore D, Tyndall M, Wood E, Kerr T. Injection drug users' access to a supervised injection facility in Vancouver, Canada: the influence of operating policies and local drug culture. Qualitative Health Research. 2011;21(6):743–756.

11. Nations M. Epidemiological research on infectious disease: quantitative rigor or rigor mortis?: Insights from ethnomedicine. In: Janes C, Stall R, Gifford S, eds. Anthropology and Epidemiology: Interdisciplinary Approaches to the Study of Health and Disease. Dordrecht: Reidel; 1986:97–123.

12. Schantz PM, Juranek DD, Schultz MG. Trichinosis in the United States, 1975: increase in cases attributed to numerous common-source outbreaks. Journal of Infectious Diseases. 1977;136(5):712–716.

13. Nelson GS. Human behavior in the transmission of parasitic disease. In: Cunning EU, Wright CA, eds. Behavioral Aspects of Parasitic Transmission. New York: Academic Press; 1972:109–121.

14. Memish ZA. The Hajj: communicable and non-communicable health hazards and current guidance for pilgrims. Euro Surveillance. 2010;15(39):19671.

15. Harris M. Cultural Materialism—The Struggle for a Science of Culture. New York: Vintage; 1979.

16. Mills E, Cooper C, Anema A, Guyatt G. Male circumcision for the prevention of heterosexually acquired HIV infection: a meta-analysis of randomized trials involving 11,050 men. HIV Medicine. 2008;9(6):332–335.

17. Brito MO, Caso LM, Balbuena H, Bailey RC. Acceptability of male circumcision for the prevention of HIV/AIDS in the Dominican Republic. PLoS One. 2009;4(11):e7687.

18. Society for Medical Anthropology. What Is Medical Anthropology. Available at: www.medanthro.net/definition.html.

19. Alland A. Adaptation in Cultural Evolution: An Approach to Medical Anthropology. New York: Columbia University Press; 1970.

20. Farmer P. Pathologies of Power: Health, Human Rights, and the New War on the Poor. Berkeley: University of California Press; 2003.

21. Goodman A, Leatherman T. Building a New Biocultural Synthesis: Political-Economic Perspectives on Human Biology. Ann Arbor: University of Michigan Press; 1998.

22. Laderman C. Malaria and progress: some historical and ecological considerations. Social Science & Medicine. 1975;9(11–12):587–594.

23. Charlwood JD, Pinto J, Ferrara PR, Sousa CA, Ferreira C, Gil V, et al. Raised houses reduce mosquito bites. Malaria Journal. 2003;2(1):45.

24. Brown P. Cultural adaptations to endemic malaria in Sardinia. Medical Anthropology. 1981;5(3):311–339.

25. Kleinman A, Benson P. Anthropology in the clinic: the problem of cultural competency and how to fix it. PLoS Medicine. 2006;3(10):e294.

26. Kleinman A. Patients and Healers in the Context of Cultures: An Exploration of the Borderland between Anthropology, Medicine, and Psychiatry. Berkeley: University of California Press; 1981.

27. Young A. The anthropologies of illness and sickness. Annual Review of Anthropology. 1982;11: 257–285.

28. Kelly JA, St Lawrence JS, Stevenson LY, Hauth AC, Kalichman SC, Diaz YE, et al. Community AIDS/HIV risk reduction: the effects of endorsements by popular people in three cities. American Journal of Public Health. 1992;82(11): 1483–1489.

29. Albrecht SA, Caruthers D, Patrick T, Reynolds M, Salamie D, Higgins LW, et al. A randomized controlled trial of a smoking cessation intervention for pregnant adolescents. Nursing Research. 2006;55(6):402–410.

30. Kawachi I, Kennedy B. The Health of Nations: Why Inequality Is Harmful to Your Health. New York: New Press; 2006.

31. Wilkinson R, Pickett K. The Spirit Level: Why Greater Equality Makes Societies Stronger. New York: Bloomsbury; 2009.

32. Skolnik R. Essentials of Global Health. Sudbury, MA: Jones and Bartlett; 2008.

33. Shain RN, Piper JM, Newton ER, Perdue ST, Ramos R, Champion JD, et al. A randomized, controlled trial of a behavioral intervention to prevent sexually transmitted disease among minority women. New England Journal of Medicine. 1999;340(2):93–100.

34. Shain RN, Piper JM, Holden AE, Champion JD, Perdue ST, Korte JE, et al. Prevention of gonorrhea and chlamydia through behavioral intervention: results of a two-year controlled randomized trial in minority women. Sexually Transmitted Diseases. 2004;31(7):401–408.

35. Singer M, Mirhej G, Santelices C, Saleheen H. From street research to public health intervention: the Hartford Drug Monitoring Project. In: Hahn R, Inhorn M,

eds. Anthropology and Public Health: Bridging Differences in Culture and Society. 2nd ed. New York: Oxford University Press; 2009:332–361.

36. Schoenberg N, Drew E, Stoller E, Kart C. Situating stress: lessons from lay discourses on diabetes. In: Hahn R, Inhorn M, eds. Anthropology and Public Health: Bridging Differences in Culture and Society. 2nd ed. New York: Oxford University Press; 2009:94–113.

Chapter 8

Evidence-Based Decision Making

Transdisciplinary Problem Solving to Improve the Health of the Public

Ross C. Brownson

Learning Objectives

- Understand how to apply an evidence-based approach to public health.
- Understand how to use transdisciplinary methods in an evidence-based approach.
- Describe the characteristics of the evidence-based approach.
- Learn how to apply the methods of the evidence-based approach.
- Understand how to develop a plan for disseminating evidence on public health.

• • •

Public health research and practice can be credited with many notable achievements, including much of the thirty-year gain in life expectancy in the United States over the twentieth century.[1] A large part of this increase can be attributed to the provision of safe water and food, sewage treatment and disposal, tobacco use prevention and cessation, injury prevention, control of infectious diseases through immunization and other means, and other population-based interventions.[2]

Despite these successes, many additional opportunities to improve the public's health remain. To achieve state and national objectives for improved population health, more widespread adoption of evidence-based strategies has been recommended.[3-8] An increased focus on evidence-based public health (EBPH) will have numerous direct and indirect benefits, including access to more and higher-quality information on what works, a higher likelihood of successful programs and policies being implemented, greater workforce productivity, and more efficient use of public and private resources.[5,9,10] As noted in the prior chapters, a hallmark of transdisciplinary problem solving that distinguishes it from other cross-disciplinary approaches is its emphasis on translation of scientific findings into practical solutions to social problems, characterized as *transdisciplinary action research*. Performing such research requires the use of evidence-based methods.

Ideally, public health practitioners should always incorporate scientific evidence in selecting and implementing programs, developing policies, and evaluating progress.[11,12] Society pays a high opportunity cost when interventions that yield the highest health return on an investment are not implemented.[13] In practice, intervention decisions are often based on perceived short-term opportunities, lacking systematic planning and review of the best evidence regarding effective approaches. These concerns were noted two decades ago when the Institute of Medicine determined that decision making in public health is often driven by "crises, hot issues, and concerns of organized interest groups."[14] Barriers to implementing EBPH include the political environment (including lack of political will) and deficits in relevant and timely research, information systems, resources, leadership, and the required competencies.[11,15-18]

Nearly every public health problem is complex,[19] requiring attention at multiple levels and among many different disciplines. Partnerships that bring together diverse people and organizations have the potential for developing new and creative ways of addressing public health issues.[20] Transdisciplinary research provides valuable opportunities to collaborate on interventions to improve the health and well-being of both individuals and communities.[21,22] For example, tobacco research efforts have been successful in facilitating cooperation among disciplines such as advertising, policy, business, medical science, and behavioral science. Research activities within these tobacco networks try to fill the gaps between scientific discovery and research translation by engaging a wide range of stakeholders.[23-25] As noted in chapter 9, transdisciplinary approaches have also shown some evidence of effectiveness in obesity prevention by engaging numerous sectors including food production, urban planning, transportation, schools, and health.[26,27]

As transdisciplinary research and practice converge, several concepts are fundamental to achieving a more evidence-based approach to public health practice. First, we need scientific information on the programs and policies that are most likely to be effective in promoting health (that is, we need to undertake evaluation research to generate sound evidence).[5,9,28,29] An array of effective interventions is now available from numerous sources, including the *Guide to Community Preventive Services (Community Guide)*,[30] the *Guide to Clinical Preventive Services*,[31] Cancer Control P.L.A.N.E.T.,[32] and the National Registry of Evidence-Based Programs and Practices.[33] Second, to translate science to practice, we need to marry information on evidence-based interventions from the peer-reviewed literature with the realities of a specific, real-world environment.[34,35] To do so, we need to better define processes that lead to evidence-based decision making, including a more transdisciplinary approach to problem solving. Finally, wide-scale dissemination of interventions of proven effectiveness must occur more consistently at state and local levels.[36]

A major goal of this chapter is to move the process of decision making toward a proactive approach that incorporates effective use of scientific evidence and data and also engages numerous sectors and partners for transdisciplinary problem solving. To accomplish this, the chapter presents five topics relevant to evidence-based decision making: (1) background issues, including a brief history, definitions, an overview of evidence-based medicine, and other concepts underlying EBPH; (2) key characteristics of an evidence-based transdisciplinary process; (3) analytical tools that enhance the uptake of EBPH and the disciplines responsible; (4) a framework for applying evidence in transdisciplinary public health practice; and (5) the barriers and opportunities that may arise as we seek widespread implementation of evidence-based approaches.

Historical Background and Core Concepts

Formal discourse on the nature and scope of evidence-based public health originated over a decade ago. In 1997, Jenicek defined EBPH as the "conscientious, explicit, and judicious use of current best evidence in making decisions about the care of communities and populations in the domain of health protection, disease prevention, health maintenance and improvement (health promotion)."[37] In 1999, scholars and practitioners in Australia[6] and the United States[11] elaborated further on the concept of EBPH. Others posed a series of questions to enhance an evidence-based approach to decision making.[5,6,11] Eventually, definitions of EBPH were broadened by a summary of many key concepts in an EBPH glossary,[38] and by the idea that decisions should take account of the perspectives of community members, which fostered a more population-centered approach.[34] There now appears to be a consensus that a combination of scientific evidence and values, resources, and context should enter into decision making (figure 8.1).[3,5,38,39] A concise definition has emerged from Kohatsu et al.: "Evidence-based public health is the process of integrating science-based interventions with community preferences to improve the health

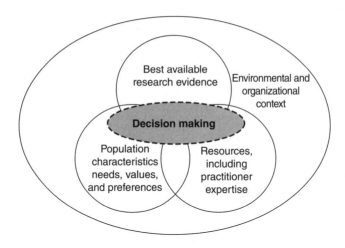

Figure 8.1. Transdisciplinary evidence-based decision making

of populations."[34] Satterfield and colleagues examined evidence-based practice and found many common challenges, including (1) how evidence should be defined, (2) how and when the patient's health or other contextual factors should enter the decision-making process; (3) how to define the roles of the experts or key stakeholders; and (4) what other variables should be considered when selecting an evidence-based practice (for example, age or social class).[38]

Defining Evidence

At the most basic level, *evidence* involves "the available body of facts or information indicating whether a belief or proposition is true or valid."[40] Ideas about evidence often derive from legal settings in Western societies, where evidence may come in the form of stories, witness accounts, police testimony, expert opinions, and forensic science.[41] Notions of evidence are also defined in large part by professional training and experience and drawn from a range of disciplinary experiences. For a public health professional, evidence is some form of data—such as epidemiological (quantitative) data, results of program or policy evaluations, and qualitative data—that can be used in making judgments or decisions[42] (figure 8.2). Public health evidence is usually the result of a complex cycle of observation, theory, and experiment.[43,44] Evidence includes medical data from patients[45] and data on patients (that is, distributional consequences),[46] and in practice settings, anecdotes sometimes trump empirical data.[47]

Several authors have defined types of scientific evidence for public health practice.[5,11,38] When moving from clinical interventions to population-level and policy interventions, context becomes more uncertain, variable, and complex.[48]

• Scientific literature in systematic reviews

• Scientific literature in one or more journal articles

• Public health surveillance data

• Program evaluations

• Qualitative data

• Community members

• Other stakeholders

• Media and marketing data

• Word of mouth

• Personal experience

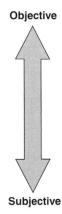

Objective

Subjective

Figure 8.2. Sources of evidence

Context highlights information needed to adapt and implement an evidence-based intervention in a particular setting or population[38] (table 8.1). The characteristics of the target population for an intervention, such as educational level and health history,[49] interpersonal variables, organizational variables,[9,50] social norms and culture, and finally, the larger transdisciplinary setting, in particular political and economic forces, affect context. For example, a high rate for a certain disease may influence a state's political will to address the issue in a meaningful and systematic way. Particularly for high-risk and understudied populations, there is a pressing need for evidence on contextual variables and ways of adapting programs and policies across settings and population subgroups. Contextual issues are being addressed more fully in the new *realist review*, which is a systematic review process that seeks to examine not only whether an intervention works but also *how* it works in a real-world setting.[51]

Challenges Related to Public Health Evidence

Evidence for public health has been described as underpopulated, dispersed, and different.[52,53] It is underpopulated because there are relatively few well-done evaluations of public health interventions (Type 2 evidence) and of the ways in which effects apply across different social groups (Type 3 evidence). Transdisciplinary information for public health decision making is also more dispersed than evidence for clinical interventions is. For example, evidence on the health effects of the built environment might be found in transportation and planning journals as well as health journals. Necessary evidence on the outcomes of clinical interventions to treat obesity might be found in health and economics journals. Finally, public health evidence is different, in part

Table 8.1. Contextual variables for intervention design, implementation, and adaptation

Category	Examples
Individual	Educational level Basic human needs[a] Personal health history
Interpersonal	Family health history Support from peers Social capital
Organizational	Staff composition Staff expertise Physical infrastructure Organizational culture
Sociocultural	Social norms Values Cultural traditions History
Political and economic	Political will Political ideology Lobbying and special interests Costs and benefits

[a]Basic human needs include food, shelter, warmth, safety; A. Maslow, "A Theory of Human Motivation," *Psychological Review*, 1943;50:370–396.

because much of the science base for interventions is derived from nonrandomized designs or so-called natural experiments, which generally take the form of observational studies in which the researcher cannot control or withhold the allocation of an intervention to particular areas or communities but where natural or predetermined variation in allocation occurs.[54]

Triangulating Evidence

Triangulation involves the accumulation of evidence from a variety of sources to gain insight into a particular topic[55] and often combines quantitative and qualitative data.[5] It generally involves the use of multiple methods of data collection or analysis to determine points of commonality or disagreement.[56] Triangulation is often beneficial because it can reveal that information from different sources is complementary. Though quantitative data provide an excellent opportunity to determine how variables are related for large numbers of people, these data provide little in the way of understanding why these relationships exist. Qualitative data, in contrast, may provide information to explain quantitative findings, thus "illuminating meaning."[56] There are many examples of the triangulation of qualitative and quantitative data to evaluate health programs and policies, including AIDS prevention programs,[57] occupational health programs and policies,[58] and chronic disease prevention programs in community settings.[59] These examples also illustrate the roles of numerous disciplines in addressing pressing public health problems.

Cultural and Geographical Differences

The tenets of EBPH have largely been developed in a Western, European American context.[60] The conceptual approach arises from the epistemological underpinnings of logical positivism,[61] which finds meaning through rigorous observation and measurement. This is reflected in a professional preference among clinicians for research designs like the randomized controlled trial. In addition, most studies in the EBPH literature are academic-based research, usually with external funding for well-established investigators. In contrast, in developing countries and in impoverished areas of developed countries, the evidence base for how best to address common public health problems is often limited, even though the scope of problem may be enormous. Cavill et al. compared evidence-based interventions across countries in Europe, showing that much of the evidence base in several areas is limited to empirical observations.[62] Even in more developed countries (including the United States), information published in peer-reviewed journals or data available through websites and official organizations may not adequately represent all populations of interest.

Transdisciplinary Audiences for EBPH

There are four overlapping user groups for EBPH, as defined by Fielding.[63] The first group consists of public health practitioners with executive and managerial responsibilities who want to know the scope and quality of evidence for alternative strategies (for example, in the form of programs or policies). In practice, however, public health practitioners frequently have a relatively narrow set of options. Funds from federal, state, or local sources are most often earmarked for a specific purpose (for example, surveillance and treatment of sexually transmitted diseases or inspection of retail food establishments). The public health practitioner has the opportunity and obligation to carefully review the evidence for alternative ways to achieve the desired health goals.

The next user group is made up of policymakers at local, regional, state, national, and international levels. They are faced with macrolevel decisions on how to allocate the public resources for which they are stewards. This group has the additional responsibility of making policies on controversial public issues. Policymakers need to be proactive in encouraging researchers to develop transdisciplinary strategies throughout their projects and to disseminate their products to the public in ways that make these products accessible. Federal policymakers have been doing this for several years, providing funds and resources to help researchers develop transdisciplinary infrastructure but also starting to develop an increasing number of funds for transdisciplinary academic degree programs.

The third group is composed of stakeholders who will be affected by any intervention. This includes the public, especially people who vote and members of interest groups formed to support or oppose specific policies, such as whether abortion should be legal, whether the community water supply should be fluoridated, or whether adults must be issued handgun licenses if they pass background checks. The final user group is composed of researchers on population health issues, such as those who evaluate the impact of a specific policy or program. They both develop and use evidence to answer research questions.

Connections among EBPH, Evidence-Based Medicine, and Transdisciplinary Work

The concept of evidence-based practice is well established in numerous disciplines, including psychology,[64] social work,[65,66] and nursing. It is probably best established in medicine. The doctrine of evidence-based medicine (EBM) was formally introduced in 1992.[67] Its origins can be traced back to the seminal work of Cochrane, who noted that many medical treatments lacked scientific effectiveness.[68] A basic tenet of EBM is to deemphasize unsystematic clinical experience and place greater emphasis on evidence from clinical research. This approach requires new skills, such as efficient literature searching and an understanding of types of evidence when evaluating the clinical literature.[69] There has been a rapid growth in the literature on EBM, contributing to its formal recognition. Using the search term *evidence-based medicine* produced 254 citations in 1990, rising to 7,331 citations in 2008. Even though the formal terminology of EBM is relatively recent, its concepts are embedded in earlier efforts such as the work on the periodic health examination in Canada[70] and the *Guide to Clinical Preventive Services* in the United States.[71]

The formal training of persons working in public health is much more variable than that of individuals in medicine or other clinical disciplines.[72] Unlike medicine, public health relies on a variety of disciplines and there is no single academic credential that "certifies" a public health practitioner, although efforts to establish credentials (via an exam) are now under way. Fewer than half of public health workers have any formal training in a public health discipline such as epidemiology or health education.[73] This high level of heterogeneity suggests the importance of transdisciplinary training, given that multiple perspectives and therefore more complexity are likely to be involved in any public health decision-making process.

Key Characteristics of Evidence-Based Decision Making and Transdisciplinary Problem Solving

It is useful to consider several overarching, common characteristics of an evidence-based approach to public health practice and transdisciplinary problem solving. Described more fully in the remainder of this section, these characteristics include

- Making decisions based on the best available peer-reviewed evidence (from both quantitative and qualitative research)
- Using data and information systems systematically
- Applying program-planning frameworks (which often have a foundation in behavioral science theory)
- Engaging the community in assessment and decision making
- Conducting sound evaluations
- Disseminating what is learned to key stakeholders and decision makers

Successfully carrying out this approach in EBPH is likely to require a synthesis of scientific skills, enhanced communication, common sense, and political acumen.

Basing Decisions on the Best Possible Evidence

When we evaluate evidence, it is useful to understand where to turn for the best possible scientific evidence. A starting point is the scientific literature and guidelines developed by expert panels. In addition, preliminary findings from researchers and practitioners are often presented at regional, national, and international professional meetings. Box 8.1 displays a summary of the large body of epidemiological studies showing the causal associations between inactivity and numerous health outcomes. This kind of information has led to the public health decision to address the lack of physical activity in youth. This large body of evidence has also led to effective intervention strategies.[74]

Using Data and Information Systems

A tried and true public health adage is "what gets measured, gets done."[75] This has typically been applied to long-term end points (for example, measuring rates of mortality makes it possible to focus on diseases most likely to lead to death). However, data for many public health end points and populations

---

Box 8.1: Engaging diverse sectors to promote physical activity in youth

---

It is now well established that regular physical activity reduces the risk of premature death and disability from a variety of conditions including coronary heart disease, diabetes, colon cancer, osteoarthritis, and osteoporosis. In spite of these benefits, data from the 2007 Youth Risk Behavior Surveillance System report that nationwide only one-third of high school students had met the recommended levels of physical activity. To address inactivity in youth, interventions have used modified curricula and policies to increase the amount of time students spend being active in physical education (PE) classes.

This can be done a variety of ways, including (1) adding new or additional PE classes, (2) lengthening existing PE classes, or (3) increasing moderate to vigorous physical activity of students during PE class without necessarily lengthening class time. Despite convincing evidence of effectiveness, there are real-world constraints to dissemination of these programs (that is, key considerations in external validity). For example, schools often feel pressure from students who want to prepare to perform well on standardized reading and math tests, which may in turn take time away from PE. However, recent data suggest that increasing time spent in PE may benefit academic achievement in math and reading. At the community level, growing attention is being focused on policies that support active transportation of youth to schools. These efforts require not only a health focus but also involvement of such diverse sectors as city planners, travel engineers, and law enforcement.

---

are not readily available at our fingertips. Data are being developed more for local-level issues (for example, the Selected Metropolitan/Micropolitan Area Risk Trends derived from the Behavioral Risk Factor Surveillance System [SMART: BRFSS]), and a few early efforts are under way to develop public health policy surveillance systems. For example, a group of federal and voluntary agencies have developed policy surveillance systems for tobacco,[76] alcohol,[77] and more recently, school-based nutrition[78] and physical education.[79]

Using Systematic Program Planning

Once an approach is decided on, a variety of planning frameworks and theories can be applied. For example, ecological, or systems, models are increasingly being used that "assume that appropriate changes in the social environment will produce changes in individuals, and that the support of individuals in the population is essential for implementing environmental changes."[80] These transdisciplinary models point to the importance of addressing problems at multiple levels and stress the interaction and integration of factors within and across all levels—individual, interpersonal, community, organizational, and governmental. The goal is to create a healthy community environment that provides health-promoting information and social support to enable people to live healthier lifestyles.[81] Effective interventions are most often grounded in health behavior theory.[44,82] As described in other chapters in this book, theory contributes to transdisciplinary approaches to public health.

Following Sound Evaluation Principles

Too often in public health, programs and policies are implemented without much attention to systematic evaluation. In addition, even when programs are ineffective, they are sometimes continued because of historical or political considerations. Evaluation plans must be laid early in program development and should include both formative and outcome evaluation. For example, Land et al. discuss an injury control program that was appropriately discontinued after its effectiveness was evaluated.[83] This program evaluation also illustrates the use of both qualitative and quantitative data in framing an evaluation.

Disseminating Results to Those Who Need to Know

Transdisciplinary approaches emphasize translation of research findings into practice to solve health problems. When a program or policy has been implemented, or when final results are known, others in public health can rely on findings from that implementation to enhance their own use of evidence in decision making. Dissemination may occur to health professionals via the scientific literature, to the general public via the media, to policymakers through personal meetings, and to public health professionals through training courses. Effective interventions are needed in a variety of settings, including schools, worksites, health care organizations, and broader community environments.

Analytical Tools and Approaches to Enhance Uptake of EBPH

Several analytical tools and planning approaches can help practitioners in answering questions such as these:

- What is the size of the public health problem?
- Are there effective transdisciplinary interventions for addressing the problem?

- What information about the local context and a particular intervention is helpful in deciding its potential use in the situation at hand?

- Is a particular program or policy worth doing (that is, is it better than alternatives), and will it provide a satisfactory return on investment, measured in monetary terms or in health impacts?

Public Health Surveillance

Public health surveillance is a critical tool for those using EBPH. It involves the ongoing systematic collection, analysis, and interpretation of specific health data, closely integrated with the timely dissemination of these data to those responsible for preventing and controlling disease or injury.[84] Public health surveillance systems should have the capacity to collect and analyze data, disseminate data to public health programs, and regularly evaluate the effectiveness of the use of the disseminated data.[85] For example, documentation of the prevalence of elevated levels of lead (a known toxicant) in the blood of the US population was used as the justification for eliminating lead from paint and then from gasoline and for documenting the effects of these actions.[86] In tobacco control, agreement on a common metric for tobacco use enabled comparisons across the states and an early recognition of the doubling and then tripling of the rates of decrease in smoking in California after state residents voted to pass Proposition 99[87] and then a quadrupling of the rate of decline in Massachusetts,[88] compared with the rates in the other forty-eight states.

Systematic Reviews and Evidence-Based Guidelines

Systematic reviews are syntheses of comprehensive collections of information on a particular topic. Reading a good review can be one of the most efficient ways to become familiar with state-of-the-art research and practice related to many specific topics in public health.[89-91] The use of explicit, systematic methods (that is, decision rules) in reviews limits bias and reduces chance effects, thus providing more reliable results upon which to make decisions.[92] One of the most useful sets of reviews for public health interventions is the *Community Guide*,[30,93] which provides an overview of current scientific literature through a well-defined, rigorous method in which available studies themselves are the units of analysis. The *Community Guide* seeks to answer these questions: (1) What interventions have been evaluated, and what have been their effects? (2) What aspects of interventions can help *Community Guide* users select an approach from the set of interventions of proven effectiveness? and (3) What might this intervention cost, and how does this cost compare with the likely health impacts? A good systematic review should allow the practitioner to understand the local contextual conditions necessary for successful implementation.[94]

Economic Evaluation

Economic evaluation is an important component of evidence-based practice as applied to transdisciplinary problem solving.[95] It can provide information for assessing the relative value of alternative expenditures on public health programs and policies. In cost-benefit analysis, all the costs and consequences of the decision options are valued in monetary terms. More often, the economic investment associated with an intervention is compared with the health impacts, such as cases of disease prevented or years of life saved. This technique, *cost-effectiveness analysis* (CEA), can suggest the relative value of alternative interventions (that is, health return on dollars invested),[95] though data to support this type of analysis are not always available, especially for possible public policies designed to improve health.[47,96]

Health Impact Assessment

Health impact assessment (HIA) is a relatively new method that seeks to estimate the probable impact on the health of the population of a policy or intervention related to a nonhealth sector important to transdisciplinary problem solving and public health issues, such as agriculture, transportation, or economic development.[97] Some HIAs have focused on ensuring the involvement of relevant stakeholders in the development of a specific project. This approach is also the basis of the environmental impact assessment required by law for many large place-based projects. Overall, the HIA, in both its forms, has been gaining acceptance as a tool because of mounting evidence that social and physical environments are important determinants of health and health disparities in populations. It is now being used to help assess the potential effects of many policies and programs on health status and outcomes.[98-100]

Participatory Approaches

Participatory approaches, core to transdisciplinary public health practice, actively involve community members in research and intervention projects[101-103] and show promise in engaging communities in EBPH.[34] Practitioners, academicians, and community members collaboratively define issues of concern, develop strategies for intervention, and evaluate the outcomes. This approach relies on *stakeholder* input,[104] builds on existing resources, facilitates collaboration among all parties, and integrates knowledge and action that it is hoped will lead to a fair distribution of the benefits of an intervention or project among all partners.[102,105] Stakeholders, or key players, are individuals or agencies that have a vested interest in the issue at hand.[106] In the development of health policies, for example, policymakers are especially important stakehold-ers.[107] Participatory approaches may also present challenges in adhering to EBPH principles, especially in reaching agreement on which approaches are most appropriate for addressing a particular health problem.[108]

An Approach to Increasing Use of Evidence in Trandisciplinary Public Health Practice

Strengthening EBPH competencies needs to take into account the diverse edu-cation and training backgrounds of the workforce. EBPH should be a common theme that connects disciplines. However, the principles of EBPH are not uni-formly taught or emphasized in all the disciplines represented in the public health workforce. For example, a public health nurse is likely to have had less training than an epidemiologist in how to locate the most current evidence and interpret alternatives. A recently graduated health educator with an MPH degree is more likely to have gained an understanding of the importance of EBPH than an environmental health specialist holding a bachelor's degree. Probably fewer than half of public health workers have any formal training in a public health discipline such as epidemiology or health education.[73] An even smaller percentage of these professionals have formal graduate training from a school of public health or other public health program. Currently, it appears that few public health departments have made continuing education about EBPH mandatory.

Even though the formal concept of EBPH is relatively new, the underlying skills are not. For example, reviewing the scientific literature for evidence or evaluating a program intervention are skills often taught in graduate programs in public health or other academic disciplines, and are building blocks of public health practice. The most commonly applied framework in EBPH is probably that of Brownson and colleagues (figure 8.3), which outlines a seven-stage, sequential process to promote greater use of evidence in day-to-day decision making.[5,50,109] The process for applying this framework is seldom a strictly prescriptive or linear one and entails numerous iterations, including the feed-back *loops* and processes that are common in many program-planning models.[110]

Competencies for more effective public health practice are becoming clearer.[111-113] For example, the skills needed to make evidence-based decisions require a specific set of competencies (table 8.2).[114] Many of the competencies on this list illustrate the value of developing partnerships and engaging with diverse disciplines in the EBPH process.

To address these and similar competencies, EBPH training programs have been developed in the United States for public health professionals in state health agencies,[50,115] local health departments, and community-based organiza-tions,[116,117] and similar programs have been developed in other countries.[109,118,119]

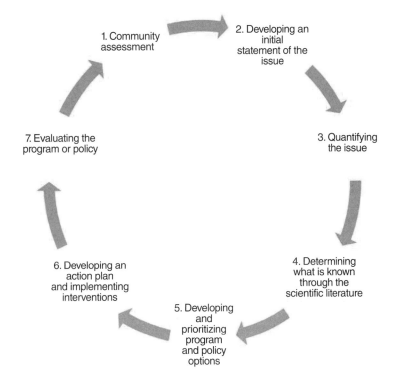

Figure 8.3. A framework for evidence-based public health
Source: R. C. Brownson et al., *Evidence-Based Public Health*, 2nd ed. (New York: Oxford University Press; 2011), p. 18.

Some programs show evidence of effectiveness.[50,117] The most common format uses didactic sessions, computer labs, and scenario-based exercises, taught by a faculty team with expertise in EBPH. Implementation of training to address EBPH competencies should take into account adult learning principles. These issues were recently articulated by Bryan and colleagues,[120] who highlighted the need to (1) know why the audience is learning, (2) tap into an underlying motivation to learn through creating a need to solve problems, (3) respect and build on individuals' previous experience, (4) design learning approaches that match individuals' backgrounds and diversity, and (5) actively involve the audience in the learning process.

Community Assessment

Community assessment typically occurs before the development of a program or policy and seeks to understand the public health issues and priorities in a given community. It also begins to identify current resources already in place

Table 8.2. Competencies in evidence-based public health

Title	Domain[a]	Level[b]	Competency
1. Community input	C	B	Understand the importance of obtaining community input before planning and implementing evidence-based interventions.
2. Etiological knowledge	E	B	Understand the relationship between risk factors and diseases.
3. Community assessment	C	B	Understand how to define the health issue at hand according to the needs and assets of the population or community of interest.
4. Partnerships at multiple levels	P/C	B	Understand how to identify and develop partnerships in order to address the issue with evidence-based strategies at multiple levels.
5. Developing a concise statement of the issue	EBP	B	Understand how to develop a concise statement of the issue in order to build support for it.
6. Grant writing need	T/T	B	Recognize the importance of grant-writing skills, including the steps involved in the application process.
7. Literature searching	EBP	B	Understand the process for searching the scientific literature and summarizing search-derived information on the health issue.
8. Leadership and evidence	L	B	Recognize the importance of strong leadership from public health professionals on the need for and importance of evidence-based interventions.
9. Role of behavioral science theory	T/T	B	Understand the role of behavioral science theory in designing, implementing, and evaluating interventions.
10. Leadership at all levels	L	B	Understand the importance of commitment from all levels of public health leadership to increase the use of evidence-based interventions.

Table 8.2. (*Continued*)

Title	Domain[a]	Level[b]	Competency
11. Evaluation in "plain English"	EV	I	Recognize the importance of translating the impacts of programs or policies into language that can be understood by communities, practice sectors, and policymakers.
12. Leadership and change	L	I	Recognize the importance of effective leadership from public health professionals when making decisions in the midst of ever-changing environments.
13. Translating evidence-based interventions	EBP	I	Recognize the importance of translating evidence-based interventions to unique real-world settings.
14. Quantifying the issue	T/T	I	Understand the importance of descriptive epidemiology (concepts of person, place, time) in quantifying the public health issue.
15. Developing an action plan for a program or policy	EBP	I	Understand the importance of developing a plan of action that describes how the goals and objectives will be achieved, what resources are required, and how the responsibility of achieving objectives will be assigned.
16. Prioritizing health issues	EBP	I	Understand how to choose and implement appropriate criteria and processes for prioritizing program and policy options.
17. Qualitative evaluation	EV	I	Recognize the value of qualitative evaluation approaches, including the steps involved in conducting qualitative evaluations.
18. Collaborative partnerships	P/C	I	Understand the importance of collaborative partnerships between researchers and practitioners when designing, implementing, and evaluating evidence-based programs and policies.

(*Continued*)

Table 8.2. (*Continued*)

Title	Domain[a]	Level[b]	Competency
19. Nontraditional partnerships	P/C	I	Understand the importance of traditional partnerships as well as those that have been considered nontraditional, such as those with planners, departments of transportation, and others.
20. Systematic reviews	T/T	I	Understand the rationale, uses, and usefulness of systematic reviews that document effective interventions.
21. Quantitative evaluation	EV	I	Recognize the importance of quantitative evaluation approaches, including the concepts of measurement validity and reliability.
22. Grant-writing skills	T/T	I	Demonstrate the ability to create a grant proposal, including an outline of the steps involved in the application process.
23. Role of economic evaluation	T/T	A	Recognize the importance of using economic data and strategies to evaluate costs and outcomes when making public health decisions.
24. Creating policy briefs	P	A	Understand the importance of writing concise policy briefs to address the issue of using evidence-based interventions.
25. Evaluation designs	EV	A	Comprehend the various designs useful in program evaluation, with a particular focus on quasi-experimental (nonrandomized) designs.
26. Transmitting evidence-based research to policymakers	P	A	Understand the importance of coming up with creative ways of transmitting what we know works (evidence-based interventions) to policymakers in order to gain interest, political support, and funding.

[a]C = community-level planning; E = etiology; P/C = partnerships and collaboration; EBP = evidence-based process; T/T = theory and analytical tools; L = leadership; EV = evaluation; P = policy.

[b]B = beginner; I = intermediate; A = advanced.

Source: Adapted from R Brownson et al., "Developing Competencies for Training Practitioners in Evidence-Based Cancer Control," *Journal of Cancer Education*, 2009;24(3):186–193.

to address the concern. Data are sometimes available through surveillance systems and national and local data sets. Other information that is useful at this stage is documentation of the context, or setting, within which the health concern is occurring, including an assessment of the social, economic, and physical environment factors. Community assessment data can be collected through quantitative (questionnaires) or qualitative (individual or group interviews) methods.

Developing an Initial Statement of the Issue

The practitioner should begin by developing a concise statement of the issue or problem being considered. To build support for any issue (with an organization, policymakers, or a funding agency), the issue must be clearly articulated. This problem definition stage has some similarities to the beginning steps in a strategic planning process, which often involve describing the mission, internal strengths and weaknesses, external opportunities and threats, and the vision for the future. It is often helpful to describe gaps between the current status of a program or organization and the desired goals. The key components of an issue statement include the health condition or risk factor being considered, the population(s) affected, the size and scope of the problem, the prevention opportunities, and the potential stakeholders.

Quantifying the Issue

After developing a working description of the public health issue of interest, it is often useful to identify sources of existing data. Such descriptive data may be available from ongoing vital statistics sources (such as birth and death records), surveillance systems, special surveys, or national studies.

Descriptive studies can take several forms. In public health, the most common type of descriptive study involves a survey of a scientifically valid sample (a representative cross section) of the population of interest. These cross-sectional studies are not intended to change health status (as an intervention would) but rather to quantify the prevalence of behaviors, characteristics, exposures, and diseases at some point (or over some period) of time in a defined population. This information can be valuable for understanding the scope of the public health problem at hand. Descriptive studies commonly provide information on patterns of occurrence according to attributes in such categories as person (for example, age, gender, ethnicity), place (for example, county of residence), and time (for example, seasonal variation in disease patterns). Additionally, under certain circumstances, cross-sectional data can provide information for use in the design of analytical studies (for example, baseline data to evaluate the effectiveness of a public health intervention).

Determining What Is Known Through the Scientific Literature

Once the issue to be considered has been clearly defined, the practitioner needs to become knowledgeable about previous or ongoing efforts to address the issue. This should include a systematic approach to identifying, retrieving, and evaluating relevant reports on scientific studies, panels, and conferences related to the topic of interest. It is important to remember that not all intervention studies will be found in the published literature.

Developing and Prioritizing Program and Policy Options

After the work of the first three steps, a variety of health program or policy options can be identified and then examined more closely. The list of options can be developed from a variety of sources. The initial review of the scientific literature can sometimes highlight various intervention options. More often, expert panels provide program or policy recommendations on a variety of issues. Summaries of available evidence are often available in systematic reviews and practice guidelines. Several considerations or contexts underlie any development of options. These considerations focus on five main issue areas: political and regulatory, economic, social values, demographic, and technological.[121]

In particular, it is important to assess and monitor the political process when developing health policy options. In doing so, stakeholder input may be useful. The stakeholder for a policy might be the health policymaker, whereas the stakeholder for a coalition-based community intervention might be a community member. In the case of health policies, supportive policymakers can frequently provide advice regarding timing of policy initiatives, methods for framing the issues, strategies for identifying sponsors, and ways to develop support among the general public. In the case of a community intervention, additional planning data may include key informant interviews, focus groups, or coalition member surveys.[122]

Developing an Action Plan and Implementing Interventions

This aspect of the process again deals largely with strategic planning issues. Once an option has been selected, a set of goals and objectives should be developed. A goal is a long-term desired change in the status of a priority health need, and an objective is a short-term, measurable specific activity that leads toward achievement of a goal. The course of action describes how the goals and objectives will be achieved, what resources are required, and how responsibility for achieving objectives will be assigned.

Evaluating the Program or Policy

In simple terms, evaluation is the determination of the degree to which program or policy goals and objectives are met. If they follow any research design, most public health programs and policies are often evaluated through *quasi-experimental* designs; that is, those lacking random assignment to intervention and comparison groups. In general, the strongest evaluation designs acknowledge the roles of both quantitative and qualitative evaluation. Furthermore, evaluation designs need to be flexible and sensitive enough to assess intermediate changes, even those that fall short of changes in behavior. Genuine change takes place incrementally over time, in ways that are often not visible to those too close to the intervention.

The seven-stage framework of evidence-based public health summarized in this chapter is similar to an eight-step approach first described by Jenicek. In Jenicek's framework, an additional logical step focuses on teaching others how to practice evidence-based public health.[37]

Barriers to EBPH and Potential Solutions

There are several barriers to more effective use of data and analytical processes in transdisciplinary decision making (table 8.3).[5,9,123,124] Possible approaches

Table 8.3. Potential barriers and their solutions in evidence-based decision making

Barrier	Potential solution
Lack of resources	Commitment to increase funding for prevention and rectifying staff shortages
Lack of leadership and instability in setting a clear and focused agenda for evidence-based approaches	Commitment from all levels of public health leaders to increase the understanding of the value of EBPH approaches
Lack of incentives for using evidence-based approaches	Identification of new ways of shaping organizational culture to support EBPH
Lack of a view of the long-term "horizon" for program implementation and evaluation	Adoption of and adherence to causal frameworks and formative evaluation plans
External (including political) pressures that drive the process away from an evidence-based approach	Systematic communication and dissemination strategies
Inadequate training in key public health disciplines	Wider dissemination of new and established training programs, including use of distance learning technologies
Lack of time to gather information, analyze data, and review the literature for evidence	Enhanced skills for efficient analysis and review of the literature, performing online searches, and using systematic reviews
Lack of evidence on the effectiveness of certain public health interventions for special populations	Increased funding for applied public health research; better dissemination of findings
Lack of information on implementation of interventions	A greater emphasis on building the evidence base for external validity

for overcoming these barriers have been discussed by others.[14,115,125] Leadership is needed from public health practitioners on the necessity for and importance of evidence-based decision making. Such leadership is evident in training programs, such as the regional leadership network for public health practitioners[126] and the efforts under way to develop and disseminate evidence-based guidelines for interventions.[30]

Summary

The successful implementation of EBPH in transdisciplinary public health practice is both a science and an art. The science is built on epidemiological, behavioral, and policy research showing the size and scope of a public health problem and identifying the interventions that are likely to be effective in addressing the problem. The art of decision making often involves knowing what information is important to a particular stakeholder at a particular time. Unlike solving a math problem, making significant decisions in transdisciplinary public health must balance science and art, because evidence-based decision making often involves choosing one alternative from among a set of rational choices. Success in public health problem solving relies on a transdisciplinary approach. By applying the concepts of EBPH outlined in this chapter, decision making and, ultimately, public health practice can be improved.

Key Terms

evidence-based public health (EBPH)	The development, implementation, and evaluation of effective programs and policies in public health through application of principles of scientific reasoning, including systematic use of data and information systems and appropriate use of behavioral science theory and program-planning models.
health impact assessment (HIA)	A relatively new method that seeks to estimate the probable impact on the health of the population of a policy or intervention related to a nonhealth sector important to transdisciplinary problem solving and public health issues, such as agriculture, transportation, or economic development.
participatory approach	An approach that actively involves community members in research and intervention projects.

public health surveillance The systematic collection, consolidation, analysis, and dissemination of data on specific diseases in public health practice.

systematic review A synthesis of a comprehensive collection of information on a particular topic.

Review Questions

1. Why are evidence-based approaches so important to public health research and practice?

2. What role do transdisciplinary research methods and team science play in the evidence-based approach?

3. What are the key characteristics and methods used for implementing the evidence-based approach?

4. What are the best methods for implementing and disseminating evidence on public health?

References

1. National Center for Health Statistics. Health, United States, 2000, with Adolescent Health Chartbook. Hyattsville, MD: Centers for Disease Control and Prevention, National Center for Health Statistics; 2000.

2. Centers for Disease Control and Prevention. Public health in the new American health system. Discussion paper. Atlanta, GA: Centers for Disease Control and Prevention; 1993.

3. Muir Gray JA. Evidence-Based Healthcare: How to Make Health Policy and Management Decisions. New York: Churchill Livingstone; 1997.

4. Brownson RC, Fielding JE, Maylahn CM. Evidence-based public health: a fundamental concept for public health practice. Annual Review of Public Health. 2009;30:175–201.

5. Brownson RC, Baker EA, Leet TL, Gillespie KN, True WR. Evidence-Based Public Health. 2nd ed. New York: Oxford University Press; 2011.

6. Glasziou P, Longbottom H. Evidence-based public health practice. Australian and New Zealand Journal of Public Health. 1999;23(4):436–440.

7. McMichael C, Waters E, Volmink J. Evidence-based public health: what does it offer developing countries? Journal of Public Health. 2005;27(2):215–221.

8. Fielding JE, Briss PA. Promoting evidence-based public health policy: can we have better evidence and more action? Health Affairs. 2006;25(4):969–978.

9. Hausman AJ. Implications of evidence-based practice for community health. American Journal of Community Psychology. 2002;30(3):453–467.

10. Kohatsu ND, Melton RJ. A health department perspective on the Guide to Community Preventive Services. American Journal of Preventive Medicine. 2000;18(1 suppl):3–4.

11. Brownson RC, Gurney JG, Land G. Evidence-based decision making in public health. Journal of Public Health Management and Practice. 1999;5:86–97.

12. McGinnis JM. Does proof matter?: why strong evidence sometimes yields weak action. American Journal of Health Promotion. 2001;15(5):391–396.

13. Fielding JE. Where is the evidence? Annual Review of Public Health. 2001;22:v–vi.

14. Institute of Medicine, Committee for the Study of the Future of Public Health. The Future of Public Health. Washington, DC: National Academy Press; 1988.

15. Anderson J. "Don't confuse me with facts . . .": evidence-based practice confronts reality. Medical Journal of Australia. 1999;170(10):465–466.

16. Baker EL, Potter MA, Jones DL, Mercer SL, Cioffi JP, Green LW, et al. The public health infrastructure and our nation's health. Annual Review of Public Health. 2005;26:303–318.

17. Haynes B, Haines A. Barriers and bridges to evidence based clinical practice. British Medical Journal. 1998;317(7153):273–276.

18. Catford J. Creating political will: moving from the science to the art of health promotion. Health Promotion International. 2006;21(1):1–4.

19. Murphy K, Wolfus B, Lofters A. From complex problems to complex problem-solving: transdisciplinary practice as knowledge translation. In: Kirst M, Schaefer-McDaniel N, Hwang S, O'Campo P, eds. Converging Disciplines: A Transdisciplinary Research Approach to Urban Health Problems. New York: Springer; 2011:111–129.

20. Roussos ST, Fawcett SB. A review of collaborative partnerships as a strategy for improving community health. Annual Review of Public Health. 2000;21:369–402.

21. Harper GW, Neubauer LC, Bangi AK, Francisco VT. Transdisciplinary research and evaluation for community health initiatives. Health Promotion Practice. 2008;9(4):328–337.

22. Stokols D. Toward a science of transdisciplinary action research. American Journal of Community Psychology. 2006;38(1–2):63–77.

23. Kobus K, Mermelstein R. Bridging basic and clinical science with policy studies: The Partners with Transdisciplinary Tobacco Use Research Centers experience. Nicotine & Tobacco Research. 2009;11(5):467–474.

24. Kobus K, Mermelstein R, Ponkshe P. Communications strategies to broaden the reach of tobacco use research: examples from the Transdisciplinary Tobacco Use Research Centers. Nicotine & Tobacco Research. 2007;9(suppl 4): S571–S582.

25. Morgan GD, Kobus K, Gerlach KK, Neighbors C, Lerman C, Abrams DB, et al. Facilitating transdisciplinary research: the experience of the Transdisciplinary Tobacco Use Research Centers. Nicotine & Tobacco Research. 2003;5(suppl 1): S11–S19.

26. Byrne S, Wake M, Blumberg D, Dibley M. Identifying priority areas for longitudinal research in childhood obesity: Delphi technique survey. International Journal of Pediatric Obesity. 2008;3(2):120–122.

27. Russell-Mayhew S, Scott C, Stewart M. The Canadian Obesity Network and interprofessional practice: members' views. Journal of Interprofessional Care. 2008;22(2):149–165.

28. Black BL, Cowens-Alvarado R, Gershman S, Weir HK. Using data to motivate action: the need for high quality, an effective presentation, and an action context for decision-making. Cancer Causes & Control 2005;16(suppl 1):15–25.

29. Curry S, Byers T, Hewitt M, eds. Fulfilling the Potential of Cancer Prevention and Early Detection. Washington, DC: National Academies Press; 2003.

30. Zaza S, Briss PA, Harris KW, eds. The Guide to Community Preventive Services: What Works to Promote Health? New York: Oxford University Press; 2005.

31. Agency for Healthcare Research and Quality. Guide to Clinical Preventive Services. Available at: www.ahrq.gov/clinic/pocketgd.htm [accessed August 15, 2011].

32. Cancer Control P.L.A.N.E.T. [Links to comprehensive cancer control resources for public health professionals.] Available at: cancercontrolplanet.cancer.gov [accessed August 15, 2011].

33. Substance Abuse & Mental Health Services Administration. National Registry of Evidence-Based Programs and Practices. Available at: www.nrepp.samhsa.gov [accessed August 15, 2011].

34. Kohatsu ND, Robinson JG, Torner JC. Evidence-based public health: an evolving concept. American Journal of Preventive Medicine. 2004;27(5):417–421.

35. Green LW. Public health asks of systems science: to advance our evidence-based practice, can you help us get more practice-based evidence? American Journal of Public Health. 2006;96(3):406–409.

36. Kerner J, Rimer B, Emmons K. Introduction to the special section on dissemination: dissemination research and research dissemination: how can we close the gap? Health Psychology. 2005;24(5):443–446.

37. Jenicek M. Epidemiology, evidence-based medicine, and evidence-based public health. Journal of Epidemiology & Community Health. 1997;7:187–197.

38. Rychetnik L, Hawe P, Waters E, Barratt A, Frommer M. A glossary for evidence based public health. Journal of Epidemiology & Community Health. 2004;58(7):538–545.

39. Satterfield JM, Spring B, Brownson RC, Mullen EJ, Newhouse RP, Walker BB, et al. Toward a transdisciplinary model of evidence-based practice. Milbank Quarterly. 2009;87(2):368–390.

40. McKean E, ed. The New Oxford American Dictionary. 2nd ed. New York: Oxford University Press; 2005.

41. McQueen DV. Strengthening the evidence base for health promotion. Health Promotion International. 2001;16(3):261–268.

42. Chambers D, Kerner J. Closing the gap between discovery and delivery. Paper presented at: Dissemination and Implementation Research Workshop: Harnessing Science to Maximize Health; 2007; Rockville, MD.

43. McQueen DV, Anderson LM. What counts as evidence?: issues and debates. In: Rootman I, ed. Evaluation in Health Promotion: Principles and Perspectives. Copenhagen: World Health Organization; 2001:63–81.

44. Rimer BK, Glanz DK, Rasband G. Searching for evidence about health education and health behavior interventions. Health Education & Behavior. 2001;28(2):231–248.

45. Mulrow CD, Lohr KN. Proof and policy from medical research evidence. Journal of Health Politics, Policy and Law. 2001;26(2):249–266.

46. Sturm R. Evidence-based health policy versus evidence-based medicine. Psychiatric Services. 2002;53(12):1499.

47. Brownson RC, Royer C, Ewing R, McBride TD. Researchers and policymakers: travelers in parallel universes. American Journal of Preventive Medicine. 2006;30(2):164–172.

48. Dobrow MJ, Goel V, Upshur RE. Evidence-based health policy: context and utilisation. Social Science & Medicine. 2004;58(1):207–217.

49. Maslow A. A theory of human motivation. Psychological Review. 1943;50:370–396.

50. Dreisinger M, Leet TL, Baker EA, Gillespie KN, Haas B, Brownson RC. Improving the public health workforce: evaluation of a training course to enhance evidence-based decision making. Journal of Public Health Management and Practice. 2008;14(2):138–143.

51. Pawson R, Greenhalgh T, Harvey G, Walshe K. Realist review—a new method of systematic review designed for complex policy interventions. Journal of Health Services Research & Policy. 2005;10(suppl 1):21–34.

52. Millward L, Kelly M, Nutbeam D. Public Health Interventions Research: The Evidence. London: Health Development Agency; 2003.

53. Petticrew M, Roberts H. Systematic reviews—do they "work" in informing decision-making around health inequalities? Health Economics, Policy and Law. 2008;3(pt 2):197–211.

54. Petticrew M, Cummins S, Ferrell C, Findlay A, Higgins C, Hoy C, et al. Natural experiments: an underused tool for public health? Public Health. 2005;119(9):751–757.

55. Tones K. Beyond the randomized controlled trial: a case for "judicial review." Health Education Research. 1997;12(2):i–iv.

56. Steckler A, McLeroy KR, Goodman RM, Bird ST, McCormick L. Toward integrating qualitative and quantitative methods: an introduction. Health Education Quarterly. 1992;19(1):1–8.

57. Dorfman LE, Derish PA, Cohen JB. Hey Girlfriend: An evaluation of AIDS prevention among women in the sex industry. Health Education Quarterly. 1992;19(1):25–40.

58. Hugentobler M, Israel BA, Schurman SJ. An action research approach to workplace health: integrating methods. Health Education Quarterly. 1992;19(1):55–76.

59. Goodman RM, Wheeler FC, Lee PR. Evaluation of the Heart to Heart Project: lessons from a community-based chronic disease prevention project. American Journal of Health Promotion. 1995;9:443–455.

60. McQueen DV. The evidence debate. Journal of Epidemiology & Community Health. 2002;56(2):83–84.

61. Suppe F. The Structure of Scientific Theories. 2nd ed. Urbana: University of Illinois Press; 1977.

62. Cavill N, Foster C, Oja P, Martin BW. An evidence-based approach to physical activity promotion and policy development in Europe: contrasting case studies. Promotion & Education. 2006;13(2):104–111.

63. Fielding JE. Foreword. In: Brownson RC, Baker EA, Leet TL, Gillespie KN, eds. Evidence-Based Public Health. New York: Oxford University Press; 2003:v–vii.

64. Presidential Task Force on Evidence-Based Practice. Evidence-Based practice in psychology. American Psychologist. 2006;61(4):271–285.

65. Gambrill E. Evidence-based practice: sea change or the emperor's new clothes? Journal of Social Work Education. 2003;39(1):3–23.

66. Mullen E, Bellamy J, Bledsoe S, Francois J. Teaching evidence-based practice. Research on Social Work Practice. 2007;17(5):574–582.

67. Evidence-Based Medicine Working Group. Evidence-based medicine: a new approach to teaching the practice of medicine. JAMA. 1992;17:2420–2425.

68. Cochrane A. Effectiveness and Efficiency: Random Reflections on Health Services. London: Nuffield Provincial Hospital Trust; 1972.

69. Guyatt G, Cook D, Haynes B. Evidence based medicine has come a long way. British Medical Journal. 2004;329(7473):990–991.

70. Canadian Task Force on the Periodic Health Examination. The periodic health examination. Canadian Medical Association Journal. 1979;121(9):1193–1254.

71. US Preventive Services Task Force. Guide to Clinical Preventive Services: An Assessment of the Effectiveness of 169 Interventions. Baltimore, MD: Williams & Wilkins; 1989.

72. Tilson H, Gebbie KM. The public health workforce. Annual Review of Public Health. 2004;25:341–356.

73. Turnock BJ. Public Health: What It Is and How It Works. 3rd ed. Gaithersburg, MD: Aspen Publishers, Inc.; 2004.

74. Kahn EB, Ramsey LT, Brownson RC, Heath GW, Howze EH, Powell KE, et al. The effectiveness of interventions to increase physical activity. A systematic review. American Journal of Preventive Medicine. 2002;22(4 suppl 1): 73–107.

75. Thacker SB. Public health surveillance and the prevention of injuries in sports: what gets measured gets done. Journal of Athletic Training. 2007;42(2): 171–172.

76. Chriqui JF, Frosh MM, Brownson RC, Stillman FA. Measuring policy and legislative change. In: Evaluating ASSIST: A Blueprint for Understanding State-level Tobacco Control. Tobacco Control Monograph No. 17. Bethesda, MD: National Cancer Institute; 2006:87–110.

77. National Institute on Alcohol Abuse and Alcoholism. Alcohol Policy Information System. Available at: alcoholpolicy.niaaa.nih.gov [accessed August 15, 2011].

78. Masse LC, Frosh MM, Chriqui JF, Yaroch AL, gurs-Collins T, Blanck HM, et al. Development of a school nutrition-environment state policy classification system (SNESPCS). American Journal of Preventive Medicine. 2007;33(4 suppl 1): S277–S291.

79. Masse LC, Chriqui JF, Igoe JF, Atienza AA, Kruger J, Kohl HW, 3rd, et al. Development of a physical education-related state policy classification system (PERSPCS). American Journal of Preventive Medicine. 2007;33(4 suppl 1): S264–S276.

80. McLeroy KR, Bibeau D, Steckler A, Glanz K. An ecological perspective on health promotion programs. Health Education Quarterly. 1988;15:351–377.

81. Stokols D. Translating social ecological theory into guidelines for community health promotion. American Journal of Health Promotion. 1996;10(4):282–298.

82. Glanz K, Bishop DB. The role of behavioral science theory in the development and implementation of public health interventions. Annual Review of Public Health. 2010;31:399–418.

83. Land G, Romeis JC, Gillespie KN, Denny S. Missouri's Take a Seat, Please!, and program evaluation. Journal of Public Health Management and Practice. 1997;3(6):51–58.

84. Thacker SB, Berkelman RL. Public health surveillance in the United States. Epidemiologic Reviews.1988;10:164–190.

85. Thacker SB, Stroup DF. Public health surveillance. In: Brownson RC, Petitti DB, eds. Applied Epidemiology: Theory to Practice. 2nd ed. New York: Oxford University Press; 2006:30–67.

86. Annest JL, Pirkle JL, Makuc D, et al. Chronological trend in blood lead levels between 1976 and 1980. New England Journal of Medicine. 1983;308: 1373–1377.

87. Tobacco Education and Research Oversight Committee for California. Confronting a Relentless Adversary: A Plan for Success: Toward a Tobacco-free California, 2006–2008. Sacramento, CA: California Department of Health Services; 2006.

88. Biener L, Harris JE, Hamilton W. Impact of the Massachusetts tobacco control programme: population based trend analysis. British Medical Journal. 2000;321(7257):351–354.

89. Hutchison BG. Critical appraisal of review articles. Canadian Family Physician. 1993;39:1097–1102.

90. Milne R, Chambers L. Assessing the scientific quality of review articles. Journal of Epidemiology & Community Health. 1993;47(3):169–170.

91. Mulrow CD. The medical review article: state of the science. Annals of Internal Medicine. 1987;106(3):485–488.

92. Oxman AD, Guyatt GH. The science of reviewing research. Annals of the New York Academy of Sciences. 1993;703:125–133; discussion: 133–134.

93. Mullen PD, Ramirez G. The promise and pitfalls of systematic reviews. Annual Review of Public Health. 2006;27:81–102.

94. Waters E, Doyle J. Evidence-based public health practice: improving the quality and quantity of the evidence. Journal of Public Health Medicine. 2002;24(3):227–229.

95. Gold MR, Siegel JE, Russell LB, Weinstein MC. Cost-Effectiveness in Health and Medicine. New York: Oxford University Press; 1996.

96. Carande-Kulis VG, Maciosek MV, Briss PA, Teutsch SM, Zaza S, Truman BI, et al. Methods for systematic reviews of economic evaluations for the Guide to Community Preventive Services. Task Force on Community Preventive Services. American Journal of Preventive Medicine. 2000;18(1 suppl): 75–91.

97. Harris P, Harris-Roxas B, Harris E, Kemp L. Health Impact Assessment: A Practical Guide. Sydney: Centre for Health Equity Training, Research and Evaluation, University of New South Wales; 2007.

98. Cole BL, Wilhelm M, Long PV, Fielding JE, Kominski G, Morgenstern H. Prospects for health impact assessment in the United States: new and improved environmental impact assessment or something different? Journal of Health Politics, Policy and Law. 2004;29(6):1153–1186.

99. Kemm J. Health impact assessment: a tool for healthy public policy. Health Promotion International. 2001;16(1):79–85.

100. Mindell J, Sheridan L, Joffe M, Samson-Barry H, Atkinson S. Health impact assessment as an agent of policy change: improving the health impacts of the mayor of London's draft transport strategy. Journal of Epidemiology & Community Health. 2004;58(3):169–174.

101. Cargo M, Mercer SL. The value and challenges of participatory research: strengthening its practice. Annual Review of Public Health. 2008;29: 325–350.

102. Israel BA, Schulz AJ, Parker EA, Becker AB. Review of community-based research: assessing partnership approaches to improve public health. Annual Review of Public Health. 1998;19:173–202.

103. Green LW, George MA, Daniel M, Fankish CJ, Herbert CJ, Bowie WR, et al. Review and Recommendations for the Development of Participatory Research in Health Promotion in Canada. Vancouver, BC: The Royal Society of Canada; 1995.

104. Green LW, Mercer SL. Can public health researchers and agencies reconcile the push from funding bodies and the pull from communities? American Journal of Public Health. 2001;91(12):1926–1929.

105. Leung MW, Yen IH, Minkler M. Community based participatory research: a promising approach for increasing epidemiology's relevance in the 21st century. International Journal of Epidemiology. 2004;33(3):499–506.

106. Soriano FI. Conducting Needs Assessments: A Multidisciplinary Approach. Thousand Oaks, CA: Sage Publications; 1995.

107. Sederburg WA. Perspectives of the legislator: allocating resources. MMWR. 1992;41(suppl):37–48.

108. Hallfors D, Cho H, Livert D, Kadushin C. Fighting back against substance abuse: are community coalitions winning? American Journal of Preventive Medicine. 2002;23(4):237–245.

109. Brownson RC, Diem G, Grabauskas V, Legetic B, Potemkina R, Shatchkute A, et al. Training practitioners in evidence-based chronic disease prevention for global health. Promotion & Education. 2007;14(3):159–163.

110. Tugwell P, Bennett KJ, Sackett DL, Haynes RB. The measurement iterative loop: a framework for the critical appraisal of need, benefits and costs of health interventions. Journal of Chronic Diseases. 1985;38(4):339–351.

111. Birkhead GS, Davies J, Miner K, Lemmings J, Koo D. Developing competencies for applied epidemiology: from process to product. Public Health Reports. 2008;123(suppl 1):67–118.

112. Birkhead GS, Koo D. Professional competencies for applied epidemiologists: a roadmap to a more effective epidemiologic workforce. Journal of Public Health Management and Practice. 2006;12(6):501–504.

113. Gebbie K, Merrill J, Hwang I, Gupta M, Btoush R, Wagner M. Identifying individual competency in emerging areas of practice: an applied approach. Qualitative Health Research. 2002;12(7):990–999.

114. Brownson R, Ballew P, Kittur N, Elliott M, Haire-Joshu D, Krebill H, et al. Developing competencies for training practitioners in evidence-based cancer control. Journal of Cancer Education. 2009;24(3):186–193.

115. Baker EA, Brownson RC, Dreisinger M, McIntosh LD, Karamehic-Muratovic A. Examining the role of training in evidence-based public health: a qualitative study. Health Promotion Practice. 2009;10(3):342–348.

116. Maxwell ML, Adily A, Ward JE. Promoting evidence-based practice in population health at the local level: a case study in workforce capacity development. Australian Health Review. 2007;31(3):422–429.

117. Maylahn C, Bohn C, Hammer M, Waltz E. Strengthening epidemiologic competencies among local health professionals in New York: teaching evidence-based public health. Public Health Reports. 2008;123(suppl 1): 35–43.

118. Oliver KB, Dalrymple P, Lehmann HP, McClellan DA, Robinson KA, Twose C. Bringing evidence to practice: a team approach to teaching skills required for an informationist role in evidence-based clinical and public health practice. Journal of the Medical Library Association. 2008;96(1):50–57.

119. Pappaioanou M, Malison M, Wilkins K, Otto B, Goodman RA, Churchill RE, et al. Strengthening capacity in developing countries for evidence-based public health: the Data for Decision-making project. Social Science & Medicine. 2003;57(10):1925–1937.

120. Bryan RL, Kreuter MW, Brownson RC. Integrating adult learning principles into training for public health practice. Health Promotion Practice. 2008;10(4):557–563.

121. Ginter PM, Duncan WJ, Capper SA. Keeping strategic thinking in strategic planning: macro-environmental analysis in a state health department of public health. Public Health. 1992;106:253–269.

122. Florin P, Stevenson J. Identifying training and technical assistance needs in community coalitions: a developmental approach. Health Education Research. 1993;8:417–432.

123. Robeson P, Dobbins M, DeCorby K, Tirilis D. Facilitating access to pre-processed research evidence in public health. BMC Public Health. 2010;10:95.

124. Jacobs JA, Dodson EA, Baker EA, Deshpande AD, Brownson RC. Barriers to evidence-based decision making in public health: a national survey of chronic disease practitioners. Public Health Reports. 2010;125(5):736–742.

125. Institute of Medicine, Committee on Public Health. Healthy Communities: New Partnerships for the Future of Public Health. Washington, DC: National Academy Press; 1996.

126. Wright K, Rowitz L, Merkle A, Reid WM, Robinson G, Herzog B, et al. Competency development in public health leadership. American Journal of Public Health. 2000;90(8):1202–1207.

Part 3

Transdisciplinary Practice: Case Studies in Domestic Health

Transdisciplinary Methods in the Prevention and Control of Maternal-Child Obesity

Debra Haire-Joshu

Learning Objectives

- Apply the principles of transdisciplinary problem solving to population-based obesity prevention and treatment.
- Design a transdisciplinary problem-solving framework for addressing obesity prevention and treatment.
- Assess obesity as a public health problem through analysis of evidence and health outcomes.
- Illustrate methods for measuring individual, family, sociocultural, and community determinants of obesity.
- Develop innovative, population-based approaches that include core elements of obesity prevention across all levels, from cellular to environmental and policy levels.
- Describe approaches that can enhance translation of obesity research to practice and dissemination of these findings.

•••

It is critical to develop an understanding of transdisciplinary perspectives and apply systematic problem-solving approaches to complex health problems.

This is apparent in the foundation provided in parts 1 and 2 of this book, addressing instructional methods for applying transdisciplinary education in public health degree programs (chapters 2, 3, and 4) as well as the importance of transdisciplinary constructs for understanding poverty (chapter 5), law and policy (chapter 6), culture (chapter 7), and evidence-based practice (chapter 8) in relation to public health. Similarly, it has become apparent that answers to complex questions about obesity and chronic disease will require a transdisciplinary problem-solving approach, with public health practitioners analyzing perspectives from diverse fields, and coming together to integrate knowledge across these disciplines.[1-7] This chapter describes a course I have taught that addresses transdisciplinary methods in the prevention and control of maternal-child obesity. This course included exposure to perspectives from diverse disciplines (biology, communication science, economics, engineering, epidemiology, law, medicine, nursing, nutrition, policy, psychology, urban planning, and social work), a breadth of knowledge that is needed to ensure the design and development of new approaches, models, and methods to address today's obesity epidemic.[8] Application of this learning through a systematic problem-solving process can lead to solutions to the multilevel causes of obesity.

This course was divided into four sections: (1) introduction to transdisciplinary problem solving and collaborative learning; (2) transdisciplinary problem analysis, addressing obesity from a *cells to society* perspective; (3) transdisciplinary solution analysis, and (4) presentation of solutions to collaborators and stakeholders. The course pedagogy reflected active learning through collaborative learning techniques.[8] Students were encouraged to take more control of their learning and to develop the skills necessary to be successful lifelong learners. This was supported by applying such techniques as collaborative learning with peers, regular peer review, frequent interaction with and support from faculty in diverse disciplines, real-world learning activities, and routine feedback at individual and team levels. Learning activities were designed around transdisciplinary objectives; students were encouraged to contribute and participate together on problem-solving tasks, sharing the workload equally.

The class was also structured for extensive interaction with experts from various disciplines, allowing opportunity for integration of content from a variety of scientific perspectives. Time was also allotted for student-led discussions incorporating relevant readings on the topic of interest selected by both faculty and students. Finally, students were divided into teams of five to six participants and a significant portion of each class was dedicated to transdisciplinary problem-solving teamwork. Teams were crafted by the instructor so that the members of each team displayed some variation in educational background, experience, and demographics. Each team was charged with solving a real-world public health problem.

Application to Real-World Problems

The key value of a transdisciplinary methodology in public health is a broader understanding of real-world problems, leading to more appropriate and effective solutions.[6] The real-world problem to be addressed in this course was prevention and control of maternal-child obesity. Our partner in this effort was Parents as Teachers, Inc. (PAT), an award-winning, national parent education and home visiting program serving families from pregnancy until the last child in the home enters kindergarten.[9,10] The premise of PAT is that positive child development outcomes will result from a program that empowers parents as their child's first and most influential teachers. PAT is supported through federal and state funds and is a universal program, with all visits provided free of charge to high-needs parents. The program is delivered by parent educators who reside in the communities they serve and typically stay with families over time. Parent educators complete training in order to be certified to deliver the evidence-based curriculum, and maintain this certification through annual continuing education. The curriculum is delivered through regular home visits and group meetings. Children are also screened for developmental progress. At the time of the course discussed in this chapter, PAT had programs across all fifty states, reaching over 250,000 parents and children nationally. The program also has an international presence.[9]

As a result of their real-world practice, PAT educators have an acute awareness of the burgeoning obesity epidemic, particularly among young children. However, obesity prevention and control is not a focus of PAT, whose charge is to promote parent education, child development, and school readiness. At the time of this course, funding streams were not available to address the linkage between obesogenic behaviors and child development. However, recent federal initiatives supported through health reform efforts did recognize the importance of agencies reaching parents in the home as a first step in preventing obesity. PAT was positioned to expand its reach and to assume the added role of a model home visiting program to prevent and control maternal-child obesity. The challenge to the students in this course was to make recommendations for positioning PAT as a model program for prevention and control of maternal-child obesity.

Course Section 1: Introduction to Transdisciplinary Problem Solving

The first class addressed the transdisciplinary problem-solving process. Students were presented with the definition of transdisciplinary science, the history of this approach, and the scientific basis for transdisciplinary approaches.[3,6,7,11] A careful review of key concepts, as presented in chapter 1, was summarized. As noted in box 9.1, discussion also included the differentiation of participatory approaches from transdisciplinary methods.

Box 9.1: Defining concepts and the process of knowledge production in integrative research

Disciplinary

- Within one academic discipline.
- Disciplinary goal setting.
- No cooperation with other disciplines.
- Development of new disciplinary knowledge and theory.

Multidisciplinary

- Involves multiple disciplines.
- Multiple disciplinary goals set under one thematic umbrella.
- Loose cooperation of disciplines for exchange of knowledge.
- Disciplinary theory development.

Participatory

- Involves academic researchers and nonacademic participants.
- Exchange of knowledge but knowledge bodies are not integrated.
- May be disciplinary or multidisciplinary.
- Not necessarily research; the goal may be academic or not.

Interdisciplinary

- Crosses disciplinary boundaries.
- Common goal setting.
- Integration of disciplines.
- Development of integrated knowledge and theory.

Transdisciplinary

- Crosses disciplinary and scientific or academic boundaries.
- Common goal setting.
- Integration of disciplinary and nonacademic participants.
- Development of integrated knowledge and theory among participants representing science and those representing society.

Students were next presented with steps to guide transdisciplinary problem and solution analysis. The three steps in problem analysis were to define the problem, measure the magnitude of the problem, and develop a conceptual framework or logic model for understanding the key determinants of the problem. The four steps of the solution analysis were to identify and develop strategies, set priorities and recommend solutions, implement solutions and evaluate outcomes, and develop a translation and dissemination strategy. The unique aspect of this approach was that students had to demonstrate how perspectives from multiple disciplines informed each step.

Teams were challenged to integrate transdisciplinary perspectives into a richer understanding of obesity prevention and control and to propose new solutions that drew on the contributions of a range of appropriate disciplines necessary for assessing the topic. Each team was responsible for identifying and recommending positions for real-world issues, and documenting its work in a product for use by the community at large.

Course Section 2: Transdisciplinary Problem Analysis

The second section of the course began with an overview of a multilevel model of childhood obesity (see figure 9.1). The purpose was to provide an

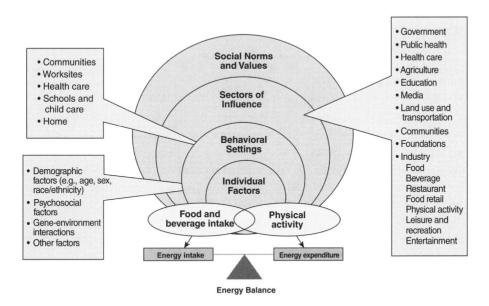

Figure 9.1. A framework to prevent and control overweight and obesity
Source: Adapted from J. P. Koplan, C. T. Liverman, and V. I. Kraak, eds., Committee on the Prevention of Obesity in Children and Youth, *Preventing Childhood Obesity: Health in the Balance* (Washington, DC: National Academies Press; 2004).

organizational framework for the initial conceptualization of childhood obesity, which could then serve as a basis for connecting cells to society discussions across various disciplines. Selected content was then organized to present information on the influence of multiple factors on maternal-child obesity, including information about the epidemiology of maternal-child obesity; the intrapersonal, interpersonal, physical, and communication environments; and the economics of obesity and obesity policy. Readings supplemented information relevant to other identified sectors of influence.

Epidemiology of Maternal-Child Obesity

Students were introduced to the problem of obesity by a nutritional epidemiologist. From an epidemiological perspective, obesity is an energy imbalance between calories consumed and calories expended through daily activity. It is a major public health problem in the United States and many other countries because of its high prevalence, causal relationship with serious medical illnesses, and economic impact. Among women, weight change in young adulthood, often initiated during pregnancy and maintained after the postpartum period, can affect lifelong risk for obesity.[12] Students were presented with data from the most recent National Health and Nutrition Examination Survey (NHANES), which showed that among adult women the prevalence of obesity was 35.3 percent. Women twenty to thirty-five years old have the fastest increase in weight and are at highest risk for obesity during specific periods of the life cycle.

The burden of obesity is borne disproportionately by some ethnic groups. For example, almost half of non-Hispanic black women ages twenty to seventy-four are obese, compared with 40 percent of Hispanic women and 30 percent of non-Hispanic white women.[13-17] Moreover, the prevalence of obesity is higher in African American women with a socioeconomic disadvantage than in those without.[13,18,19] Obesity affects not only the woman but her offspring, almost from the moment of conception.[20-25] Adverse pregnancy outcomes associated with obesity include higher rates of stillbirth, neonatal death, miscarriage, congenital malformations, preeclampsia, gestational diabetes, preterm birth, macrosomia, and cesarean delivery.[22-24,26-38] In addition, offspring born to obese women have a greater risk of neurodevelopmental delay, atypical neurodevelopment, becoming obese, becoming insulin resistant or diabetic, and having earlier cardiovascular disease than do those born to healthy, lean women.[20-22,28,30,31,34,37,39,40-42]

Obesity affects the quality of life of the young mother and is associated with impairment of physical functioning, general health, and social functioning and also with twice the rate of depression found among men.[25] Women tend to be less active than men and perceive their parenting role as a barrier to activity. Lack of time, fatigue, lack of child care, and competing roles and responsibilities are major deterrents to activity. These same barriers are associated with increased intake of convenience or takeaway foods, resulting in additional caloric intake.[25] Women are also more likely to live in poverty than men and to have less education than men.[14,18,43–45] These income disparities affect diet quality; healthier diets may cost more whereas energy dense foods may cost less.

Among children, rates of obesity have tripled since 1980 and have left American children and teenagers on track to have poor health throughout their adult lives.[46] Even the youngest children in the United States are at risk of becoming obese. Today, almost 10 percent of infants and toddlers carry excess weight for their length, and slightly more than 20 percent of children between the ages of two and five are already overweight or obese. Most excess weight that is gained by five years of age tracks predictably into later years, with little additional excess gain.[46] Because early obesity can track into adulthood, efforts to prevent obesity should begin long before a child enters school. If current trends persist, obesity could cause this generation's life expectancy to be lower than that of their parents.

Collaborative problem-solving exercises. Student teams were given group rules for engaging in collaborative problem-solving exercises, in order to ensure the involvement of each member (see box 9.2). Students then engaged in two exercises guided by these group rules of operation. For the first exercise, team members worked to answer a series of data-driven questions regarding obesity in the local region. These questions directly reflected information presented by the nutritional epidemiologist and found in readings provided for the course. Discussion centered on epidemiological methods and ways that this information might be used to address the class's real-world problem with the community partners for the course. The questions challenged students to address causal relationships between nutrition and obesity; to examine assumptions, conclusions, or interpretations related to causal factors; and to prioritize the meanings of the scientific findings.

Box 9.2: Group rules: each week, members rotate roles on the team

Facilitator. Moderates all team discussions, keeps team on task for each assignment, ensures appropriate share of work, encourages participation of all members with respect.

Recorder. Records assigned activities, takes notes, and keeps all records.

Reporter. Serves as team spokesperson.

Timekeeper. Monitors and informs group of time constraints.

The second exercise, titled "Walk the Talk," included a self-assessment of diet and activity behaviors for the members of each team. This was an important tool to ensure that students were self-aware in understanding the challenges of behavior change and realistic in any solutions proposed. Each week one of the teams identified a nutrition and activity challenge to be completed by members of all the teams over the next week. The challenge focused on some aspect of the nutrition and physical activity guidelines. Pedometers and online food trackers were provided for self-assessment. Self-reported results were calculated and reported the following week. The supports and barriers encountered in meeting the challenges, and the ways in which these experiences might inform solutions for the class's real-world problem, were discussed.

Intrapersonal Environment

Students were next exposed to the problem of obesity as it focuses on the individual. The scientific basis of obesity was presented, from perspectives of the disciplines of cellular biology, genetics, and medicine. Readings provided by faculty and students broadened their understanding of individual determinants. Questions initiated to guide student learning included the following: What role does biology or genetics play in body weight? How do these mechanisms alter understanding of body weight from a population perspective? How should these perspectives influence an understanding of obesity as it relates to public health interventions?

Biology of Maternal-Child Obesity: Gut Microbia

The purpose of the material on gut microbia, presented by a scientist and physician engaged in basic cellular science, was to introduce students to the biological environment, the potential influence of this environment on obesity, and the ways that these findings might influence public health interventions. Interactions among microorganisms in the gut appear to affect nutrient acquisition and energy regulation, suggesting an important role in host energy homeostasis.[47-50] Gut microbiota in lean animals and humans have been found to differ from those in obese ones. Metabolic activities of the gut microbiota may facilitate the extraction and storage of calories from dietary substances in adipose tissue for later use.[47] There is also evidence for a role of gut microbes in obesity-related type 2 diabetes.[50] This suggests that changes in gut microbiota may provide an alternative means for treating people who are overweight or obese.[48]

Genetics of Taste and Food Preferences

The purpose of this content, presented by a nutrition geneticist, was for students to recognize the genetic influence of the prenatal environment on postnatal, obesity-related behaviors, and how this might shape real-world messages to pregnant women and young mothers.[26,31] For example, many flavors in the maternal diet appear to be present in amniotic fluid.[51-54] This means that taste and smell are already functional during fetal life due to fetal swallowing of amniotic fluid. This also means that the first experiences with flavors of food occur prior to birth.[55-59] Shortly after birth, infants express preferences for sweet tastes and reject those that are sour and bitter, suggesting flavor preferences are initially maintained postnatally.[52,54]

Initial taste preferences can be unlearned after birth with repeated exposures to other flavors. Laboratory studies confirm that young children form preferences for flavors associated with energy-rich foods, which may promote energy intake in abundant dietary environments.[53,60] New foods may need to be offered to preschool-aged children ten to sixteen times before acceptance occurs. Understanding this concept of neophobia is important in dealing with parents who are concerned that their child is not eating enough.[60] Awareness of this normal course of food acceptance is important because approximately one-quarter of parents with infants and toddlers draw conclusions about their child's preference for foods prematurely, after two or fewer exposures.[60-62]

Finally, interaction with other environments can also influence the development of child taste preferences. Children decide their food likes and dislikes by eating, and also by associating food flavors with the social contexts and the physiological consequences of consumption.

Metabolic Abnormalities

The purpose of this content, presented by physician scientists, was for students to learn about obesity and its association with a constellation of serious metabolic abnormalities. Students explored influences on the obesogenic prenatal environment and whether these influences can increase the likelihood of obesity in the offspring through epigenetic effects. In turn, learning about the biological risk factors promotes an understanding of linkages between the environment and metabolic systems and the effects of these linkages on behavior and health.[63]

Obesity in pregnant women and excessive gestational weight gain increase the risk for alterations in maternal metabolism, including dyslipidemia, glucose intolerance and insulin resistance, hyperleptinemia, and inflammation.[23,33,64] Obesity and weight gain are also associated with an increased incidence of gestational diabetes during pregnancy, which leads to infant macrosomia.[20,37] In addition, infants born to obese and insulin resistant women are at greater risk for increased adiposity, insulin resistance, dyslipidemia, and increased plasma concentrations of leptin and inflammatory markers.[20,21,33,54] Dysregulated maternal lipid metabolism can also have adverse consequences in offspring health and is associated with increased neonatal birth weight and adiposity and cardiovascular disease risk later in life.[36,37,54,60,64]

Additionally, students learned that maternal obesity was associated with abnormal neurodevelopment in children and that higher than recommended gestational weight gain was a significant negative predictor of IQ at age five.[35,36] Other studies have suggested associations between higher prepregnancy body mass index (BMI), higher than recommended gestational weight gain, and increased levels of attention deficit/hyperactivity disorder (ADHD) symptoms.[42]

Collaborative problem-solving exercises. Following each class, students were challenged to incorporate new learning into "redefining" the problem of maternal-child obesity. Questions of interest, generated by the teams, were developed. Each team then passed its questions to another team for discussion. Active listening and analysis of content across teams was encouraged by this round-robin approach. Select questions were then anchored through the use of a case study describing an obese woman's challenges with weight control prior to pregnancy, during pregnancy, and postpartum. Each team used problem-solving steps to analyze the case study and discuss how different disciplines might answer the question of interest from their conceptual perspectives. Additionally, students were asked to think through and apply the disciplinary perspectives to the development of real-world interventions.

Interpersonal Environment

The purpose of presenting information about the interpersonal environment was for the student to be able to describe the parent or caregiver interactions with the child that influence the child's food intake and the relationship of this environment to obesity prevention and control. This content was presented by experts from several disciplines, including education, educational psychology, nursing, and social work. Questions to guide this section included: What influence does the mother have on child intake? How do maternal-child interactions affect short- and long-term body weight?

Child Development and Communication

Students were exposed to extensive literature showing that obesity runs in families, with parental overweight being the major familial factor contributing to child overweight.[31] Traditional feeding practices of parents, especially those who are obese, can promote overeating and weight gain in children.[60,61,65,66] These child feeding practices include specific behavioral strategies parents employ (such as using food as a reward) to control what, how much, or when their children eat. As noted previously, a child develops food preferences by responding to what he or she is fed, observing adults, and reacting to the availability of food in the immediate environment. Because food consumed by young children is determined by caregivers, every effort needs to be made to introduce children to healthy foods and lifestyle habits from the beginning of infancy onward. Children who have early experiences with healthy foods and eating practices are more likely to prefer and consume those foods and to have dietary patterns that promote healthy growth and weight throughout life.[46,60]

Behavioral Science: Parental Modeling

The psychology of behavior and the how's and why's of what we do are critical to understanding influences on obesity. The means by which we learn our eating and activity behavioral patterns are particularly relevant to obesity, as they cross generations. Students were exposed to this science through the concept of parental modeling. Parents are models of substantial relevance and credibility and have increasing influence on development of parent-child concordance in food intake and activity over time.[46,60,61] Parental modeling is defined as a process in which the behavior of the parent acts as a stimulus for similar behavior for the child, helping to shape children's values, beliefs, and behaviors.[46,67,68] Several studies suggest that strong modeling influences occur via several factors, including observational learning, when young children learn what and how to eat by watching their parents' intake and reactions to foods; response facilitation, the frequency of the behavior being modeled; and reinforcement, verbal and nonverbal responses to eating new foods. Evidence-based lifestyle strategies may have the potential to influence the parent's construction of the child's food and activity environment.[46] The desire to be a good parent and role model may be a conceptual motivator for a mother to improve her health behaviors and achieve weight loss.

Collaborative problem-solving exercises. Each team was provided a case study on the development of obesity in a young postpartum woman and her child. Teams analyzed the role of behavioral science in explaining the development of obesity, and considered how this might affect their construction of the problem of maternal-child obesity. Team members discussed their interpretation of disciplinary perspectives regarding obesity among themselves and across groups. How these perspectives influenced interpretations related to the case study and problem identification were addressed. Each team then presented the problem it had identified, followed by a debate across teams. This was facilitated by instructor prompts (for example, How do you know? What is the evidence? How reliable is the evidence? From what viewpoint or perspective?).

Other Environmental Influences

Students were challenged to broaden their scientific perspective on factors influencing maternal-child obesity. The initial sessions examined the complex interaction of individual and interpersonal factors related to dietary intake and physical activity. The next sessions broadened this perspective by introducing the science suggesting the influence of the physical environment and communication environment. Community urban planners presented information on the built environment; health communication scientists addressed the media environment and its role in obesity. Readings supplemented other learning.

Built Environment

Students were introduced to the concept of the environment, defined as all that is external to individuals, and environmental influences on behaviors that contribute to energy balance.[69-72] Access to areas for play or recreation and walking trails and also the degree of residential density, sidewalk access, and sprawl suggest the environmental influence on the development of obesity.[73-76] In the food environment, lack of access to grocery stores with healthy foods versus access to fast-food restaurants and the numbers of food outlets are associated with obesity.[77-80] Objective components of the physical environment are interpreted by the individual based on sociocultural features he or she attributes to those components. Studies have suggested that an individual's perceptions of safety and distance have relevance in decisions that influence body weight. For example, the presence of safe walking trails in communities is associated with increased physical activity.[81]

Communication Environment

The American population lives in a media-saturated environment in which marketing is pervasive across any number of venues (for example, television, digital devices, video games, the Internet).[46,82] The majority of marketing promotes brands and food products high in calories, fats, sugars, and salt. The dietary intake modeled by food marketing is inconsistent with a healthy diet—even at dosages smaller than those generally available for those products. Food marketing works especially effectively on young children.[83-85] It influences their food beliefs and preferences, purchase requests to parents, short-term consumption, and usual dietary intake. From a behavioral perspective, TV viewing alone is a risk factor for overweight in childhood and adulthood and is associated with inactivity, decreased metabolic rate, and increased snacking.[46,86] Limiting total screen time has been recommended by many health organizations as a means to reduce exposure of young children to food and beverage marketing and decrease the likelihood of early childhood obesity.[46]

Collaborative problem-solving exercises. Teams were challenged to expand on their prior case studies on the development of obesity in a young postpartum woman and her child. They were asked to analyze the role of the environment and consider how this analysis might influence their construction of the problem of maternal-child obesity. Team members discussed their ideas about this process among themselves and across groups.

Obesity Policy: Influences across Settings

The multiple sectors and facets of the obesity epidemic were initially addressed in the groundbreaking Institute of Medicine (IOM) report *Preventing Childhood Obesity: Health in the Balance*.[87] The importance given to policies that support healthy eating and activity behaviors, implemented consistently across these multiple settings, was notable. Policy recommendations were suggested for the multiple settings where children spend time (such as health care, child-care, school, and community settings) and also the home setting, where parental interactions and behaviors play a critical role. For this part of the course, students were challenged to examine and define the role of evidence-based policy as it related to maternal-child obesity. Disciplinary perspectives from health policy, economics, and political science were presented.

Policy and Energy Balance Strategies

Policy is recognized as a powerful instrument for influencing public health and an important strategy for preventing obesity.[82,88] Policies can enhance health by mitigating the negative effects of the multiple environments that influence the lives of individuals. Several lessons have been learned about the use of public policy as a strategy for reducing health threats such as tobacco use, and these lessons can be applied to obesity prevention. For example, policies can directly deter behavior by altering the cost of personal choices known to negatively affect health (for instance, smoking has been reduced through increases in tobacco pricing). Similarly, policies can promote or establish social norms that indirectly influence behavior (by eliminating smoking in workplaces, for example).[91] Obesity policies are now being initiated to limit serving sizes or to increase taxes on sugary drinks and restrict sales of certain energy drinks.[88-91] Such approaches may provide a means of addressing health disparities by ensuring socioeconomic or physical environmental conditions that serve as deterrents to unhealthy eating behaviors. Anticipating and addressing the unintended consequences of policies, due to lack of evidence-based content or systematic evaluation, is critical to ensuring that the policy goal, such as the goal of energy balance, is reached and maintained.

Economics of Obesity

Students were introduced to the role of economics in policy development and implementation and provided with a foundation for understanding the economic challenge presented by obesity. Obese children are two to three times more likely to be hospitalized and are about three times more costly to care for and treat than the average insured child. Childhood obesity alone is estimated to cost $14 billion annually in direct health expenses.[92] These costs will increase over time as obese children move to adulthood and will have a negative influence on governmental budgets at all levels over the long term.[93,94] The need for evidence-based policy, and for better evaluations of the cost implications of such policies, was discussed.

Governmental Role in Policy

Students were exposed to the varying views on the role of government in obesity prevention and control. Government has an interest in preventing obesity, given the rise in medical expenditures that burden the health care system as a result of obesity. However, there are differing perspectives as to the appropriate federal role in establishing policies that address obesity. One view is that government should have a very limited role because obesity is the ultimate result of lifestyle choices falling within the purview of individual and personal responsibility.[94] This perspective encourages policies and programs designed to improve individual awareness and knowledge through education. In contrast, proponents of a more active governmental role point to evidence that obesity causes harm not only to the individual but to the public at large and is the result of negative health influences in multiple areas: behavioral, environmental, and genetic.

Students learned about current governmental structure and the numerous federal agencies and private organizations that have issued guidelines and reports advising Americans on strategies to address obesity.[94-96] Most of strategies tend to focus on interventions and actions for individuals, and the evidence supporting the recommendations is either not clear or highly variable. At the same time, there has been an exponential growth in the attention that this condition has received from policymakers at the state and federal levels, and some have called for substantial involvement by government at all levels and across multiple sectors.[97]

Current Policy Initiatives: School Settings

More than 95 percent of American youth aged five to seventeen are enrolled in school, and no other institution has as much continuous and intensive contact with children during their first two decades of life.[98] Schools can promote good nutrition, physical activity, and healthy weight among children through appropriate nutrition, physical activity, and health education. Nutrition policies that encourage access to healthy foods show promise for weight control. The evidence supporting physical activity policies that promote multiple opportunities for students to be physically active, in addition to physical education, is abundant. Recommendations for activity programs include providing students with the knowledge and skills necessary to remain physically strong and healthy, providing opportunities for students to be active during the school day, and motivating students to be active every day.

Collaborative problem-solving exercises. Teams were first challenged to review current federal, state, or local policy databases and also to select and evaluate the evidence-based content of specific obesity policies. They then discussed their findings and how these results might influence their definition of the problem noted in the case study on the development of obesity in a young postpartum woman and her child. Finally, teams generated questions they thought relevant to policy and the real-world challenge they faced. They then organized meetings with the PAT partners to collect relevant information to inform their problem identification.

Course Section 3: Transdisciplinary Solution Analysis

This part of the course focused on applying transdisciplinary learning to solutions for maternal-child obesity. Students were now asked to draw from the initial conceptual model that guided organization of the content (figure 9.1) and to incorporate two new concepts: systems model building to identify solutions, and dissemination and implementation of new solutions to the population at large. This section included presentations by engineers and public health scientists.

A Systems Approach to Obesity

Obesity is a multilevel health concern, and the prevention and control of obesity requires multipronged interventions. At the individual level, biological factors influence body weight. At the interpersonal level, maternal behavior influences child behavior. For example, improvements in the mother's intake at home yield improvements in the intake of her preschool child.[67] At the environmental level, the availability of healthy and affordable food options, the quality of the built environment, the social and cultural attitudes around body weight, and the level of access to quality settings all play a role in obesity prevalence.[91] Any efforts to address obesity moving forward must account for all these factors, since incremental changes will only marginally reduce rates of obesity. Students were next introduced to a systems-oriented approach to promote research capacity building. Consistent with the work of Huang et al., and the transdisciplinary focus of the course, obesity is approached by first looking at the entire interaction across the multiple environments (biological, physical, economic, and so forth).[63] The application of systems modeling approaches, to better understand the exact levers contributing to obesity, was presented. Students were also encouraged to develop an understanding of the multiple influences on the systems and to consider intervening at various leverage points to yield energy balance behaviors and outcomes. A discussion of examples of how model building best depicts associations with obesity prevention and control was conducted.

Translating What Works: Dissemination and Implementation Science

Limited practical trial research, addressing the impact and sustainability of evidence-based weight loss approaches translated to natural settings,[99,100] is critical because many individuals who lose weight with diet and exercise regain most of that lost weight over time. To conceptualize how this research might inform their solutions, students were exposed to the RE-AIM (*Reach, Efficacy, Adoption, Implementation, Maintenance*) framework. RE-AIM is the leading framework for evaluating the potential of an intervention to be applied and sustained in practice settings.[100-104] *Reach* refers to the number, proportion, and representativeness of those who participate in the intervention relative to all persons in the target population. *Efficacy* (and *effectiveness*, when measured) identifies effects of an intervention on not only clinical outcomes but also in terms of positive and negative program consequences, quality of life, satisfaction as perceived by the participants, and economic factors. *Adoption* refers to the absolute number, proportion, and representativeness of settings (in this case, PAT sites) and agents (parent educators) that agree to implement the intervention. Adoption is influenced by such core elements as consistency with the organization's mission and such characteristics as relative advantage, compatibility, complexity, trialability, and observability. *Implementation* involves delivering the intervention as intended (that is, it addresses consistency, fidelity, and adaptation). *Maintenance* refers not only to sustained behavior change over time among participants but also to integration of the intervention within an organization's standard practices.[100,104]

Applying Transdisciplinary Solutions

Team members developed and presented a series of projects that, cumulatively, proposed a roadmap for the development of intergenerational obesity prevention strategies and programs to affect the home environment, offered a systematic evaluation of the proposed strategies, and suggested mechanisms for disseminating findings to real-world practice. Two teams addressed interventions to increase physical activity; two teams focused on the food environment. Strategies were multilevel and included policy initiatives. Each proposal offered clear, specific aims and provided a planned solution, incorporating multiple disciplinary perspectives while clearly establishing the magnitude of the problem. A conceptual model mapped the approach in addressing the problem and outcome. One or more potential solutions were noted as were implementation plans and costs. Benchmarks for success included cost effectiveness.

Course Section 4: Presentation of Team Solutions to Partners and Stakeholders

Each team of students developed a detailed proposal documenting solutions to the challenge. Each team then conducted a fifteen-minute presentation, highlighting key elements of its proposal. PAT partners, stakeholders, and school and faculty members were invited to attend the presentation. Active questioning of each proposal then ensued. Box 9.3 highlights the core ideas presented during this process. There is also an epilogue to these efforts; the partner organization is actively engaged in implementing several of the student recommendations. Thus there is the potential of national impact for this coursework.

Box 9.3: Suggested team solutions

Based on a transdisciplinary problem-solving approach, the teams' suggestions for the partnering organization were as follows:[8]

- Review, update, and implement evidence-based nutrition and physical activity organizational policies.
- Institute as a national requirement for certification that all parent educators be trained on determinants of maternal-child obesity, its impact on child development, and evidence-based obesity prevention and control strategies.
- Target high-needs obese women and children, and develop a curriculum that translates evidence-based obesity treatment strategies to this group.
- Partner with urban planning and parks and recreation groups so parent educators can facilitate linkages between parents and environments supportive of physical activity.
- Evaluate, on a systematic and regular basis, the cost and impact of changes in the organization's obesity prevention policies and programming.
- Implement a communication strategy to ensure the dissemination of information on policy changes to parents, educators, policymakers, and funders of obesity prevention approaches.

Systematic Evaluation Methods

Systematic and frequent evaluation is critical to transdisciplinary learning and the learning process.[8] Evaluation was divided equally between individual and team assignments. Individual assignments accounted for 50 percent of each student's grade and included addressing student discussion questions from readings, participation in class, and completion of policy and case study analysis of obesity-related topics. Ten percent of this 50 percent was determined by peer evaluation.

Team assignments accounted for the other 50 percent of the grade and included the team transdisciplinary problem-solving project paper and oral presentation of the project to stakeholders. Twenty percent of this fifty percent was determined by team members evaluating each other for team efforts and contributions. Team evaluation occurred four times during the semester. The evaluation allotted a total number of points for such specific teamwork criteria as preparation, completion of assigned tasks, and quality and timeliness of efforts. These total points had to be distributed across team members in accordance with the value assigned to their individual efforts. Students were provided with their peer scores after each evaluation. Students were encouraged to work with their team members to address any concerns with the scores. Faculty members monitored or facilitated these discussions as needed.

Summary

Transdisciplinary problem-solving approaches teach public health practitioners to address complex problems with outside-the-box perspectives. This approach also requires that learning takes place and that findings have an impact on real-world situations. In this course, students were exposed to multiple perspectives on maternal-child obesity and were able to apply these perspectives in developing solutions to a real-world problem. The kind of potential this course provided for long-term impact on our partner organization and the mothers and children it interacts with nationally is critical to transdisciplinary science and approaches. It is also critical to training the next generation of public health practitioners and scientists.

Key Terms

body mass index (BMI)	A number calculated from height and weight in order to categorize an adult's weight as underweight, normal, overweight, or obese. BMI is used because, for most people, it correlates with their amount of body fat.

built environment	All the human-made surroundings that provide the setting for human activity, from buildings and parks to neighborhoods and cities; it may include supporting infrastructure, such as the water supply.
food environment	Everything that influences food choices and quality, such as presence of and access to food through store or restaurant proximity, food prices, food and nutrition assistance programs, and community characteristics.
gut microbiota	An assortment of microorganisms inhabiting the gastrointestinal tract. The composition of this microbial community is host specific, evolves throughout an individual's lifetime, and is involved in aspects of physiology, including nutritional status.
overweight and obesity	Labels for ranges of weight that are greater than is generally considered healthy for a person of a given height; that is, they increase the likelihood of certain diseases and other health problems. For an adult, a BMI between 25 and 29.9 is considered overweight; a BMI of 30 or higher is considered obese. A child's weight status is determined using an age- and sex-specific percentile for BMI. Overweight is defined as a BMI at or above the 85th percentile and lower than the 95th percentile for children of the same age and sex; obesity is defined as a BMI at or above the 95th percentile for children of the same age and sex.
parental modeling	A process in which the behavior of the parent acts as a stimulus for similar behavior in the child; such modeling can shape children's values and beliefs as well as behaviors.

Review Questions

1. What is the significance of a multilevel model of childhood obesity?
2. What does the influence of multiple environments on maternal-child obesity mean for problem solving efforts?

3. What is the role of gut microbia in maternal-child obesity?

4. How are taste preferences influenced by the interaction of genetics and behavior?

5. What are the factors in the communication environment that may influence childhood obesity?

6. What is RE-AIM, and how does it apply to maternal-child obesity interventions?

This publication was made possible by Grant Number 1P30DK092950 from the NIDDK, and its contents are solely the responsibility of the authors and do not necessarily represent the official views of the NIDDK.

References

1. Colditz GA, Emmons KM, Viswanath K, Kerner JF. Translating science to practice: community and academic perspectives. Journal of Public Health Management and Practice. 2008;14(2):144–149.

2. Conrad PA, Mazet JA, Clifford D, Scott C, Wilkes M. Evolution of a transdisciplinary "one medicine-one health" approach to global health education at the University of California, Davis. Preventive Veterinary Medicine. 2009;92(4):268–274.

3. Grey M, Connolly CA. "Coming together, keeping together, working together": interdisciplinary to transdisciplinary research and nursing. Nursing Outlook. 2008;56(3):102–107.

4. Hiatt RA. Epidemiology: key to translational, team, and transdisciplinary science. Annals of Epidemiology. 2008;18(11):859–861.

5. Juster RP, Bizik G, Picard M, Arsenault-Lapierre G, Sindi S, Trepanier L, et al. A transdisciplinary perspective of chronic stress in relation to psychopathology throughout life span development. Development and Psychopathology. 2011;23(3):725–776.

6. Kessel F, Rosenfield PL. Toward transdisciplinary research: historical and contemporary perspectives. American Journal of Preventive Medicine. 2008;35(2 suppl):S225–S234.

7. Klein JT. Evaluation of interdisciplinary and transdisciplinary research: a literature review. American Journal of Preventive Medicine. 2008;35(2 suppl):S116–S123.

8. Barkley E, Cross KP, Major CH. Collaborative Learning Techniques: A Handbook for College Faculty. San Francisco: Jossey-Bass; 2005.

9. Parents as Teachers National Center I. Born to Learn Annual Report Program Summary: 2008–2009. St. Louis, MO: Parents as Teachers; 2009.

10. Zigler E, Pfannenstiel JC, Seitz V. The Parents as Teachers program and school success: a replication and extension. Journal of Primary Prevention. 2008;29(2):103–120.

11. Stokols D. Toward a science of transdisciplinary action research. American Journal of Community Psychology. 2006;38(1–2):63–77.

12. Walker LO, Sterling BS, Kim M, Arheart KL, Timmerman GM. Trajectory of weight changes in the first 6 weeks postpartum. Journal of Obstetric, Gynecologic, and Neonatal Nursing. 2006;35(4):472–481.

13. Baker EA, Schootman M, Barnidge E, Kelly C. The role of race and poverty in access to foods that enable individuals to adhere to dietary guidelines. Preventing Chronic Disease. 2006;3(3):A76.

14. Drewnowski A, Darmon N. The economics of obesity: dietary energy density and energy cost. American Journal of Clinical Nutrition. 2005;82(1 suppl): 265S–273S.

15. Gordon-Larsen P, Nelson MC, Page P, Popkin BM. Inequality in the built environment underlies key health disparities in physical activity and obesity. Pediatrics. 2006;117(2):417–424.

16. Hedley AA, Ogden CL, Johnson CL, Carroll MD, Curtin LR, Flegal KM. Prevalence of overweight and obesity among US children, adolescents, and adults, 1999–2002. JAMA. 2004;291(23):2847–2850.

17. Kurian AK, Cardarelli KM. Racial and ethnic differences in cardiovascular disease risk factors: a systematic review. Ethnicity & Disease. 2007;17(1):143–152.

18. Delisle HF. Poverty: the double burden of malnutrition in mothers and the intergenerational impact. Annals of the New York Academy of Sciences. 2008;1136:172–184.

19. Klohe-Lehman DM, Freeland-Graves J, Clarke KK, Cai G, Voruganti VS, Milani TJ, et al. Low-income, overweight and obese mothers as agents of change to improve food choices, fat habits, and physical activity in their 1-to-3-year-old children. Journal of the American College of Nutrition. 2007;26(3):196–208.

20. Catalano PM, Presley L, Minium J, Hauguel-de Mouzon S. Fetuses of obese mothers develop insulin resistance in utero. Diabetes Care. 2009;32(6):1076–1080.

21. Chiavaroli V, Giannini C, D'Adamo E, de Giorgis T, Chiarelli F, Mohn A. Insulin resistance and oxidative stress in children born small and large for gestational age. Pediatrics. 2009;124(2):695–702.

22. Chu SY, Kim SY, Lau J, Schmid CH, Dietz PM, Callaghan WM, et al. Maternal obesity and risk of stillbirth: a metaanalysis. American Journal of Obstetrics and Gynecology. 2007;197(3):223–228.

23. Doherty DA, Magann EF, Francis J, Morrison JC, Newnham JP. Pre-pregnancy body mass index and pregnancy outcomes. International Journal of Gynecology & Obstetrics. 2006;95(3):242–247.

24. Gould Rothberg BE, Magriples U, Kershaw TS, Rising SS, Ickovics JR. Gestational weight gain and subsequent postpartum weight loss among young, low-income, ethnic minority women. American Journal of Obstetrics and Gynecology. 2011;204(1):52 e1–e11.

25. Johnson DB, Gerstein DE, Evans AE, Woodward-Lopez G. Preventing obesity: a life cycle perspective. Journal of the American Dietetic Association. 2006;106(1):97–102.

26. Durand EF, Logan C, Carruth A. Association of maternal obesity and childhood obesity: implications for healthcare providers. Journal of Community Health Nursing. 2007;24(3):167–176.

27. Kinnunen TI, Pasanen M, Aittasalo M, Fogelholm M, Weiderpass E, Luoto R. Reducing postpartum weight retention—a pilot trial in primary health care. Nutrition Journal. 2007;6:21.

28. Lapolla A, Bonomo M, Dalfra MG, Parretti E, Mannino D, Mello G, et al. Prepregnancy BMI influences maternal and fetal outcomes in women with isolated gestational hyperglycaemia: a multicentre study. Diabetes & Metabolism. 2010;36(4):265–270.

29. Mamun AA, O'Callaghan M, Callaway L, Williams G, Najman J, Lawlor DA. Associations of gestational weight gain with offspring body mass index and blood pressure at 21 years of age: evidence from a birth cohort study. Circulation. 2009;119(13):1720–1727.

30. Neggers YH, Goldenberg RL, Ramey SL, Cliver SP. Maternal prepregnancy body mass index and psychomotor development in children. Acta Obstetricia et Gynecologica Scandinavica. 2003;82(3):235–240.

31. Oken E. Maternal and child obesity: the causal link. Obstetrics and Gynecology Clinics of North America. 2009;36(2):361–377, ix–x.

32. Phelan S, Phipps MG, Abrams B, Darroch F, Schaffner A, Wing RR. Randomized trial of a behavioral intervention to prevent excessive gestational weight gain: the Fit for Delivery Study. American Journal of Clinical Nutrition. 2011;93(4):772–779.

33. Ramsay JE, Ferrell WR, Crawford L, Wallace AM, Greer IA, Sattar N. Maternal obesity is associated with dysregulation of metabolic, vascular, and inflammatory pathways. Journal of Clinical Endocrinology & Metabolism. 2002;87(9):4231–4237.

34. Rasmussen SA, Chu SY, Kim SY, Schmid CH, Lau J. Maternal obesity and risk of neural tube defects: a metaanalysis. American Journal of Obstetrics and Gynecology. 2008;198(6):611–619.

35. Rooney BL, Schauberger CW, Mathiason MA. Impact of perinatal weight change on long-term obesity and obesity-related illnesses. Obstetrics & Gynecology. 2005;106(6):1349–1356.

36. Schack-Nielsen L, Michaelsen KF, Gamborg M, Mortensen EL, Sorensen TI. Gestational weight gain in relation to offspring body mass index and obesity from infancy through adulthood. International Journal of Obesity. 2010;34(1):67–74.

37. Sewell MF, Huston-Presley L, Super DM, Catalano P. Increased neonatal fat mass, not lean body mass, is associated with maternal obesity. American Journal of Obstetrics and Gynecology. 2006;195(4):1100–1103.

38. Yun S, Kabeer NH, Zhu BP, Brownson RC. Modifiable risk factors for developing diabetes among women with previous gestational diabetes. Preventing Chronic Disease. 2007;4(1):A07.

39. Boney CM, Verma A, Tucker R, Vohr BR. Metabolic syndrome in childhood: association with birth weight, maternal obesity, and gestational diabetes mellitus. Pediatrics. 2005;115(3):e290–e296.

40. Keim SA, Branum AM, Klebanoff MA, Zemel BS. Maternal body mass index and daughters' age at menarche. Epidemiology. 2009;20(5):677–681.

41. Rodriguez A. Maternal pre-pregnancy obesity and risk for inattention and negative emotionality in children. Journal of Child Psychology and Psychiatry. 2010;51:134–143.

42. Rodriguez A, Miettunen J, Henriksen TB, Olsen J, Obel C, Taanila A, et al. Maternal adiposity prior to pregnancy is associated with ADHD symptoms in offspring: evidence from three prospective pregnancy cohorts. International Journal of Obesity. 2008;32(3):550–557.

43. Burdette HL, Whitaker RC. Neighborhood playgrounds, fast food restaurants, and crime: relationships to overweight in low-income preschool children. Preventive Medicine. 2004;38(1):57–63.

44. Candib LM. Obesity and diabetes in vulnerable populations: reflection on proximal and distal causes. Annals of Family Medicine. 2007;5(6):547–556.

45. Dinour LM, Bergen D, Yeh MC. The food insecurity-obesity paradox: a review of the literature and the role Food Stamps may play. Journal of the American Dietetic Association. 2007;107(11):1952–1961.

46. Birch L, Parker L, Special Committee on Obesity Prevention Policies. Obesity Prevention Policies for Young Children. Washington, DC: Institute of Medicine; 2011.

47. Delzenne NM, Cani PD. Interaction between obesity and the gut microbiota: relevance in nutrition. Annual Review of Nutrition. 2011;31:15–31.

48. Diamant M, Blaak EE, de Vos WM. Do nutrient-gut-microbiota interactions play a role in human obesity, insulin resistance and type 2 diabetes? Obesity Reviews. 2011;12(4):272–281.

49. Ley RE, Turnbaugh PJ, Klein S, Gordon JI. Microbial ecology: human gut microbes associated with obesity. Nature. 2006;444(7122):1022–1023.

50. Musso G, Gambino R, Cassader M. Interactions between gut microbiota and host metabolism predisposing to obesity and diabetes. Annual Review of Medicine. 2011;62:361–380.

51. Bayol SA, Farrington SJ, Stickland NC. A maternal "junk food" diet in pregnancy and lactation promotes an exacerbated taste for "junk food" and a greater propensity for obesity in rat offspring. British Journal of Nutrition. 2007;98(4):843–851.

52. Beauchamp GK, Mennella JA. Flavor perception in human infants: development and functional significance. Digestion. 2011;83(suppl 1):1–6.

53. Beauchamp GK, Mennella JA. Early flavor learning and its impact on later feeding behavior. Journal of Pediatric Gastroenterology and Nutrition. 2009;48(suppl 1):S25–S30.

54. Shalev U, Tylor A, Schuster K, Frate C, Tobin S, Woodside B. Long-term physiological and behavioral effects of exposure to a highly palatable diet during the perinatal and post-weaning periods. Physiology & Behavior. 2010;101(4):494–502.

55. Mennella JA. Flavour programming during breast-feeding. Advances in Experimental Medicine and Biology. 2009;639:113–120.

56. Mennella JA, Forestell CA, Morgan LK, Beauchamp GK. Early milk feeding influences taste acceptance and liking during infancy. American Journal of Clinical Nutrition. 2009;90(3):780S–788S.

57. Mennella JA, Ventura AK. Early feeding: setting the stage for healthy eating habits. Nestlé Nutrition Workshop Series Paediatric Programme. 2011;68:153–163; discussion 164–168.

58. Mennella JA, Lukasewycz LD, Castor SM, Beauchamp GK. The timing and duration of a sensitive period in human flavor learning: a randomized trial. American Journal of Clinical Nutrition. 2011;93(5):1019–1024.

59. Mennella JA, Pepino MY, Lehmann-Castor SM, Yourshaw LM. Sweet preferences and analgesia during childhood: effects of family history of alcoholism and depression. Addiction. 2010;105(4):666–675.

60. Savage JS, Fisher JO, Birch LL. Parental influence on eating behavior: conception to adolescence. Journal of Law, Medicine & Ethics. 2007;35(1):22–34.

61. Faith MS, Scanlon KS, Birch LL, Francis LA, Sherry B. Parent-child feeding strategies and their relationships to child eating and weight status. Obesity Research. 2004;12(11):1711–1722.

62. Francis LA, Hofer SM, Birch LL. Predictors of maternal child-feeding style: maternal and child characteristics. Appetite. 2001;37(3):231–243.

63. Huang TT, Drewnosksi A, Kumanyika S, Glass TA. A systems-oriented multilevel framework for addressing obesity in the 21st century. Preventing Chronic Disease. 2009;6(3):A82.

64. Stewart FM, Freeman DJ, Ramsay JE, Greer IA, Caslake M, Ferrell WR. Longitudinal assessment of maternal endothelial function and markers of inflammation and placental function throughout pregnancy in lean and obese mothers. Journal of Clinical Endocrinology & Metabolism. 2007;92(3):969–975.

65. Campbell KJ, Hesketh KD. Strategies which aim to positively impact on weight, physical activity, diet and sedentary behaviours in children from zero to five years: A systematic review of the literature. Obesity Reviews. 2007;8(4):327–S38.

66. Faith MS, Berkowitz RI, Stallings VA, Kerns J, Storey M, Stunkard AJ. Parental feeding attitudes and styles and child body mass index: prospective analysis of a gene-environment interaction. Pediatrics. 2004;114(4):e429–e436.

67. Haire-Joshu D, Elliott MB, Caito NM, Hessler K, Nanney MS, Hale N, et al. High 5 for Kids: The impact of a home visiting program on fruit and vegetable intake of parents and their preschool children. Preventive Medicine. 2008;47(10):77–82.

68. Haire-Joshu D, Fleming C. An ecological approach to understanding contributions to disparities in diabetes prevention and care. Current Diabetes Reports. 2006;6(2):123–129.

69. Berke EM, Koepsell TD, Moudon AV, Hoskins RE, Larson EB. Association of the built environment with physical activity and obesity in older persons. American Journal of Public Health. 2007;97(3):486–492.

70. Committee on Physical Activity, Health, Transportation, and Land Use, Transportation Research Board and Institute of Medicine. Does the Built Environment Influence Physical Activity? Examining the Evidence. Washington, DC: National Academies Press; 2005.

71. Eyler AA, Brownson RC, Doescher MP, Evenson KR, Fesperman CE, Litt JS, et al. Policies related to active transport to and from school: a multisite case study. Health Education Research. 2008;23(6):963–975.

72. Handy S, Clifton K. Planning and the built environment: implications for obesity prevention. In: Kumanyika S, Brownson R, eds. Handbook of Obesity Prevention: A Resource for Health Professionals. New York: Springer; 2007:167–188.

73. Dunton GF, Kaplan J, Wolch J, Jerrett M, Reynolds KD. Physical environmental correlates of childhood obesity: a systematic review. Obesity Reviews. 2009;10(4):393–402.

74. Ewing R, Brownson RC, Berrigan D. Relationship between urban sprawl and weight of United States youth. American Journal of Preventive Medicine. 2006;31(6):464–474.

75. Joshu CE, Boehmer TK, Brownson RC, Ewing R. Personal, neighbourhood and urban factors associated with obesity in the United States. Journal of Epidemiology & Community Health. 2008;62(3):202–208.

76. Lopez R. Urban sprawl and risk for being overweight or obese. American Journal of Public Health. 2004;94(9):1574–1579.

77. Block JP, Scribner RA, DeSalvo KB. Fast food, race/ethnicity, and income: a geographic analysis. American Journal of Preventive Medicine. 2004;27(3):211–217.

78. Forsyth A, Lytle L, Mishra N, Noble P, Van Riper, D. Environment, Food, + Youth: GIS Protocols, Version 1.1, work in progress; Minnesota University, Transdisciplinary Research on Energics and Cancer (TREC); May 2007.

79. Hayne CL, Moran PA, Ford MM. Regulating environments to reduce obesity. Journal of Public Health Policy. 2004;25(3–4):391–407.

80. Oakes JM, Masse LC, Messer LC. Work group III: Methodologic issues in research on the food and physical activity environments: addressing data complexity. American Journal of Preventive Medicine. 2009;36(4 suppl):S177–S181.

81. Ball K, Timperio A, Salmon J, Giles-Corti B, Roberts R, Crawford D. Personal, social and environmental determinants of educational inequalities in walking: a multilevel study. Journal of Epidemiology & Community Health. 2007;61(2):108–114.

82. Story M, Kaphingst KM, Robinson-O'Brien R, Glanz K. Creating healthy food and eating environments: policy and environmental approaches. Annual Review of Public Health. 2008;29:253–272.

83. Harris JL, Pomeranz JL, Lobstein T, Brownell KD. A crisis in the marketplace: how food marketing contributes to childhood obesity and what can be done. Annual Review of Public Health. 2009;30:211–225.

84. Wilde P. Self-regulation and the response to concerns about food and beverage marketing to children in the United States. Nutrition Review. 2009;67(3):155–166.

85. Zimmerman FJ. Using marketing muscle to sell fat: the rise of obesity in the modern economy. Annual Review of Public Health. 2011;32:285–306.

86. Bowman SA. Television-viewing characteristics of adults: correlations to eating practices and overweight and health status. Preventing Chronic Disease. 2006;3(2):A38.

87. Koplan JP, Liverman CT, Kraak VI, eds.; Committee on the Prevention of Obesity in Children and Youth. Preventing Childhood Obesity: Health in the Balance. Washington, DC: National Academies Press; 2004.

88. McKinnon RA, Orleans CT, Kumanyika SK, Haire-Joshu D, Krebs-Smith SM, Finkelstein EA, et al. Considerations for an obesity policy research agenda. American Journal of Preventive Medicine. 2009;36(4):351–357.

89. Dodson EA, Fleming C, Boehmer TK, Haire-Joshu D, Luke DA, Brownson RC. Preventing childhood obesity through state policy: qualitative assessment of enablers and barriers. Journal of Public Health Policy. 2009;30(suppl 1): S161–S176.

90. Boehmer T, Luke DA, Haire-Joshu DL, Bates H, Brownson R. Preventing childhood obesity through state policy: predictors of bill enactment. American Journal of Preventive Medicine. 2008;34(4):333–340.

91. Brownson RC, Haire-Joshu D, Luke DA. Shaping the context of health: a review of environmental and policy approaches in the prevention of chronic diseases. Annual Review of Public Health. 2006;27:341–370.

92. Pelone F, Specchia ML, Veneziano MA, Capizzi S, Bucci S, Mancuso A, et al. Economic impact of childhood obesity on health systems: a systematic review. Obesity Reviews. 2012;13(5):431–440.

93. Robroek SJ, Bredt FJ, Burdorf A. The (cost-)effectiveness of an individually tailored long-term worksite health promotion programme on physical activity and nutrition: design of a pragmatic cluster randomised controlled trial. BMC Public Health. 2007;7:259.

94. Haire-Joshu D, Fleming C, Schermbeck R. The role of government in preventing obesity. In: Kumanyika SK, Brownson RC, eds. Handbook of Obesity Prevention. New York: Springer; 2008:129–170.

95. Haire-Joshu D, Yount BW, Budd EL, Schwarz C, Schermbeck R, Green S, et al. The quality of school wellness policies and energy-balance behaviors of adolescent mothers. Preventing Chronic Disease. 2011;8(2):A34.

96. Haire-Joshu D, Elliott M, Schermbeck R, Taricone E, Green S, Brownson RC. Surveillance of obesity-related policies in multiple environments: the Missouri Obesity, Nutrition, and Activity Policy Database, 2007–2009. Preventing Chronic Disease. 2010;7(4):A80.

97. Trust for America's Health and Robert Wood Johnson Foundation. F as in Fat: How Obesity Threatens America's Future 2011. Washington, DC: Trust for America's Health; 2011.

98. Pekruhn C. Preventing Childhood Obesity: A School Health Policy Guide. Washington, DC: National Association of State Boards of Education; 2011.

99. Glasgow RE, Emmons KM. How can we increase translation of research into practice? Types of evidence needed. Annual Review of Public Health. 2007;28:413–433.

100. Jilcott S, Ammerman A, Sommers J, Glasgow RE. Applying the RE-AIM framework to assess the public health impact of policy change. Annals of Behavioral Medicine. 2007;34(2):105–114.
101. Glasgow RE, Klesges LM, Dzewaltowski DA, Estabrooks PA, Vogt TM. Evaluating the impact of health promotion programs: Using the RE-AIM framework to form summary measures for decision making involving complex issues. Health Education Research. 2006;21(5):688–694.
102. Glasgow RE, Green LW, Klesges LM, Abrams DB, Fisher EB, Goldstein MG, et al. External validity: we need to do more. Annals of Behavioral Medicine. 2006;31(2):105–108.
103. Green LW, Glasgow RE. Evaluating the relevance, generalization, and applicability of research: issues in external validation and translation methodology. Evaluation & the Health Professions. 2006;29(1):126–153.
104. Glasgow RE, Nelson CC, Strycker LA, King DK. Using RE-AIM metrics to evaluate diabetes self-management support interventions. American Journal of Preventive Medicine. 2006;30(1):67–73.

Transdisciplinary Approaches to Violence and Injury Prevention and Treatment among Children and Youth

Melissa Jonson-Reid   Brett Drake
Nancy Weaver   John Constantino

Learning Objectives

- Apply the transdisciplinary problem-solving perspective to violence and injury prevention among children and youth.
- Describe the major causes and consequences of injury among children and youth.
- Identify and frame problems in a transdisciplinary manner within an ecological, developmental, and systems of service context.
- Discuss the general systems and approaches used to address violence and injury among children and youth, including primary, secondary, and tertiary prevention approaches.
- Apply transdisciplinary problem solving and solution analysis and evaluation to injury among children and youth.
- Discuss key issues in disseminating knowledge in a transdisciplinary manner.

•••

Violence and injury among children are linked to a large number of contributory factors, from possible genetic predispositions in parents and children to learned behaviors and poverty to social policies and cultural norms. As noted in chapter 1, answers to such complex problems require a transdisciplinary problem-solving approach that can synthesize information from multiple disciplines and integrate it with appropriate input from community members and service providers to effect change. The previous chapter, by Haire-Joshu, demonstrated application of a transdisciplinary approach to the current public health problem of obesity. In this chapter, we draw on educational, research, and theoretical perspectives from multiple disciplines to illustrate how this approach can be used to prevent intentional injury (violence) and unintentional injury to children and youth.

Some readers may be puzzling over why we are addressing both intentional and unintentional injury. While there are important differences, there are also significant similarities in risk and protective factors that can lead to children being simultaneously vulnerable to injury from violence and from accidents. Excluding one or the other misses important crossover concepts that can lead to better strategies for improving the health and well-being of children. Having stated a broad purpose, we intentionally limited the types of injury and violence discussed in order to cover the issues within the bounds of a single chapter. Chapter foci include household and motor vehicle injury, chosen from the unintentional injury literature, and youth violence and child maltreatment, chosen from the violence literature.

Finally this chapter addresses improving prevention from both a practice and an educational standpoint. Although this topic is not the primary focus of the chapter, many of the same factors that matter to prevention are important to research and evaluation as well. Case examples of real-world community-based projects follow discussion of the risks, protective factors, developmental influences, and methodological considerations. We also discuss the utility of transdisciplinary courses in the areas of violence and injury to prepare future public health practitioners. Readers of this chapter will understand and be able to describe the transdisciplinary problem-solving perspective as it applies to violence and injury prevention among children and youth.

Overview and Rationale

Injury, victimization, and violence perpetration are far too common among children, adolescents, and their families. Throughout the world, about 2,000 children die from injury each day.[1] Although US rates of childhood fatalities from unintentional injuries by most causes have decreased over the last twenty years,[2] injuries remain the biggest health threat to children. While unintentional injury is more prevalent, fatalities due to intentional injury are also high. For example, somewhat fewer than 2,000 children die in the United States each year due to known abuse and neglect.[3] Most intentional and unintentional incidents, however, result in nonfatal cognitive, physical, or socioemotional harm, which results in significant costs to individuals and society. In 2000, the total lifetime costs (medical expenses and productivity loss) of unintentional injuries among children ages zero to fourteen were estimated to be over \$50 billion[4] and one study estimated that the cost of severe child maltreatment alone is over \$100 billion.[5] The need to fully address intentional and unintentional injury was recognized as one of seven national priorities in the National Prevention Strategy: America's Plan for Better Health and Wellness,[3] and the National Center for Injury Prevention and Control has articulated research priorities to advance injury control efforts in both areas.[6]

Pediatric violence and injury prevention are best understood through careful attention to the environmental and developmental contexts in which they are embedded.[7] While many theoretical approaches have been applied to injury prevention,[8] probably the most notable framework is the Haddon matrix. This matrix sets the targets for prevention and the timing of interventions along a two-dimensional continuum.[9] The prevention targets are the interacting host, agent, and environment. The *host* is the person being injured or at risk, the *agent* is the vector or energy that is transmitted during the injury event, and the *environment* consists of the sociocultural and physical contexts in which the injury occurs. We amend this framework slightly by adding that the influence of various environmental contexts may operate differently according to the developmental stage of the child (see figure 10.1). A child moves from being influenced primarily by the family context to being increasingly influenced directly by the larger community as he or she moves through adolescence. In this framework special attention is paid to distinguishing situations in which approaches to unintentional injury and intentional injury can and cannot be similar.

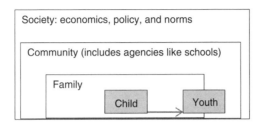

Figure 10.1. An ecodevelopmental perspective

Definitions

According to Stokols and colleagues,[10] the hallmark of transdisciplinary science, which includes *transdisciplinary problem solving*, is *intellectual integration*. Violence and injury prevention requires substantial understanding and integration of knowledge generated from multiple disciplines to arrive at real-world solutions that transcend the contribution of any one discipline. Classroom settings and training programs offer a structured opportunity for such integration, building skills that will encourage this approach in the field. Those without such training, however, can still transcend disciplinary bounds by drawing on the unique perspectives of a variety of professions and community experts to solve social problems.

Injuries can be defined generally as damage that occurs during energy transfer, as in the crash of an automobile, or when energy is prevented from transferring, as in the case of suffocation or drowning. Injuries are commonly classified by their severity, setting, mechanism, intent, and type and by activity performed when the injury occurred.[11] These labels suggest opportunities for intervention. Among *unintentional injuries*, we pay particular attention in this chapter to motor vehicle injury and household injury prevention.

- *Motor vehicle injury* is the most common cause of unintentional fatality among children,[12] and addressing this area has required efforts from multiple disciplines. An adolescent hospitalized for a nonfatal motor vehicle injury may incur costs exceeding $467,000; adding up to about $9 billion across all such injuries.[13]

- *Household injury* for young children is our second concern here because it typically involves a family focus and because some of the antecedents of such injuries bear similarities to intentional harm, as in child abuse and neglect.[14]

Definitions of *intentional injury* vary somewhat by discipline. For example, law enforcement considers intentionality from a criminal justice point of view, with an emphasis on planned harm; a doctor may attempt to assess from medical evidence whether an injury could have been caused accidentally; and social services may examine the level of harm and ongoing risk of harm through assessment of the family or social context. This chapter focuses on youth violence and child abuse and neglect.

- *Child maltreatment* (CM) involves harm to children by a parent or other care provider, generally characterized as sexual, physical, or emotional abuse or as neglect. Reports grew exponentially from the "discovery" of child abuse in 1962[15] through about 1992, but the rate of allegations has since leveled off.[16] According to the National Child Abuse and Neglect Data System, around three million reports

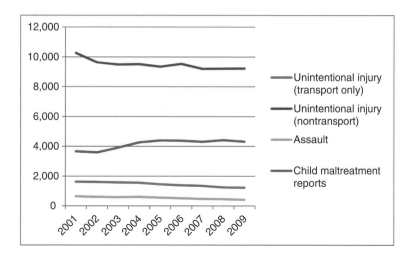

Figure 10.2. Trends in intentional and unintentional injury rates per 100,000 children, 2001–2009

of child abuse and neglect receive some type of investigation per year.[17] Individual and societal costs include immediate physical injury and longer-term consequences like poor physical health and mental health, violent criminality, and further victimization.[18,19]

- *Youth violence* may include bullying, dating violence, assault, and gang behaviors. In 2007, homicide was the second leading cause of death for young people ages ten to twenty-four years old.[20] In a 2009 national survey, about 31 percent of high school students reported being in a physical fight in the prior twelve months.[20] About 25 percent of adolescents report abuse from a dating partner.[20]

Trends for selected intentional and unintentional injury rates for the first decade of this century, according to hospital records and official reports of child maltreatment, are provided in figure 10.2. These trends reveal modest and continuing reductions in hospital records of nonfatal assaults and unintentional injuries. Child maltreatment report rates increased somewhat during the first few years of the decade but have since stabilized.

Although we illustrate incidence separately, there is ample reason to believe that there is significant overlap between unintentional and intentional injury over time. One study using children's visits to the emergency department (ED) as the reference found that children with two or more injury-related ED visits in one year were substantially more likely to be reported for child maltreatment.[21] A New Zealand study found that an infant who had a medically attended injury was nine times more likely to have a child maltreatment report than a noninjured child.[22] Another study noted that lack of parental supervision (a type of child neglect) was associated with pediatric injury even after controlling for child behaviors.[14] Studies have found an increased tendency toward serious delinquency and youth violence to be associated with maltreatment.[23-26] Bina, Graziano, and Bonino found an association between antisocial behavior in teens and risky driving, which in turn can lead to a greater incidence of motor vehicle crashes.[27] In part this overlap may be due to common risk antecedents,[28] such as social environments, parenting approaches, and stressful life events, a notion that has not yet been fully explored.

Developmental Approaches

Vulnerability to and potential buffers from various types of injuries, victimization, or violence perpetration changes from birth through adolescence. For example, during infancy a child is fully dependent on his or her primary caregiver(s), and injury or victimization at this age can have a range of consequences, from disruption of attachment and cognitive development to long-term emotional, physical, or mental disability or even death. Protective factors at this early stage include good medical care; an educated, nurturing, and watchful caregiver; safe housing; good nutrition; and so forth. Approaches to securing these protective factors include improving health coverage and access, providing effective parenting education, and providing resources like housing assistance, food, and safety devices (like car seats). For young children, modifying risk through product design has been put forward as the most effective means of preventing household and motor vehicle injury.[28] Of course, such improved products must then be used.[29]

In contrast, during adolescence young people become vulnerable to injury that is caused by their own behaviors, such as using poor driving skills, engaging in risky behaviors, or joining peer groups that tend toward violence. Consequences range from poor peer interaction and school failure to health problems, long-term disability, and even death. Protective factors at this stage still include good medical care and an educated nurturing caregiver but expand to include things like positive coping and social skills, other positive adult role models, safe and good-quality schools, adequate healthy recreational opportunities, and preparation for a productive, healthy adulthood. Approaches to securing protective factors in adolescence include engaging positive adult role models other than parents, receiving social and health skills training directed to the youth themselves, having positive safe places for recreation, and having access to resources that will enable youth to make positive transitions to continued productivity in young adulthood.

There are several widely accepted approaches to reducing motor vehicle injuries, set in place by several disciplines. For children, this includes restricting the seat a child is allowed to ride in to certain types at certain ages, ensuring universal availability of seat belts, and having age- and weight-appropriate car seats.[30–32] Car seats and seat belts must be adjusted as a child grows in order to continue the protective benefit. These products are developed by engineers and then are put into place through market forces that require car manufacturers to include the equipment needed to use them. Public policy outlines sanctions for adults if they do not use proper safety equipment for young children in cars, and these sanctions are enforced by the legal system. Research indicates that parent education by pediatricians is a key factor in safety equipment use.[33] Pediatricians, however, often have limited skill and knowledge to support such an approach (see, for example, Brixey and Guse[34]).

In contrast, the target for motor vehicle injury prevention for teenagers is primarily the adolescent. Mandated driver's training and safety instruction is designed to develop driving behaviors that reduce the likelihood of a traffic crash. Age-specific policies outline permissible driving hours and limits on passengers to reduce vulnerability from distraction due to peer behaviors, sleepiness, or driving home late from parties. Sanctions include legal penalties as well as economic sanctions in the form of insurance costs. Research indicates that these protective measures are effective in reducing traffic fatalities among teen drivers.[35]

These findings vary in some respects for intentional injury. In pediatric motor vehicle injury, the constellation of risk factors changes quickly throughout the child's development. It is highly related to physical development, temperament, and other personal factors, and is also strongly moderated by parenting and environmental factors. In contrast, while vulnerability to physical injury from child abuse or neglect changes rapidly as the child develops, the family factors giving rise to maltreatment may be persistent across time. There is some evidence to suggest that risk of physical or sexual abuse is more likely to decline than is neglect.[36] It is therefore possible to reduce the risk of physical injury in a maltreating home without reducing the rate of ongoing maltreatment or the negative downstream effects.

Injury Prevention, Causes, and Impacts

There is a growing recognition that intentional injury and unintentional injury during childhood and adolescence have some similar antecedents. For example, a parent who has a sufficient understanding of child development is more likely to take adequate steps to protect his or her child from hazards in the home and also more likely to understand how to avoid maltreating behaviors.[37] An adolescent who has been traumatized by violence in the home may engage in more risky behaviors than his or her peers do, which in turn may lead to unintentional injury like motor vehicle crashes.[27] The reader should note the overlap in the following discussion.

Overview of Unintentional Injury Risk Factors

Leading causes of death among children are motor vehicle crashes, drowning, suffocation, fires and burns, and pedestrian-related injuries.[2] Generally, male children and children of either sex who are younger than four have a greater risk of unintentional death. Children living in poverty are more likely than children in better-off families to sustain an injury or to die from injury, primarily owing to the greater likelihood of an unsafe living environment.[38] Children with developmental disabilities or living with parents with cognitive delays have been found to have higher risk of pediatric injury than children who do not face these challenges.[22,39]

Risk for unintentional injury changes substantially as a child grows.[14] Because of the need to take physiological changes in a child's size into account, children under age two are placed in a rear-facing car seat, but after that age, they transition to a five-point, front-facing harness seat.[31,40] Children's propensity to take risks may also increase injury rates, but this may be offset by parenting practices. For example, in one study risk-taking behavior in preschool children was found to predict greater injury but not when the children had adequate supervision.[14] While parental supervision in early childhood has been long touted as a strategy for prevention, other research suggests this remains protective in later years as well.[41] Examples of matching development to prevention strategies are provided in table 10.1.

Table 10.1. Connecting age and developmental levels to prevention strategies

	Developmental capacity	Matching strategy	References
Infancy to age 4	Dependent on parent or caregiver	Parental supervision and environmental modifications	Morrongiello et al.[14]
Age 4+	Able to self-regulate to some extent	Parental supervision along with clear household safety rules and environmental modifications	Alho et al.[42]
Age 10+	Increasing ability to prevent injury by making safe choices	Educational programs in schools	Turner et al.[43]

The ability to self-protect may increase from early childhood to school-age, but the transition to adolescence also confers further risks. Some of the "normative" increases in risk-taking behavior during adolescence also increase the risk of injury.[44] Those youth who engage in more risk-taking behaviors have a higher rate of injury.[26] The suggested differences in brain development among teens as compared to adults have prompted what some people call social scaffolding approaches, to attempt to provide environmental controls to limit exposure to dangerous or unproductive situations.[45]

Overview of Intentional Injuries (Child Maltreatment) and Risk Factors

Child maltreatment, the most common kind of intentional injury to children, has traditionally been tracked and approached in a manner somewhat consistent with unintentional injury efforts. In most states, medical, social service, educational, and law enforcement professionals are mandated to report maltreatment, but reports may also be made by nonmandated citizens. As with unintentional injury, very young children have a greater risk of injury, with children under the age of three accounting for nearly 81 percent of fatal child maltreatment cases.[3] Poverty is also a significant risk factor for abuse and neglect. At the geographical level, more than half the variance in local child maltreatment rates can be explained by income or poverty level.[46] In addition to poverty, other broad areas of risk include parental incapacity due to mental health issues, substance abuse, or other limits to capacity;[19] family structure (young parents and single parents present a higher risk); and stress.[47] Compared to nonabusive parents, abusive parents have been found to perceive parenting as more burdensome, to be more likely to assign hostile intent to their child's behavior, and to have less social support.[48,49] Domestic abuse is also a common risk factor for maltreatment.[48,50] However, research suggests that it is cumulative risk that is of greatest concern.[49,50]

As with unintentional injury, the primary reason that very young children make up the vast majority of fatal maltreatment cases is their physical vulnerability. For example, so-called shaken baby syndrome is a common reason for death among child maltreatment cases, due to the unique features of the brain and skull during infancy.[51] Children with disabilities have also been found to be at higher risk for maltreatment.[52,53] Risk for certain forms of maltreatment may also change over time. For example, research suggests that children ages seven to thirteen have the highest risk for sexual abuse.[54] Children who begin to display mental health and behavioral problems have been found to be at greater risk for maltreatment.[55,56] Abuse of adolescents is understudied in comparison to that of younger children, and reported incidents are more likely to include mutual parent and child assault.[57] Earlier research pointed to increased vulnerability when the adolescent desire for autonomy conflicts with parental roles and causes strain that precipitates maltreating behaviors.[58]

As discussed here, there are several common antecedents to unintentional injury and intentional injury. Poverty is clearly a common risk factor. The age and risk-taking tendencies of a child are also of import when considering risk of injury. Finally, caregiver impairment influences both intentional and unintentional child injury.

Common Downstream Impacts for Child Injury and Maltreatment

In many ways the downstream impact of intentional and unintentional injury are similar. We have divided impacts into three categories, rather than review all the possible outcomes. Even with this imposed limitation, one can see that outcomes, like risk and protective factors, transcend disciplinary boundaries.

1. There may be easily observable physical or mental effects, such as scarring or reductions in physical or mental capabilities secondary to the injury. In the case of unintentional injury, the consequent damage is solely physiological. In the case of child maltreatment, long-term cognitive deficits may also arise due to lack of necessary stimulation required for brain development.[40,59,60] Such effects may require intervention informed by the health, education, and social service disciplines in order to meet the child's rehabilitative and long-term needs. Such effects may also necessitate supportive equipment and changes in recreation and family life that require additional forms of expertise.

2. There may be psychosocial effects from both types of injury. These may take the form of diagnosable entities, such as post-traumatic stress disorder.[61,62] Other impacts may include effects on social interactions, such as increased peer rejection due to disfigurement or poor social interaction skills.[63,64] Such effects may require intervention informed by the education, law enforcement, mental health, pharmacology, social service, and law enforcement professions. These services may be required at the individual or family level.

3. Emerging research is pointing to a new class of physical effects of trauma that may not be easily observed and that may manifest in an apparently psychological, behavioral, or physiological manner. Research on subtle physical effects (epigenetic effects, alterations in telomere length, enduring changes to information processing, and emotional dysregulation[65]) requires the integration of multiple scientific fields to understand this process and then translate that knowledge into prevention and intervention approaches.

As even this brief summary illustrates, unintentional and intentional injury can result in problems that clearly transcend the knowledge base of one or even two disciplines. Although in practice intervention may be piecemeal, in an ideal world transdisciplinary approaches would create seamless and accessible supportive care.

A Caveat on Differences and Similarities

Even though there are many similarities in risk factors and outcomes associated with both intentional and unintentional injury, readers should be careful not to assume this means that problem-solving approaches are identical. Most families in which pediatric injury occurs are not families in which violence occurs. Families in which intentional violence occurs are likely to be characterized by not one but multiple risks accruing over time.[49] Whereas teaching a mother to use a car seat correctly may address a situation in which the issue is a knowledge deficit, education alone is unlikely to prevent the types of behaviors in a high-risk maltreating home. What is clear, however, is that prevention of both forms of injury requires attention to the developmental age, the family, and the socioenvironmental context.

Problem Identification and Structuring

We have already discussed how the issues of injury, violence, and victimization cannot be understood absent their environmental and developmental contexts. In addition, these problems cannot be fully appreciated without a full understanding of the vast array of existing systems designed to mitigate or control them. Haddon distinguished injury prevention strategies in terms of when they would have their impact: the time before an injury occurs (pre-event strategies), the time during the injury (event strategies), and the time after the injury (post-event strategies), corresponding to primary, secondary, and tertiary prevention, respectively.[9] Primary prevention must be transdisciplinary in order to address the variety of risks and the approaches necessary to mitigate those risks. Likewise, intervention following unintentional or intentional injury, in order to prevent further harm (tertiary prevention), may involve a wide range of disciplines. Typically, prevention needs are met by different entities, organizations, or teams of experts rather than by employing an overarching strategy. Failure to think about how these supports can be integrated and prioritized can cause duplication of services, can overwhelm families and others with services coming from multiple directions, can result in provision of tools that cannot be used by the target population because of other barriers, and can make it difficult to assess whether the approach is ultimately helpful.

For example, there are evidence-based, psychosocial violence prevention programs available to use in a school setting. Typically, such programs provide children with a set of tools to help them with relationships, communication, and risk avoidance. If children targeted by such a program are experiencing violence in their homes, lack safe places to play and participate in prosocial activities, or feel compelled to engage in violence for self-protection, it is unlikely that this approach will work. A transdisciplinary planning approach would assess the problem from all angles. In addition to offering skills training at school, a transdisciplinary plan might engage family services agencies to address violence in the home, law enforcement to help improve neighborhood safety, public health educators to communicate violence prevention messages to the surrounding adult community, and community planners to address the recreational and economic structures in the area.

Understanding Systems Designed to Prevent Injury, Violence, and Victimization

An almost endless number of professionals have something to offer in the quest to reduce child injury. Some are specifically tasked by policy or professional mandates to address factors related to intentional and unintentional injury. Others are engaged through their creation of safety devices. Still others provide educational, social, and mental health services to mitigate risk. Businesses and community organizations can provide recreational and even employment opportunities for young people that can help to prevent their engagement in risky behaviors. Finally, policymakers can create the structures and allocate the resources needed for an effective prevention approach. Table 10.2 compares and contrasts a few of these disciplines.

While many disciplines are involved in this work, that is not to say that all the same disciplines are, or should be, involved in all cases of unintentional and intentional injury prevention. Although unintentional injury prevention may rely heavily on engineering, policies enforcing use of safety devices, and parental education, solutions to youth violence require a different constellation of approaches. Gun safety devices, storage of ammunition separate from the weapon, and gun control legislation, in isolation, have not been found to have much of an impact on youth violence.[66] Instead most approaches now target broader issues: creating community engagement (community members), addressing past trauma and social skills deficits (mental health professionals, social workers), providing other forms of education (public health educators, teachers), and providing supporting efforts by community police.[66–68]

Arguably, it is important to map out the various engaged professions according to their mandated or voluntary roles for each problem to be solved. This list of contributors should be dynamic, expanding in innovative ways to address new challenges as organizations and communities move from planning to implementation to evaluation and sustainability. For instance, economists may play a vital role in understanding the relative costs and benefits of a given approach. Such information is critical to informing policymakers who may be needed to allocate funds or provide incentives to use evidence-based

Table 10.2. Roles and expertise of selected disciplines in injury prevention and intervention

	Mandate	Intervention	Prevention	Policy	Environment
Medical professionals	Report threats of harm to others, self-harm, and maltreatment.	Treatment of injury.	Disseminate safety and health information in medical setting.	NA	NA
Teachers	Report threats of harm to others, self-harm, and maltreatment.	Primarily, refer to others.	Implement safety and school health curricula.	NA	NA
Social services	Report threats of harm to others, self-harm, and maltreatment.	Provide risk assessment, counseling, and provision of resources.	Provide violence prevention programs.	Engage in advocacy.	Support community development efforts.
Public health	Various, depending on function.	Provide information about resources.	Provide or promote injury and violence prevention education, assessment, evaluation.	Engage in advocacy; provide data on trends; provide assurance.	Provide safety equipment; promote community access to information.
Law enforcement	Report threats of harm to others, self-harm, and maltreatment.	Arrest; place individuals in protective custody; fine individuals for failure to use safety equipment.	Provide violence prevention and firearm safety programs.	NA	Provide community policing.
Engineers	NA	NA	Design safety equipment.	NA	Create community designs for health and safety.
Business	NA	NA	Support education about and marketing of safety equipment.	Provide financial backing for advocacy efforts.	Fund community development and youth employment.

Note: NA = not applicable.

approaches. A second goal would be to identify the best and most feasible approaches to integrating stakeholders, given the developmental age of the target population, community acceptance, and the capacity of the organizations that must deliver and sustain services.[69] Doing this requires time and both horizontal communication (among providers) and vertical communication (from policymakers to service providers) so that people in different disciplines can overcome the barriers raised by discipline-specific terminology, methods, and professional traditions.

Operationalizing Problems from a Transdisciplinary Perspective: Barriers and Opportunity

Several calls have been made to move from interdisciplinary (defined as collaboration between or training in two disciplines) to transdisciplinary approaches to violence and injury prevention. Transdisciplinary approaches are better able to address the many determinants of violence and injury in order to create more effective prevention strategies, but there are challenges. The first and most important part of responding to any issue is identifying the problem to be solved. This may be relatively simple for some problems (for example, preventing child cranial injury due to falls) but dauntingly difficult for others. For example, legislative definitions of *child maltreatment* vary radically from state to state.[70] A state that defines substance exposure prior to birth as a type of maltreatment may more actively involve prenatal care practitioners and substance abuse professionals in prevention, whereas a state that does not may have different priorities. Even when the outcomes of interest are seemingly clearly defined, the scope of the problem may be understood differently by different disciplines.

Once consensus about a problem definition is achieved, the second challenge is to identify potential conflicts in approaches and gaps in services. For example, overlaps between services and needs related to domestic violence on the one hand and child abuse on the other are well known,[71] but ongoing collaborative approaches to redress the policy, funding, and service issues have proved difficult to implement and sustain.[72] Some US counties and states have changed their definitions to include exposure to domestic violence as a form of child abuse because of potential harm to the child.[73,74] Some professionals in the area of domestic violence argue that this approach is unfair to the adult victim, who may fear seeking services because of the risk of losing the children.[75] Ultimately, Minnesota repealed this change in its child maltreatment definition because inadequate planning and funding made it impossible for existing systems to adequately address reports made.[74]

The third essential consideration is the method of service delivery that best fits the situation. Most would agree that effective parent education is key to the proper use of safety precautions for young children.[76] Yet there is considerable disagreement as to the best method. Some advocate universal or near-universal home visitation after birth, provided by paraprofessionals, through education systems, or by nurses (see, for example, Nurses for Newborns[77]). Others advocate an increased role for pediatricians in counseling about injury prevention.[78] Still others are seeking ways of using technology to reach parents in collaboration with medical professionals.[29,79]

Finally, after using a transdisciplinary perspective to plan, it is important to avoid dropping that perspective when accountability and sustainability are considered. While school-based youth violence prevention programming may be an effective approach, that does not mean that education should adopt sole responsibility for ending youth violence. Indeed, when research related later outcomes for youth with their prior histories with child welfare at an early age, there was concern that these outcomes would be seen as the sole responsibility of the child welfare system, even though services needed to address many of the outcome issues were outside the child welfare system.[80] Complex problems are likely to require complex solutions, with different parties playing complementary roles.

Problem Identification

Identifying the locus of the problem can be a counterintuitive process. Although child injury implies a focus on children, the problem is generally located in other domains. The physical construction of the environment (for example, toy designs, cupboard safety mechanisms, pool fencing) might be specified as the problem. Parental behavior is very commonly specified as the target for intervention (for example, parents may need to increase supervision, take CPR training, or use smoke detectors). In other cases a problem may be located across systems. For example, youth violence might be seen as a function of some combination of adolescent behavior, parenting practices, insufficient enforcement of laws, lack of community resources for youth development, and underperforming schools.

Identifying key modifiable contributing or risk factors can also pose challenges. Without such an identification, our ability to provide preventive services or create effective policy is dramatically limited. Again, purely physical systems may allow easier operationalization (for example, reducing the number of components of children's toys that can be swallowed is a straightforward goal), whereas many psychosocial factors related to intentional violence (such as stress, efficacy, and poverty) remain difficult to disentangle. Arguably, we must target risk factors that can feasibly be changed. For example, poverty is a risk factor for both violence and unintentional home injury, but the eradication of poverty may well be beyond the capacity of a given prevention effort.

Identifying key issues related to uptake and adaptation is essential because even after understanding the problem and identifying risk factors, we still need an effective solution. For many issues, best practices in injury and violence prevention are available through various clearinghouses (for example, the California Evidence-Based Clearinghouse for Child Welfare, the Cochrane Collaboration, the National Registry of Evidence-Based Programs and Practices, *The Guide to Community Preventive Services*, and the Wisconsin Clearinghouse for Prevention Resources). Sometimes, however, implementation of best practices is far from easy. Safer car seats (physical problem resolution) are useful only when they are used properly (behavioral problem resolution) and when people have the resources to obtain them (societal problem resolution). The solution to the problem of "unsafe car seats" may involve increasing the use, or *reach*, of what we know to be effective. In other cases, an evidence-based practice may not have been adapted to a given population or setting. Glasgow and Emmons[81] identify several factors that are key impediments to implementation of evidence-based approaches. Among these are understanding the feasibility given the setting and the acceptability to and effectiveness with a given target population. Even when efficacious programs are offered to interested organizations, the integration of these programs may be suboptimal; changes in organizational culture or processes to support and sustain the approach may take a long time to realize.[79]

Without transdisciplinary input, a number of serious problems can occur at this stage. A problem might be defined in such a way as to exclude key systems. Structuring identification of the problem with an understanding of how this definition may affect other systems is a key concern. Understanding the particular context of the problem is critical to understanding whether or not there is already an appropriate and feasible evidence-based practice or whether innovation is required. For instance, manufacturers can design safer car seats, but without the support of retail organizations and pediatric interest groups, the uptake of these car seats may be limited. Moreover, a child with a disability may require adaptations in the equipment and parental behaviors in order to be kept safe.

Solution Analysis and Evaluation: Case Examples

Obviously, it is best not to reinvent the wheel when an effective tactic exists for a given situation. It is outside the scope of the present chapter to provide a summary of effective approaches to pediatric unintentional and intentional injury. Instead we focus here on some examples of innovations. According to Saul and colleagues[82] *innovation* refers to knowledge that could be useful to prevention efforts but that is currently not known to the potential users. Each case described here involved problem identification from a transdisciplinary perspective, engagement of disciplines in nontraditional ways or engagement of new disciplines, enhancing work already occurring, and monitoring the implementation to better inform sustainability and replication. Although cost effectiveness is not addressed in these case scenarios, we would argue that innovation should also attend to this issue, including costs related to intended and unintended consequences.

Case 1: Primary prevention of household injuries and child maltreatment

---

The Problem

Communication theory can be used to develop highly relevant materials for promoting a variety of health behaviors, including childhood injury prevention. When communication materials are developed to address the specific needs or interests of a target audience, it is more likely that members of that audience will respond favorably to the content of the materials. *Message tailoring*, a particular communication approach, uses specific information assessed about an audience member to provide individually customized information,[83] as in the case of the Safe N' Sound Injury Prevention Program, a program that has been used to successfully promote unintentional injury prevention.[29,84] Even though randomized controlled trials had previously shown Safe N' Sound to result in the desired outcomes in a clinical setting, transdisciplinary planning has allowed the program to be (1) expanded for use in home visitation programs, (2) strategically disseminated to children's hospitals nationwide, and (3) expanded with the aim of reducing child abuse and neglect.

Transdisciplinary Planning

Several critical partnerships were forged to form synergies between complementary sciences. First, home visitation nursing staff from Nurses for Newborns were engaged to develop clinical guidelines for home risk assessments.[77] This allowed the team to address injury risks in the context of other immediate child and parent needs and to involve skilled nursing expertise in injury control efforts. Building on two evidence-based programs stemming from social work, nursing, and public health is expected to result in increased use of car seats, safe sleep environments, smoke detectors, and other precautions—although this is yet to be tested.

(*Continued*)

Second, business partners, including health informatics and clinical management experts, were involved to position injury prevention counseling as a billable pediatric service. Consistent with the recommendations of the American Academy of Pediatrics,[78,85] Safe N' Sound has been provided as part of the anticipatory guidance parents receive specific to the developmental stage of their child. Integrating Safe N' Sound into the accepted context of the clinic setting addressed an organizational barrier that can be a challenge to the adoption of innovative programs. Similarly, the program's evidence base allowed injury prevention community outreach efforts to be advanced as part of the community benefit provided by nonprofit hospital organizations. Further, guided by theories of translation and dissemination[86] (such as RE-AIM[87]), a partnership was formed with the National Association of Children's Hospitals and Related Institutions to evaluate factors related to the adoption of the injury prevention program.[88]

In order to extend Safe N' Sound to provide positive parenting messages to reduce the risk of child abuse and neglect, researchers used elements from the Triple P—Positive Parenting Program [89–91] and conducted extensive formative research with pediatricians, nurses, and office staff to develop the program content and delivery approach. This blend of psychology, social work, behavioral science, and communication principles allowed meaningful information to be delivered in an appropriate setting to a targeted audience. For instance, a parent who reported challenges with meal time, toileting, or sleep habits was given tailored, age-appropriate tools for increasing her self-efficacy for parenting in this high-stress situation. She could then review the provided information with her pediatrician and connect with community resources as needed.

Resolution

In order to both widely disseminate and conceptually expand the Safe N' Sound program, it was critical to involve a wide array of professionals and leverage the assets of their disciplines. The immediate project teams include biostatisticians, psychologists, nurses, public health researchers, and professionals and business partners. Community and federal grants were received specifically to promote the work of the academic, community, medical, and national partnerships. Working across disciplines has advanced the collective science of injury control and has resulted in injury risk reductions that would not have been actualized without transdisciplinary approaches.

Case 2: Prevention of poor outcomes and injury after maltreatment

The Problem

Most young children placed in foster care will return home, but their ongoing safety and well-being is not always secure.[59,92] When children are subjected to continued maltreatment and repeated spells in care, their risk of later poor outcomes like youth violence is greatly increased.[80,93,94] Their families typically have multiple problems and are engaged with at least two systems at the time of foster care placement, the juvenile court system and social services. Family support teams are designed to bring multiple disciplines together to make effective case plans. However, the juvenile court and social service specialists tasked with bringing recommendations to such teams struggle with decisions about whether to reunite maltreated children with their parents of origin. The specialists' respective caseloads are high, and their training and education regarding the mental health and development of infants and toddlers is insufficient to allow them to confidently determine the parameters of the risk, assess prospective caregivers and the quality of their interactions with young children, develop comprehensive intervention plans, or articulate appropriate contingencies and surveillance plans for reunification. Another barrier to effective reunification is the insufficient availability of mental health personnel in the community to assist with assessment and services and a lack of sufficient connections with community resources to provide ongoing support.

Transdisciplinary Planning

Representatives from the juvenile court (including the family court judge) and from social services and the head of child and adolescent psychiatry at the local university met to discuss these issues. Given the continued high caseload and lack of appropriate background of many of the juvenile court and social services staff, it was not feasible to train them to provide comprehensive child development and caregiver mental health screening. At the policy level, the recent passage of a state tax to support mental health services for children made funds available to support innovation. The academic was aware of a model that addressed similar needs in the state of Louisiana. The collaborative group applied for funds to replicate an adaptation of the model.

(Continued)

Resolution

For cases in which the specialists are concerned about (1) the viability of a reunification being considered by the court or (2) a possible untreated or inadequately addressed developmental or mental health disorder in a young foster child or his or her parent, the team now invites the participation of a doctoral-level expert in infant mental health and development (generally a child psychiatrist or child psychologist) to assess the child, child-caregiver relationship, and capacity of the caregiver to meet the ongoing needs of the child. The brief report addresses the strengths and vulnerabilities of the child, the caregiver, and their relationship. The strategy for addressing identified needs integrates the mandates and capacity of a number of professionals as well as the preferences of the family, when possible. The results of the assessment are shared with the family support team and directly inform the articulation of a comprehensive set of recommendations communicated to the court. The viability of reunification is serially reassessed, advancing the involvement of the parent as meaningful progress toward milestones is made. Continued teamwork allows timely cultivation of alternate caregiving arrangements if the reunification is nonviable. Social work students, supervised by a social work professor with evaluation expertise, assist with data collection and identification of community services that can better support families. Ultimately, the program will require a rigorous evaluation that includes weighing the benefits to the children served and the possible time savings for the court against the costs of sustaining the consultation services.

Dissemination of Findings

Researchers and academics from multiple disciplines can help to identify effective prevention and intervention approaches, train future practitioners in such approaches, and work with other professionals to disseminate this information. Dissemination can be passive or active. Effective dissemination needs to consider the community or organizational factors that will allow adoption and sustainability. One means of disseminating information and improving use of transdisciplinary approaches to synthesizing information is the implementation of transdisciplinary education. The authors of this chapter have been involved in the creation of three courses specifically aimed at educating students from multiple disciplines to address injury and violence prevention. Some lessons learned are provided in the remainder of this section.

Training future practitioners in the area of violence and injury prevention, as we have conceived it, involves transdisciplinary educational approaches. As previously mentioned, children live in families that live in communities that are nested in broader areas or political units (counties, states, provinces, countries, and so forth). The broader sociopolitical units have relevance in determining regulations for safety and sanctions for violence as well as distribution of resources to certain groups. Families may also exist within cultural boundaries that have prescriptions regarding child rearing and appropriate treatment of others. The community surrounding a family also contributes to the issue by the level of supportive resources it offers (such as available employment, parks, adequate housing, and the like), its level of safety, and its level of cohesiveness. Then within the family itself there are various predisposing factors and inhibiting factors that lead toward more positive or negative behaviors. Finally the individual brings his or her own set of risk and protective factors in the form of cognitive capacity, physical health, and personality. So one of the first challenges in transdisciplinary education is to help students understand and accept the complex nature of the issue.

The second challenge is to expose students to the perspectives of the disciplines that are currently engaged in the issue. It is particularly important that students come away with an understanding of how involved disciplines, outside their own, approach and act on particular problems. This understanding can be achieved in a number of ways. The simplest, but arguably insufficient, way is to assign academic readings from various disciplines. Such readings are necessary but are limited in impact. First of all, scientific articles tend toward similarity, regardless of the disciplines of the authors. Research methods, generally speaking, are shared across disciplines, and the consistent structure of research articles (introduction, approach, results, discussion) also tends to minimize differences. Of course, readings can and should also draw on the professional literature in the form of practice guidelines and policy statements that may be more idiosyncratic to a given discipline. Beyond readings, assignments can be structured with a transdisciplinary focus embedded in the selection of issues to be addressed, in the problem-solving goals of the assignments (by ensuring that proposed solutions address multiple perspectives, for example), and ideally, in the composition of student groups. Finally, and most important, we believe there is no real substitute for exposure to professionals from different disciplines. For example, in a course on child maltreatment prevention, we invited judges, emergency room medical staff, heads of social service agencies, genetics researchers, and others to speak and answer student questions. Some of our most successful experiences have been when such speakers are invited to speak on panels where the substantive issue is common to all participants but the disciplines or agencies represented are diverse (juvenile court, foster care, law enforcement, psychological treatment, and so forth). True transdisciplinary learning happens when students are able to fully *integrate* across familiar and less familiar academic foundations.

There are many other ways transdisciplinary training can be achieved. For example, we have not talked at all about field education, in a clinic, practicum, or research site. The selection of such sites, the tasks assigned at the site, and the persons worked with all provide opportunities for enhancing a student's transdisciplinary experience. Even small things, like requiring a transdisciplinary committee to review a thesis or culminating experience, can add value to the student's efforts and shape an educational experience that is more responsive to the needs of the transdisciplinary environments than most of our students will find themselves entering upon graduation.

Measures of Collaboration and Change

There is a need to understand whether the transdisciplinary perspective in violence and injury prevention is a necessary and effective force for improving injury control efforts. The measures of collaboration will not be different from measures of collaboration in other areas, but the connection to outcomes is both critical and complex. Violence and injury have multiple determinants so it is important to have logic models that link implementation across disciplines to measurable outcomes. We must structure evaluation so that we understand whether community policing with youth development is equally as effective as youth development alone for reducing youth violence. It is also important to carefully measure the geography of impact. If a youth development program reaches only a small number of youth then it may be more challenging to understand whether the broader community policing effort or the more concentrated and smaller youth program actually altered youth violence. As difficult as this challenge may be, it is critical to informing the sustainability of collaborative efforts.

Ongoing Needs

Dissemination of prevention information and methods must become transdisciplinary. Pediatric approaches to injury or violence prevention are largely disseminated through medical journals. Social services approaches tend to be published by area; for example, there are at least three major journals in this field devoted to child abuse and neglect. School-based approaches to prevention will be largely found in education journals. Public health approaches will be found in public health journals. Sometimes the latest work in an area is published in the "gray" literature produced by various think tanks. Relying on such information silos is counterproductive for the organization seeking best practices or even the researcher attempting to understand the current state of knowledge to move the field forward. Clearinghouses for evidence-based practices, such as the ones listed earlier in this chapter, are one way to address the need for a broad range of thought and practice. Sometimes, however, even these resources fail to adequately highlight the appropriateness of a practice to a given setting.

There are also tremendous gaps in understanding the effectiveness of existing services and policies. Even though we know vulnerable children often engage multiple systems, we know relatively little about the receipt of the usual care services that form the backdrop or platform for many of the interventions we hope to implement.[95] Only recently has there been a concerted, rigorous effort to compare injury rates for child safety seats to rates for seat belts for older children. It is imperative that evaluation approaches quantify the extent to which existing processes have the desired long-term outcomes and at what costs. Transdisciplinary approaches allow us to consider not only the systems that may mount prevention programs but also the larger question of how systems may work together to achieve a common goal.

While transdisciplinary training may be an ideal way to move forward, there are complications here as well. Each discipline has its own curriculum framework and accreditation guidelines. Courses designed for students from multiple disciplines need to be attuned to the requirements of their profession. For example, in medicine it can be difficult to find space in the students' schedule to provide training on the social issues related to intentional and unintentional injury. For medical students, training may need to come in the form of discrete programs with clinical follow-up.

Transdisciplinary work hinges on successful collaboration between diverse, vested partners, and partnerships take time and effort to develop. Organizations typically do not allot time for collaboration outside individual client referral. Funders of services may not reimburse for the time a professional spends to work with someone from another discipline to meet the client's needs. So for example, a pediatrician may find it difficult to bill for time spent trying to connect a family to services or providing prevention education. Organizational goals may not be conducive to innovation. A school teacher trying to attend to organizational demands to raise test scores may not see a clear means of integrating violence prevention into the lesson plan.

Summary

It is perhaps ironic that a chapter on prevention of injury should end with a section that attempts the dangerous task of predicting the future. Nonetheless, we see several reasons why we believe transdisciplinary work is here to stay in the area of child injury. First of all, many sciences are finding that siloed research is hitting a rather low ceiling in terms of ability to explain outcomes.

For example, early optimistic predictions regarding the ability of genetic mapping to predict behavior and mental illness have had to be modified as we learn that many key mechanisms are, in fact, epigenetic, meaning that genetic expression is fundamentally changeable, perhaps intergenerationally, due to environmental conditions.[96,97] For another example, it appears that environmental or biological interactions may hold promise for explaining substantial variance in response to early stressors.[98] In short, the illusion that siloed science can be truly explanatory is dissipating.

Additionally technological advances in information sciences are making us accustomed to rapid knowledge generation and dissemination. This creates both an expectation and the means for science to be more responsive. Data sources from different disciplines are becoming increasingly available for merging and combination. For example, official child maltreatment reports in the United States and Canada are increasingly merged with health, economic, geographical, or other forms of data to help inform prevention efforts in a more rapid and responsive fashion.[19] Some jurisdictions (for example, South Carolina and British Columbia) are now *designing* information systems with transdisciplinary applications as the guiding principle.

Finally, a fair amount of the low-hanging fruit in injury prevention has already been plucked. What remains is often more complex and requires the contribution of a range of professionals and streams of knowledge. It seems unlikely that the multiple and distinct approaches to injury prevention of the past will be adequate to advance science and practice. Beyond this, however, we find that transdisciplinary practice once begun is mutually reinforcing for the professions involved as they see new avenues to decreasing violence and injury among children.

Key Terms

child maltreatment	Emotional, physical, or sexual abuse by a child's primary caregiver or neglect of care that places the child at risk of harm.
ecodevelopmental framework	A framework in which the likelihood of child injury is influenced by nested contexts of family, community, and society and in which the relative influence of these factors changes as a child ages.
Haddon matrix	A three-by-four matrix wherein the cells represent various intersections of injury phases and prevention targets.
injury	Damage that occurs during energy transfer, as in the crash of an automobile, or when energy

is prevented from transferring, as in the case of suffocation or drowning.

intentional injury Injury to a child or adolescent that is characterized by knowing commission of an act or omission of the care reasonably expected of a caregiver and that results in cognitive, emotional, or physical harm.

unintentional injury Injury to a child or adolescent that is characterized by a lack of intent or a lack of awareness of a safety risk and that results in cognitive, emotional, or physical harm.

youth violence Intentional acts committed by youth toward youth that could potentially result in harm.

Review Questions

1. What are the risk factors that are common to intentional and unintentional injury? Name at least two.

2. Why is a developmental perspective important in transdisciplinary prevention of pediatric violence and injury?

3. How would you describe the potential contributions of at least three disciplines to the prevention of motor vehicle injury in children and youth? How would the target of the activities change according to age?

4. What are at least two of the three categories of potential outcomes of violence and injury presented here? How might intervention following the initial injury (post-event) benefit from a transdisciplinary perspective?

5. What are two barriers to successfully employing a transdisciplinary approach to prevention in the area of violence and injury?

References

1. World Health Organization. World Report on Child Injury Prevention. Geneva: World Health Organization; 2008.
2. Safe Kids, USA. Report to the Nation: Trends in Unintentional Childhood Injury Mortality and Parental Views on Child Safety. Washington, DC: Safe Kids, USA; 2008.
3. US Department of Health and Human Service, Children's Bureau. Child Maltreatment 2010. Washington, DC: US Department of Health and Human Services; 2011.

4. National Research Council, Committee on Evaluation of Children's Health. Children's Health, The Nation's Wealth: Assessing and Improving Child Health. Washington, DC: National Academies Press; 2004.

5. Wang C, Holton JK. Total Estimated Cost of Child Abuse and Neglect in the United States. Chicago: Prevent Child Abuse America; 2007.

6. Centers for Disease Control and Prevention. CDC Research Agenda, 2009–2018. Atlanta, GA: Centers for Disease Control and Prevention, National Center for Injury Prevention and Control; 2009.

7. Belsky J. Child maltreatment: an ecological integration. American Psychologist. 1980;35(4):320–335.

8. Sleet D, Gielen A, Diekman S, Ikeda R. Preventing unintentional injury: a review of behavior change theories for primary care. American Journal of Lifestyle Medicine. 2010;4(1):25–31.

9. Haddon W. Advances in the epidemiology of injuries as a basis for public policy. Public Health Reports. 1980;98(5):411–421.

10. Stokols D, Fuqua J, Gress J, Harvey R, Phillips K, Baezconde-Garbanati L, et al. Evaluating transdisciplinary science. Nicotine & Tobacco Research. 2003;5(suppl 1):S21–S39.

11. McClure R. The Scientific Basis of Injury Prevention and Control. Melbourne: IP Communications; 2004.

12. Borse N, Gilchrist J, Dellinger A, Rudd R, Ballesteros M, Sleet D. CDC Childhood Injury Report: Patterns of Unintentional Injuries among 0–19 Year Olds in the United States, 2000–2006. Atlanta, GA: Centers for Disease Control and Prevention, National Center for Injury Prevention and Control; 2008.

13. Children's Safety Network. Promoting Teen Driving Safety: Strategies and Tools for Community Programs. Waltham, MA: Children's Safety Network; 2008.

14. Morrongiello BA, Klemencic N, Corbett M. Interactions between child behavior patterns and parent supervision: implications for children's risk of unintentional injury. Child Development. 2008;79(3):627–638.

15. Kempe CH, Silverman FN, Steele BF, Droegemueller W, Silver HK. The battered-child syndrome. JAMA. 1962;181:17–24.

16. Finkelhor D, Jones L. Why have child maltreatment and child victimization declined? Journal of Social Issues. 2006;62(4):685–716.

17. Child Welfare Information Gateway. Child Abuse and Neglect Fatalities 2009: Statistics and Interventions. Washington, DC: US Department of Health and Human Services, Children's Bureau; 2011.

18. Horwitz AV, Widom CS, McLaughlin J, White HR. The impact of childhood abuse and neglect on adult mental health: a prospective study. Journal of Health and Social Behavior. 2001;42(2):184–201.

19. Jonson-Reid, Drake MB, Kohl P. Is the overrepresentation of the poor in child welfare caseloads due to bias or need? Children and Youth Services Review. 2009;31:422–427.

20. Centers for Disease Control and Prevention. Web-based Injury Statistics Query and Reporting System (WISQARS) [Online]. Available at: www.cdc.gov/injury/wisqars/index.html [accessed October 16, 2012].

21. Spivey MI, Schnitzer PG, Kruse RL, Slusher P, Jaffe DM. Association of injury visits in children and child maltreatment reports. Journal of Emergency Medicine. 2009;36(2):207–214.

22. Pratt J. Injured or Abused Children Less Than One Year of Age: Are They the Same Sub-population? Brisbane, Australia: Queensland University of Technology; 2007.

23. Widom CS. Posttraumatic stress disorder in abused and neglected children grown up. American Journal of Psychiatry. 1999;156(8):1223–1229.

24. Jonson-Reid M, Way I. Adolescent sexual offenders compared to other incarcerated delinquents: childhood maltreatment, serious emotional disturbance, and offending histories. American Journal of Orthopsychiatry. 2001;71(1):1–11.

25. Widom CS. Does violence beget violence?: a critical examination of the literature. Psychological Bulletin. 1989;106(1):3–28.

26. Spano R, Bolland J. Disentangling the effects of violent victimization, violent behavior, and gun carrying for minority inner-city youth living in extreme poverty. Crime & Delinquency. 2010;57(4):1–23.

27. Bina M, Graziano F, Bonino S. Risky driving and lifestyles in adolescence. Accident Analysis & Prevention. 2006;38(3):472–481.

28. Peterson L, Brown D. Integrating child injury and abuse-neglect research: common histories, etiologies, and solutions. Psychological Bulletin. 1994;116(2):293–315.

29. Weaver NL, Williams J, Jacobsen HA, Botello-Harbaum M, Glasheen C, Noelcke E, et al. Translation of an evidence-based tailored childhood injury prevention program. Journal of Public Health Management and Practice. 2008;14(2):177–184.

30. Doyle JJ, Levitt SD. Evaluating the effectiveness of child safety seats and seat belts in protecting children from injury. Economic Inquiry. 2010;48(3):521–536.

31. Henary B, Sherwood CP, Crandall JR, Kent RW, Vaca FE, Arbogast KB, et al. Car safety seats for children: rear facing for best protection. Injury Prevention. 2007;13(6):398–402.

32. Rice TM, Anderson CL. The effectiveness of child restraint systems for children aged 3 years or younger during motor vehicle collisions: 1996 to 2005. American Journal of Public Health. 2009;99(2):252–257.

33. Cooley D, Coren J. Child safety seats: 2010 educational update. Osteopathic Family Physician. 2011;3(1):30–39.

34. Brixey SN, Guse CE. Knowledge and behaviors of physicians and caregivers about appropriate child passenger restraint use. Journal of Community Health. 2009;34(6):547–552.

35. Shope JT, Molnar LJ. Graduated driver licensing in the United States: evaluation results from the early programs. Journal of Safety Research. 2003;34(1):63–69.

36. Drake B, Jonson-Reid M, Way I, Chung S. Substantiation and recidivism. Child Maltreatment. 2003;8(4):248–260.

37. Knox M, Burkhart K, Hunter K. ACT Against Violence Parents Raising Safe Kids program: effects on maltreatment-related parenting behaviors and beliefs. Journal of Family Issues. 2011;32(1):55–74.

38. Laflame L, Hasselberg M, Burrows S. Years of research on socioeconomic inequality and children's unintentional injuries: understanding the cause-specific evidence at hand. International Journal of Pediatrics [online]. 2010.

39. Lee LC, Harrington RA, Chang JJ, Connors SL. Increased risk of injury in children with developmental disabilities. Research in Developmental Disabilities. 2008;29(3):247–255.

40. Developmental surveillance and screening of infants and young children. Pediatrics. 2001;108(1):192–196.

41. Morrongiello BA, Kane A, Zdzieborski D. "I think he is in his room playing a video game": parental supervision of young elementary-school children at home. Journal of Pediatric Psychology. 2011;36(6):708–717.

42. Alho E, Piotrowski C, Briggs G. Child injury at home: exploring a connection between household rules about safety, sibling harm and child injury. Injury Prevention. 2010;16(suppl 1):A182.

43. Turner HA, Finkelhor D, Ormrod R. Family structure variations in patterns and predictors of child victimization. American Journal of Orthopsychiatry. 2007;77(2):282–295.

44. Ramon C, Boyce J, Pickett K. Associations between adolescent risk behaviors and injury: the modifying role of disability journal of school health. Journal of School Health. 2008;79(1):8–16.

45. Johnson S, Sudhinaraset M, Blum R. Neuromaturation and adolescent risk taking: why development is not determinism. Journal of Adolescent Research. 2009;25(1):4–23.

46. Drake B, Pandey S. Understanding the relationship between neighborhood poverty and specific types of child maltreatment. Child Abuse & Neglect. 1996; 20(11):1003–1018.

47. Gibbs DA, Martin SL, Kupper LL, Johnson RE. Child maltreatment in enlisted soldiers' families during combat-related deployments. JAMA. 2007;298(5):528–535.

48. Asawa LE, Hansen DJ, Flood MF. Early childhood intervention programs: opportunities and challenges for preventing child maltreatment. Education & Treatment of Children. 2008;31(1):73–110.

49. MacKenzie M, Kotch J, Lee L. Toward a cumulative ecological risk model for the etiology of child maltreatment. Children and Youth Services Review. 2011;33(9):1638–1647.

50. Parrish JW, Young MB, Perham-Hester KA, Gessner BD. Identifying risk factors for child maltreatment in Alaska: a population-based approach. American Journal of Preventive Medicine. 2011;40(6):666–673.

51. Blumenthal I. Shaken baby syndrome. Postgraduate Medical Journal. 2002;78:732–735.

52. Sobsey D. Exceptionality, education, and maltreatment. Exceptionality. 2002;10(1):29–46.

53. Sullivan P. Violence against children with disabilities: prevention, public policy, and research implications. Paper presented at: National Conference on Preventing

and Intervening with Violence Against Children and Adults with Disabilities; 2002; Washington, DC.

54. Finkelhor D. Current information on the scope and nature of child sexual abuse. The Future of Children. 1994;4(2):31–53.

55. Whipple EE, Webster-Stratton C. The role of parental stress in physically abusive families. Child Abuse & Neglect. 1991;15(3):279–291.

56. Haskett M, Portwood S, Lewis K. Physical child abuse. In: Ferguson CJ, ed. Violent Crime: Clinical and Social Implications. Los Angeles: Sage; 2009: 207–228.

57. Rees G, Stein M. Abuse of adolescents. Children & Society. 1997;11(1): 63–70.

58. Doueck HJ, Ishisaka AH, Greenaway KD. The role of normative development in adolescent abuse and neglect. Family Relations. 1988;37(2):135–139.

59. Jonson-Reid M, Drake B, Kim J, Porterfield S, Han L. A prospective analysis of the relationship between reported child maltreatment and special education eligibility among poor children. Child Maltreatment. 2004;9(4):382–394.

60. Strathearn L, Gray PH, O'Callaghan MJ, Wood DO. Childhood neglect and cognitive development in extremely low birth weight infants: a prospective study. Pediatrics. 2001;108(1):142–151.

61. Daviss WB, Mooney D, Racusin R, Ford JD, Fleischer A, McHugo GJ. Predicting posttraumatic stress after hospitalization for pediatric injury. Journal of the American Academy of Child & Adolescent Psychiatry. 2000;39(5):576–583.

62. DeBellis M, Thomas L. Biologic findings of post-traumatic stress disorder and child maltreatment. Current Psychiatry Reports. 2003;5(2):108–117.

63. Lawrence JW, Rosenberg L, Mason S, Fauerbach JA. Comparing parent and child perceptions of stigmatizing behavior experienced by children with burn scars. Body Image. 2011;8(1):70–73.

64. Trickett PK, Negriff S, Juye J, Peckins M. Child maltreatment and adolescent development. Journal of Research on Adolescence. 2011;21(1):3–20.

65. Wilson KR, Hansen DJ, Li M. The traumatic stress response in child maltreatment and resultant neuropsychological effects. Aggression & Violent Behavior. 2011;16(2):87–97.

66. Makarios M, Pratt T. The effectiveness of policies and programs that attempt to reduce firearm violence: a meta-analysis. Crime & Delinquency. 2008;58(2):222–244.

67. Crooks CV, Scott K, Ellis W, Wolfe DA. Impact of a universal school-based violence prevention program on violent delinquency: distinctive benefits for youth with maltreatment histories. Child Abuse & Neglect. 2011;35(6):393–400.

68. Kunkel P, Thomas CJ, Seguin C, Dereczyk D, Rajda C, Brandt MM. A hospital-based violence prevention tour: a collaborative approach to empower youth. Journal of Trauma. 2010;68(2):289–293.

69. Flaspohler P, Duffy J, Wandersman A, Stillman L, Maras MA. Unpacking capacity: an intersection of research-to-practice models and community-centered models. American Journal of Community Psychology. 2008;41(3–4):182–196.

70. US Department of Health and Human Services, Administration for Children & Families. State Statutes Search. Available at: www.childwelfare.gov/systemwide /laws_policies/state [accessed October 16, 2012].

71. Hamby S, Finkelhor D, Turner H, Ormrod R. The overlap of witnessing partner violence with child maltreatment and other victimizations in a nationally representative survey of youth. Child Abuse & Neglect. 2010;34(10): 734–741.

72. Banks D, Dutch N, Wang K. Collaborative efforts to improve system response to families who are experiencing child maltreatment and domestic violence. Journal of Interpersonal Violence. 2008;23(7):876–902.

73. Black T, Trocme N, Fallon B, MacLaurin B. The Canadian child welfare system response to exposure to domestic violence investigations. Child Abuse & Neglect. 2008;32(3):393–404.

74. Edleson JL, Gassman-Pines J, Hill MB. Defining child exposure to domestic violence as neglect: Minnesota's difficult experience. Social Work. 2006;51(2):167–174.

75. Magen RH. In the best interests of battered women: reconceptualizing allegations of failure to protect. Child Maltreatment. 1999;4(2):127–135.

76. Gielen AC, McKenzie LB, McDonald EM, Shields WC, Wang MC, Cheng YJ, et al. Using a computer kiosk to promote child safety: results of a randomized, controlled trial in an urban pediatric emergency department. Pediatrics. 2007;120(2):330–339.

77. Nurses for Newborns. Available at: www.nfnf.org/missouri [accessed October 18, 2012].

78. Gardner HG. Office-based counseling for unintentional injury prevention. Pediatrics. 2007;119(1):202–206.

79. Weaver N, Nansel T, Williams J, Tse J, Botello-Harbaum M, Willson K. Reach of a kiosk based pediatric injury prevention program. Translational Behavioral Medicine. 2011;1(4):515–522.

80. Barth R, Jonson-Reid M. Probation foster care as an outcome for children exiting child welfare foster care. Social Work. 2000;48(3):348–361.

81. Glasgow RE, Emmons KM. How can we increase translation of research into practice?: types of evidence needed. Annual Review of Public Health. 2007;28:413–433.

82. Saul J, Wandersman A, Flaspohler P, Duffy J, Lubell K, Noonan R. Research and action for bridging science and practice in prevention. American Journal of Community Psychology. 2008;41(3–4):165–170.

83. Kreuter M. Tailoring Health Messages: Customizing Communication with Computer Technology. London: Taylor & Francis; 2008.

84. Nansel TR, Weaver N, Donlin M, Jacobsen H, Kreuter MW, Simons-Morton B. Baby, be safe: the effect of tailored communications for pediatric injury prevention provided in a primary care setting. Patient Education and Counseling. 2002;46(3):175–190.

85. Cohen LR, Runyan CW, Downs SM, Bowling JM. Pediatric injury prevention counseling priorities. Pediatrics. 1997;99(5):704–710.

86. Fixsen DL, Naoom SF, Blasé KA, Friedman RM. Implementation Research: A Synthesis of the Literature. Tampa, FL: University of South Florida, Louis de la Parte Florida Mental Health Institute, The National Implementation Research Network; 2005.

87. Dzewaltowski DA, Glasgow RE, Kiesges LM, Estabrooks PA, Brock E. RE-AIM: evidence-based standards and a web resource to improve translation of research into practice. Annals of Behavioral Medicine. 2004;28(2):75–80.

88. National Association of Children's Hospitals and Related Institutions. Available at: www.childrenshospitals.net.

89. Child Welfare Information Gateway. Promoting healthy families in your community: 2008 resource packet. Washington, DC: US Department of Health and Human Services; 2008.

90. Horton C. Protective Factors Literature Review: Early Care and Education Programs and the Prevention of Child Abuse and Neglect. Washington, DC: Center for the Study of Social Policy; 2003.

91. Sanders MR, Ralph A, Thompson R, Sofronoff K, Gardiner P, Bidwell K. Every Family: A Public Health Approach to Promoting Children's Wellbeing. Brisbane, Australia: University of Queensland; 2005.

92. Connell CM, Vanderploeg JJ, Katz KH, Caron C, Saunders L, Tebes JK. Maltreatment following reunification: predictors of subsequent Child Protective Services contact after children return home. Child Abuse & Neglect. 2009;33(4):218–228.

93. Jonson-Reid M, Barth RP. From maltreatment report to juvenile incarceration: the role of child welfare services. Child Abuse & Neglect. 2000;24(4):505–520.

94. Ryan J, Testa M. Child maltreatment and juvenile delinquency: investigating the role of placement and placement instability. Children and Youth Services Review. 2004;27:227–247.

95. Jonson-Reid M. Disentangling system contact and services: a key pathway to evidence-based children's policy. Children and Youth Services Review. 2011;33:598–604.

96. Champagne FA. Epigenetic mechanisms and the transgenerational effects of maternal care. Frontiers in Neuroendocrinology. 2008;29(3):386–397.

97. Jonson-Reid M, Presnall N, Drake B, Fox L, Bierut L, Reich W, et al. Effects of child maltreatment and inherited liability on antisocial development: an official records study. Journal of the American Academy of Child & Adolescent Psychiatry. 2010;49(4):321–332; quiz 431.

98. Caspi A, McClay J, Moffitt TE, Mill J, Martin J, Craig IW, et al. Role of genotype in the cycle of violence in maltreated children. Science. 2002;297(5582):851–854.

Chapter 11

Transdisciplinary Problem Solving for Integrating Public Health and Social Service Systems to Address Health Disparities

Matthew W. Kreuter
Debbie Pfeiffer

Learning Objectives

- Describe approaches to simulating transdisciplinary teams in short-term student learning projects.
- Explain how transdisciplinary solutions apply not just to academicians and scientists but also to practitioners and a range of nonacademic public and community agencies.
- Discuss the concept that transdisciplinary work should be focused on practical solutions to social problems.
- Explain shared model building as a key skill for transdisciplinary work.
- Explore the use of case studies of cross-disciplinary collaborations as available and valuable tools for teaching about the transdisciplinary process.

•••

Much of the recent focus on transdisciplinary work has centered on the activity of scientists—what they do, how they do it, and how they organize themselves to do it. Yet as Stokols and colleagues describe in chapter 1, transdisciplinary approaches can also include partnerships among practitioners in nonacademic fields and can seek to improve practice by changing the way governmental and community organizations, agencies, and systems think about and carry out their core tasks and goals. This chapter describes a graduate course in which graduate students in public health and social work were asked to apply transdisciplinary thinking to a practical challenge: better coordinating the fragmented efforts of public agencies to help eliminate health disparities.

The chapter begins with a brief description of the challenge students were asked to address, followed by an overview of the pedagogical approach and process that guided the course. Next, it offers more detailed descriptions of specific course activities undertaken by students. The chapter concludes with lessons learned and an epilogue about the project undertaken by the students.

The Challenge

As it has been for decades, smoking remains the greatest preventable cause of premature death in the United States.[1] But unlike in decades past, today's smokers are disproportionately concentrated in the lower socioeconomic strata. Among adult Americans who did not complete high school or who earned a GED, 28 to 41 percent smoke cigarettes; by comparison, only 11 percent of those with a bachelor's degree smoke and just 6 percent of those with a graduate degree smoke.[2] Smoking rates are also higher among those with lower incomes. About one in three adults in poor families and those living below the federal poverty level smoke, compared to roughly one in five adult Americans with higher levels of income.[2,3] As a result of the shifting demographics of smoking, it is critical that public health and tobacco control leaders find ways to reach disadvantaged populations with policies and programs that can reduce the uptake of smoking by nonsmokers and help current smokers quit.

One of the population-based strategies for doing this is telephone tobacco quitlines. Quitlines are available in all fifty states and provide free telephone counseling, cessation aids, information resources, and other support services to help smokers quit. Smokers can initiate the call to a quitline or, through a third party, can consent to be contacted by a quitline. During the initial quitline contact, smokers arrange a series of telephone counseling sessions to be initiated by the quitline and delivered over a two- to three-month period. Quitlines are administered by state health agencies.

Telephone counseling for smoking cessation is an evidence-based intervention that is recommended in both clinical and community practice guidelines.[4-6] Unlike many behavioral interventions, telephone counseling for smoking cessation has been tested and found to be effective in real-world settings, through existing quitline services.[7,8] Studies show six-month abstinence rates of 10 to 13 percent among quitline users who receive multisession counseling, and up to 28 percent when counseling is accompanied by nicotine replacement therapy.[6,8,9] Because quitlines offer population-wide free access to smoking cessation, they have the potential to reach a diverse cross section of American smokers.

Increasing the use of tobacco quitlines among low-income and low-education smokers is a major priority for US health agencies.[10] In particular, there is a need to develop new and sustainable community outreach strategies to supplement and extend the reach of quitline referrals available through traditional channels like health care organizations.[11] One approach is to partner with social service agencies and public assistance programs that serve a large proportion of low-income Americans. Five promising partners are the Food Stamp program, Low Income Home Energy Assistance Program, Public Housing Program, Unemployment Services programs, and 2-1-1 services. Because these federal and state systems exist in every US community and serve tens of millions of low-income Americans, the potential for population impact on smoking and smoking-related diseases is great if quitline referrals could be integrated into such systems for their program participants who smoke.

The course described in this chapter was built around this challenge. Broadly, the course required students from public health and social work to work together to generate strategies for integrating public health services into social service systems. Specifically, they were asked to integrate tobacco quitline referrals into Food Stamp offices.

The Food Stamp program—now formally known as the Supplemental Nutrition Assistance Program, or SNAP—helps poor people buy food. Because of their income and household size, many socioeconomically disadvantaged Americans qualify for Food Stamps. Eligible households receive an electronic benefits transfer card that can be used like an ATM card at authorized grocery stores or retail outlets to buy food or seeds and plants that produce food. Over forty million American currently receive Food Stamp benefits; about one in eight adults and one in four children live in a household receiving Food Stamps. Program participation has been at record levels during the current economic recession. The Food Stamp program is a US Department of Agriculture program that is administered by states through local (such as county-level) social services offices.

Nationally, surveys have shown that the smoking rate among adults in Food Stamp households is roughly double the rate found in non-Food Stamp households (40 percent versus 19 percent).[12] In St. Louis, Missouri, where this course was taught, the rates are similar. In 2009, we conducted a survey of

522 local Food Stamp program participants and found that 40 percent were smokers. High smoking rates in low-income families are particularly troubling because the cost of cigarettes not only deepens their poverty but can also lead to compromises like choosing between cigarettes and food.[13] Both children and adults in low-income households are twice as likely to experience food insecurity when there is a smoker in the household than they are when there are no smokers in the household.[14] The good news is that these smokers want to quit. In our survey, 78 percent of smokers who received Food Stamps said they were thinking about quitting, and 61 percent reported that they had tried to quit in the last year. Yet only one-third of these smokers had ever heard about the telephone quitline, and only 2 percent had ever called it.

Thus the Food Stamp program provides access to a large number of smokers who want to quit and who are experiencing serious health and financial consequences because of their smoking behavior. There is a widely available and evidence-based resource that can help them quit for free (that is, a telephone quitline), but the vast majority of smokers who receive Food Stamps don't know about it. What's more, these two programs—Food Stamps and the tobacco quitlines—are both administered by state governments, seemingly creating an opportunity for greater efficiency and more comprehensive assistance to disadvantaged populations through coordination of services.

Course Overview

The course had five main sections: (1) background on the challenge, (2) case studies in public agency collaboration and innovation, (3) conceptual model building, (4) solution workshop, and (5) presentation to stakeholders. Using the information acquired during the first three sections of the course, students worked in teams in section 4 to develop strategies to integrate screening for smoking and referrals to the Missouri Tobacco Quitline into Food Stamp offices in Missouri, and the course culminated in section 5 with the student teams presenting their strategies to key stakeholders for evaluation and feedback.

Background on the Challenge

To address the challenge, students needed to learn about and integrate perspectives from multiple disciplines. Primary among these were *public health*; *social services*, specifically service delivery programs and systems like Food Stamps and tobacco quitlines; and *organizational behavior*, specifically the ways in which public agencies make decisions, choose whether or not to collaborate with other agencies, and think about and approach innovation. Much of this information has been outlined earlier in this book.

The content was delivered through several channels. In addition to lectures, discussions, and assigned readings, the class made a field trip to the largest Food Stamp office in Missouri, meeting with and interviewing administrators, touring the facility, and walking through the same process participants follow in applying for or renewing eligibility for program participation. Similarly, tobacco control specialists from state departments of health in Missouri and Oregon visited the class to talk and be interviewed about quitline services. As Stokols et al. suggest in chapter 1, these practitioners indeed provided unique and relevant inside knowledge and experience-based points of view that helped students think about possible solutions.

In addition to these practice perspectives, students also heard from and interviewed a faculty member from the Olin Business School at Washington University in St. Louis about organizational behavior in public agencies. Separately, they learned about perspectives and opportunities from policy, economics, and technology. Although course contributors were not part of the student teams generating solutions, several of them were available to confer with teams throughout the semester. Collectively, the readings, lectures, interviews, and field trips provided students with building blocks for a transdisciplinary solution.

Case Studies in Public Agency Collaboration and Innovation

Regardless of the specific strategies students would propose for addressing the challenge, all solutions would require public agencies to work together. Thus, understanding public agency partnerships was a critical component of the course. Students were introduced to the subject through case studies of successful public agency partnerships. In a series of three assignments, students (1) critically analyzed one of seven such cases in a written paper, (2) planned and presented a brief panel discussion on their case with other students who had selected the same case, and (3) synthesized observations and lessons learned across all cases to develop a conceptual model of factors influencing public agency partnerships.

The seven cases featured public agencies at the local, state, or federal level working together with other public agencies, not-for-profit community organizations, or industry. All used innovative and cross-disciplinary approaches to address important health or social problems. Cases were identified by course instructors through a search of published news reports and peer-reviewed literature, and included the US Department of Energy and the Environmental Protection Agency's Energy Star program;[15] organ donor registries, such as Donate Life Missouri,[16] administered by state motor vehicle departments; Habitat for Humanity's Prison Partnership program with state and local departments of corrections;[17] the Oregon Solar Highway project, involving the Oregon Department of Transportation and a local utility company;[18] the Vice President's Middle Class Task Force, involving the US Departments of Labor, Education, Energy, and Housing and Urban Development;[19] the Recycle Bank's collaborations with municipal governments across the United States, such as Philadelphia Recycling Rewards;[20] and the urban fishing programs initiated by various combinations of state and federal wildlife and conservation agencies together with local municipalities, such as the program involving the Missouri Department of Conservation.[21]

The learning objective for students was to identify and understand factors associated with initiating and successfully executing innovative collaborative partnerships involving public agencies. To do this, students had to research, describe, and critically evaluate one of the cases. The primary goal of their analyses was to identify potentially generalizable principles that could be applied in developing new cross-disciplinary public agency collaborations, such as an integration of tobacco quitline referrals into Food Stamp offices. Students selected a case; gathered information about it from published sources, original interviews, and agency documents; and described its background, goals, funding, implementation, evidence for effectiveness, challenges, and keys to success. Students' papers concluded with three to five principles for effective interorganizational collaboration. These principles focused on factors that enhanced success in the initiation, execution, and funding or sustaining of the partnership.

After students had received written feedback on their case analyses, they were divided into groups so that all the students who had analyzed the same case would be working together. Each group synthesized its principles into a single set and presented them to the class through the medium of a discussion panel. The principles from all the groups were then compiled into a single document that was distributed to the students. This list became the starting point for more formal, didactic learning about theories and principles of organizational behavior in public agencies (as found, for example, in Wilson,[22] Fernandez,[23] and Rainey[24]). Fortunately (from a pedagogical perspective), many of the students' case study observations and principles closely mirrored empirical findings and expert opinions in the organizational behavior literature.

Conceptual Model Building

Integration and cross-fertilization of theoretical perspectives is a hallmark of transdisciplinary work.[25] One of the ways this is accomplished is by generating new conceptual models that reflect perspectives from different disciplines. As Stokols et al.'s definition of transdisciplinary research and practice in chapter 1 makes clear, such joint model building across disciplines is essential to the transdisciplinary process. In this course, the term *disciplines* was also applied to the practice experiences of public agencies working in different domains, engaged in different partnerships, and aiming for different goals. To develop this transdisciplinary skill, students learned about model building and then were assigned to generate their own conceptual model of successful public agency partnerships, using their list of principles from the case studies and literature on organizational behavior.

The goal of model building for this course was to capture the complexity of building public agency partnerships but also to reflect it clearly and simply by focusing on its essential elements. Students learned a general four-step model-building process: (1) specifying the phenomena to be modeled, (2) mapping the phenomena into constructs, (3) describing the relationships between constructs, and (4) reviewing and refining the model. They learned that within these steps it was important to clearly define the scope of inquiry, specify the outcomes or outputs of the model, deconstruct the process into key concepts or principles, and arrange or group related concepts accordingly. In addition, they needed to hypothesize causal direction or temporal sequence, indicate the relative importance of difference concepts and how each might lead to different outcomes of interest, and identify gaps in the model not explained by currently available information. Students were exposed to different types of models from a range of domains that illustrated how this general approach could be translated into multiple forms and visual designs.

For their assignment of developing a conceptual model of factors influencing public agency partnerships, students had to consider a diverse range of factors that influence agency partnerships and integrate these in a way that improved understanding of how partnerships succeed. Students worked in teams of four or five. Team members created a visual illustration of their model, described its key components and the relationships among them, and critiqued the model's strengths and weaknesses. In formal presentations, each team shared its model with the class and fielded questions about it. Each team also submitted a written assignment describing its model. The models varied in scope (for example, one focused on initiating partnerships and another on sustaining partnerships over time) and approach (for example, one was a temporally oriented stage model and another described a cyclical process), but all were thoughtful and thorough.

Solution Workshop

For the remainder of the course, students applied these conceptual models—along with their new knowledge about cigarette smoking in low-income populations, telephone tobacco quitlines, and the Food Stamp program—to generate strategies for integrating quitline referrals into local Food Stamp offices. The in-class format for this work was modeled after the design studio approach used in architectural training. Design studio work is characterized by its focus on time-limited projects (the usual time is one semester) that address "complex and open-ended problems" through a "rapid iteration of design solutions" informed by frequent formal and informal critiques from peers and instructors.[26] This work is also influenced by precedent and therefore may involve examining past solutions to problems deemed relevant to the current project.

During each of the last five weeks of the course, students spent sixty to ninety minutes of class time working in preselected teams (described later) on their solutions. During these periods, course instructors would meet with each team, providing feedback and suggestions and offering an informed perspective on the feasibility of specific strategies. Instructors also met with each team separately outside class at least once during this period. The teams also presented their ideas to each other during each class session, taking questions and suggestions from their classmates. Teams spent much more time working on their solutions *outside* class than in class, but the design studio approach guaranteed that they received regular feedback throughout the development process.

The course instructors preselected the students for each team in order to maximize the variation in disciplinary backgrounds represented on each team and to ensure that all teams possessed, across their members, all the skills required for project success. In addition to students' current status as public health or social work degree students, the instructors had obtained information about their disciplinary backgrounds as undergraduates, and on the first day of the course all students had completed a self-assessment in which they rated their own skills and experience in nine areas: developing and delivering presentations, understanding and analyzing data, conceptual thinking, leading or coordinating, working in groups, interviewing, writing, editing, and working with community organizations. This was the information used to create teams that were disciplinarily diverse and equivalent in skills. Before announcing these teams to the students, we also had course instructors from the previous semester evaluate each team's membership to make sure there were no concerns about group dynamics or strong personality conflicts.

The teams functioned well and produced interesting and diverse solutions. One proposed a technology-based strategy linked to a forthcoming system to help low-income families in Missouri apply for Food Stamps online. After users had completed their application, the system would ask up to three questions: (1) Does anyone in your household smoke cigarettes?; (2) IF YES: Is that person interested in quitting?; and (3) IF YES: Is it okay to have the Missouri Tobacco Quitline call that person to help them quit smoking? Answering these questions would take less than one minute, and contact information for respondents answering yes to all three questions would be forwarded to the quitline, which would then have a quit smoking counselor initiate contact and cessation support.

Another team proposed a technology-based solution that used text messaging to increase quitline referrals. The team observed that a large proportion of Food Stamp clients who smoke are young women, a majority of whom own cell phones and use them for text messaging. By texting "quit" to a designated number, Food Stamp clients would be letting the quitline know that they wanted to talk with a counselor about quitting. A counselor would then initiate contact with the client. Given the long wait time for clients in many Food Stamp offices, the team proposed promoting this service through materials and media placed in the waiting area. This solution was influenced in part by the recent success of another public agency partnership, the text4baby program.[27]

A third team chose not to focus on a specific solution but rather on a strategy to generate funding that would ensure ongoing support of another group's proposed solution. The team introduced state-level policy measures (for example, increased cigarette taxes) and language that would earmark a proportion of the revenue generated by these measures for the use of the tobacco quitline and for the support of partnerships with public agencies like Food Stamp programs that serve low-income populations with a high prevalence of smokers.

Presentation to Stakeholders

On the final day of the course, students presented their solutions to a group of stakeholders that included leaders from the Missouri Department of Social Services, the Missouri Department of Health and Senior Services, the Missouri Tobacco Quitline, and the Missouri Foundation for Health (which funds quitline activities), and also half a dozen state and local public health, social services, and tobacco control professionals. These stakeholders had been identified and invited to attend by course instructors. Several of them had been involved in the student projects, serving as interviewees and providing program information and data. The two-hour session included brief introductions by the stakeholders and course instructors, eighty minutes of presentations, and twenty minutes of questions from the stakeholders.

The instructors had three broad goals for the stakeholder presentations. First, students needed to develop and practice skills in preparing and effectively delivering information, ideas, and data to key decision makers. Of particular importance for a transdisciplinary approach, students had to recognize that stakeholders from a particular practice discipline may lack what Stokols and colleagues refer to as "critical awareness" (see chapter 1), a familiarity with key concepts and principles from other practice disciplines. Thus their presentations needed to include more orientation, explanation, and context than they might use for a presentation to a unidisciplinary audience. Second, feedback from the stakeholders would help the students recognize the strengths and limitations of their solutions, especially as they related to feasibility and implementation in real-world practice settings. Finally, the third goal of the presentations was translational—to give stakeholders ideas they might consider or adopt to help eliminate health disparities.

Student teams worked with course instructors to develop their presentations, and two dress rehearsals were held for students to practice their delivery, refine the content of their slides and narrative, and practice answering questions from the audience. Each team also prepared a one-page concept brief that summarized its solution. These briefs were provided to the stakeholders.

The student presentations to stakeholders were highly polished and professional. Stakeholders were impressed by the student projects. They congratulated students on their work and expressed particular enthusiasm about the fact that the students were working on a real problem affecting real agencies. Stakeholders also rated the students on eight items that assessed the quality, feasibility, and likely impact of their ideas; their knowledge of the subject matter; and the organization and presentation of their solutions. Students received high marks for presentations that were well organized (mean = 9.6 on a 1 to 10 scale ranging from "strongly disagree" to "strongly agree") and effectively delivered (9.3) and for doing a good job answering questions (9.1). Scores were slightly lower for the feasibility of their ideas (8.3) and the likelihood that these ideas would reduce smoking (7.8), although stakeholders strongly agreed that they would share the information they learned from the presentations with their colleagues (9.2).

The high point of the stakeholder presentation came during the discussion period, when a state-level leader from the Food Stamp program indicated her intention to act on the information students presented. She commented that although many of the student solutions were too large in scope for her office to implement alone or immediately, she would support distributing quitline referrals in Food Stamp offices in Missouri. She then publicly engaged the quitline director in a discussion of how to make that happen, while the students and other stakeholders looked on. The result of this discussion is briefly described in the following epilogue.

Epilogue

Nine months after the students presented their solutions to stakeholders, the Missouri Department of Social Services sent a letter to the Food Stamp managers in every office in the state ($n = 120$) encouraging them to distribute quitline referrals to their clients who smoke. Managers were given a phone number to call where they could order customized referral materials designed specifically for the populations served at their office (paying attention, for example, to race or ethnicity and whether they were urban or rural and a parent of young children or not). In four weeks, every Food Stamp office in Missouri had ordered quitline referrals, and today all those offices include quitline displays and referrals. We are working with these agencies to evaluate the impact of this solution.

Lessons Learned

As with any course offered for the first time, we learned a great deal from this attempt to teach transdisciplinary problem solving to students. Here we summarize four lessons—derived from instructor observations, formal course evaluations, and informal discussions with students—that have influenced our thinking about future iterations of the course and may be beneficial for others planning similar coursework.

1. *The real-world context appealed to students.* Students liked the practice perspective of the course. They enjoyed hearing from guest speakers who worked in public agencies, touring these agencies on field trips, and interviewing practitioners. They appreciated the chance to apply knowledge from foundational courses in real-world settings, and felt this influenced their ideas and solutions. Although hardly a surprise, this finding suggests that learning about transdisciplinary approaches should be more than an academic exercise in integrating different perspectives to gain new insights. It is important to recall that this was a class of public health and social work master's degree students. Such students might be more oriented toward practice than, say, doctoral students who are studying to become researchers and who might be (even if they shouldn't be) less interested in application.

2. *Student instincts may undermine the transdisciplinary approach.* The flip side of lesson 1 is that students' strong interest in application also manifests as a bias toward action. We noticed a tendency for students to jump to familiar solutions rather than adhere to a process that explores perspectives from different disciplines. The design studio approach helped us catch and redirect such thinking early on in the development process.

3. *Creating student teams with diverse backgrounds and skills is beneficial.* Ideally, a course like this would draw students from many disciplines across campus, not just students in public health. This is, indeed, a major goal for our transdisciplinary public health courses as they evolve and mature. In the absence of this level of variety, we attempted to construct teams whose members varied in undergraduate training, amount and type of work experience, and specific skills needed to carry out key assignments in the course. Although we do not know how things would have been different if we had used other methods of creating teams (such as self-selection by students or random assignment), there was certainly anecdotal evidence that the solutions

emerging from different teams reflected a melding of the unique perspectives represented by each team's members.

4. *Students' desire for autonomy and sense of competition challenge this learning approach.* Although students were nearly universal in liking the practice of applying what they were learning, they were divided in their level of interest in the particular topic being addressed (that is, smoking in low-income populations). Practically speaking, it would be very difficult to plan a course as applied as this one if it had addressed multiple topics, especially if the topics were not known well in advance of the course start date. A better approach is to make clear to enrolling students what the focus will be, and let those who are uninterested self-select out of the course. We also found that students' sense of competition—against other individuals and teams in the class—was initially an obstacle to the design studio process. Students didn't want to share their team's ideas publicly for fear that other teams would take the ideas. If their best ideas were not unique, they reasoned, they would lose a comparative advantage and their grades might reflect this. When we recognized this, we addressed it directly and reoriented the solution and presentation exercises as a classwide initiative to collectively provide stakeholders with the best set of ideas we could generate. This made it not just permissible, but desirable, to help every team do the best it could.

Summary

This chapter described approaches for simulating transdisciplinary teams in short-term student learning projects. It explained how transdisciplinary solutions apply to academicians, scientists, practitioners, and public and community agencies. That the process of transdisciplinary problem solving was successfully used to address a key public health problem was demonstrated in the case study. Further use of case studies of cross-disciplinary collaborations, as described in other chapters in this book, is critical to understanding and developing skills in application of the transdisciplinary process.

Key Terms

conceptual model building	A four-step process: (1) specifying the phenomena to be modeled, (2) mapping the phenomena into constructs, (3) describing the relationships between constructs, and (4) reviewing and refining the model.
design studio	An pedagogical approach with a focus on time-limited projects (the usual time is one

semester) that address "complex and open-ended problems" through a "rapid iteration of design solutions" informed by frequent formal and informal critiques from peers and instructors.

Review Questions

1. What practice and academic disciplines are important for the study of health disparities?

2. Which phases of the transdisciplinary (TD) initiative described by Stokols et al. in chapter 1 were represented in the course described in this chapter?

3. Did the transdisciplinary approach used in the course reflect horizontal integration or vertical integration, as described by Stokols et al. (chapter 1)?

4. How did the instructors simulate transdisciplinary teams among students in the course? What other strategies would you suggest to accomplish this goal?

References

1. Mokdad AH, Marks JS, Stroup DF, Gerberding JL. Actual causes of death in the United States, 2000. JAMA. 2004;291(10):1238–1245.
2. Cigarette smoking among adults and trends in smoking cessation—United States, 2008. MMWR. 2009;58(44):1227–1232.
3. Barbeau EM, Leavy-Sperounis A, Balbach ED. Smoking, social class, and gender: what can public health learn from the tobacco industry about disparities in smoking? Tobacco Control, 2004;13(2):115–120.
4. Lichtenstein E, Glasgow RE, Lando HA, Ossip-Klein DJ, Boles SM. Telephone counseling for smoking cessation: rationales and meta-analytic review of evidence. Health Education Research. 1996;11(2):243–257.
5. Stead LF, Lancaster T, Perera R. Telephone counselling for smoking cessation. Cochrane Database of Systematic Reviews. 2003(1):CD002850.
6. Fiore MC. Treating tobacco use and dependence: an introduction to the US Public Health Service Clinical Practice Guideline. Respiratory Care. 2000;45(10):1196–1199.
7. Borland R, Segan CJ, Livingston PM, Owen N. The effectiveness of callback counselling for smoking cessation: a randomized trial. Addiction. 2001;96(6):881–889.
8. Zhu SH, Anderson CM, Tedeschi GJ, Rosbrook B, Johnson CE, Byrd M, et al. Evidence of real-world effectiveness of a telephone quitline for smokers. New England Journal of Medicine. 2002;347(14):1087–1093.

9. Cummings KM, Hyland A, Fix B, Bauer U, Celestino P, Carlin-Menter S, et al. Free nicotine patch giveaway program 12-month follow-up of participants. American Journal of Preventive Medicine. 2006;31(2):181–184.

10. National Cancer Institute. The NCI Strategic Plan for Leading the Nation to Eliminate the Suffering and Death Due to Cancer. Washington, DC: US Department of Health and Human Services, National Institutes of Health; 2006.

11. McAfee TA. Quitlines a tool for research and dissemination of evidence-based cessation practices. American Journal of Preventive Medicine. 2007;33(6 suppl):S357–S367.

12. Child Trends of National Health Interview Survey data, 1998–2004. Child Trends Databank. Available at: www.childtrendsdatabank.org [accessed November 26, 2011].

13. Siahpush M, Borland R, Yong HH. Sociodemographic and psychosocial correlates of smoking-induced deprivation and its effect on quitting: findings from the International Tobacco Control Policy Evaluation Survey. Tobacco Control. 2007;16(2):e2.

14. Cutler-Triggs C, Fryer GE, Miyoshi TJ, Weitzman M. Increased rates and severity of child and adult food insecurity in households with adult smokers. Archives of Pediatrics & Adolescent Medicine. 2008;162(11):1056–1062.

15. US Environmental Protection Agency and Department of Transportation. Energy Star. Available at: www.energystar.gov [accessed November 26, 2011].

16. Donate Life Missouri. Available at: www.donatelifemissouri.com [accessed October 18, 2012].

17. Ta C. Prison partnership: it's about people. Corrections Today. 2000;62(6):114–123. Available at: www.ncjrs.gov/App/Publications/abstract.aspx?ID=185411 [accessed November 20, 2012].

18. Oregon Office of Innovative Partnerships and Alternative Funding, Innovative Partnerships Program. All about the Oregon Solar Highway. Available at: www.oregon.gov/ODOT/HWY/OIPP/pages/inn_solarhighway.aspx [accessed October 19, 2012].

19. The White House. About the Middle Class Task Force. Available at: www.whitehouse.gov/strongmiddleclass/about [accessed October 19, 2012].

20. Philadelphia Recycling Rewards. Available at: phillyrecyclingpays.com [accessed October 19, 2012]

21. Borgwordt C, Nodine B, for Missouri Department of Conservation. City slicker fishing. The Conservationist [online]. January 2, 1996 [last updated October 20, 2010]. Available at: mdc.mo.gov/conmag/1996/01/city-slicker-fishing [accessed October 19, 2012].

22. Wilson J. Bureaucracy: What Government Agencies Do and Why They Do It. New York: Basic Books; 2000.

23. Fernandez S, Rainey, HG. Managing successful organizational change in the public sector. Public Administration Review. 2006;66(2):168–176.

24. Rainey H, Steinbauer P. Galloping elephants: developing elements of a theory of effective government organizations. Journal of Public Administration Research and Theory. 1999;9(1):1–32.

25. Stokols D, Fuqua J, Gress J, Harvey R, Phillips K, Baezconde-Garbanati L, et al. Evaluating transdisciplinary science. Nicotine & Tobacco Research. 2003;5(suppl 1):S21–S39.

26. Kuhn S. Learning from the architecture studio: implications for project-based pedagogy. International Journal of Engineering Education. 2001;17(4–5): 349–352.

27. National Healthy Mothers Healthy Babies Coalition. text4baby. Available at: text4baby.org [accessed October 18, 2012].

Part 4

Transdisciplinary Practice: Case Studies in Global Health

Chapter 12

Transdisciplinary Problem Solving for Global Hunger and Undernutrition

Lora Iannotti

Learning Objectives

- Generate new conceptual frameworks representing the transdisciplinary causal pathways to hunger and undernutrition.
- Combine various methodologies and tools from different disciplines to analyze and describe hunger and undernutrition problems.
- Identify a broad set of biological, public health, and sociological determinants to the problem of undernutrition.
- Collaborate to build a consensus and capitalize on the assets across competing agendas.
- Produce practical and feasible implementation strategies that incorporate ongoing research, programming, and policy inputs and outputs, and disseminate these strategies to a broad audience.

• • •

Undernutrition remains a leading risk factor in the global burden of disease, and without innovative, transdisciplinary strategies, it is unlikely the world will meet the United Nation's first Millennium Development Goal of eradicating extreme poverty and hunger in the coming decades. This chapter illustrates the application of transdisciplinary concepts discussed by Stokols et al. in chapter 1 and provides a pedagogical approach to transdisciplinary problem solving (TPS), with the aim of motivating new ideas to significantly boost the trajectory of positive change. Its global dimension presents an opportunity both to operate in a space generally open to diversity and to find ways to address the added complexity arising from cultural, socioeconomic, and political differences across nations. The content is organized to present the rationale for applying a TPS framework to the problems of hunger and undernutrition; introduce a pedagogical approach for a graduate-level course, "TPS Global Hunger and Undernutrition," on this issue; review the critical disciplines that should serve as a foundation to TPS in hunger and undernutrition; describe three TPS working groups (in research, programming, and policy); and provide assessment methods that may be applied to critically evaluate the performance of students in the TPS course.

Worldwide, it is estimated that 925 million people are hungry, a figure now down from the startling 1.023 billion reached in 2009 after the food price crisis.[1] Prevalence of undernutrition is also unacceptably high. Nearly one-third (32 percent) of children less than five years old are stunted, and one-fifth (20 percent) are underweight. Underweight is the leading risk factor in all global burden of disease analyses, accounting for more disability-adjusted life-years (DALYs) than all other risk factors, while iron, zinc, and vitamin A deficiencies rank among the top twenty risk factors.[2] When these factors are combined, more than 10 percent of the entire global burden of disease is attributable to maternal and child undernutrition.[3]

The first part of this chapter addresses the closely linked issues of hunger and undernutrition, and the crucial nutrient intake gaps that can occur in populations and lead to serious public health consequences. Around the world, the problem is more prevalent in resource-poor populations living in developing countries, but it can also affect groups in middle- and high-income nations. The term *global* in this chapter refers to a community of societies engaging in complex interactions as they deal with similar problems and, ideally, share solutions.[4] One of the expressed tenets of global health is that it is *interdisciplinary*; it is conceptualized as a field in which many disciplines, such as biomedicine, behavioral science, economics, engineering, environmental science, history, law, social work, and public policy are coming together to provide solutions across the prevention, treatment, and care spectrum.[4]

Hunger has many definitions and must be interpreted according to context. The *gaajo* hunger experienced by a family fleeing the drought and famine of Somalia is profoundly different from the hunger one might feel in the morning before breakfast. Generally, hunger is understood to be simply the "feeling of discomfort associated with lack of food."[5] The official definition of hunger from the Food and Agriculture Organization (FAO) of the United Nations (UN) is consumption of fewer than 1,800 kilocalories a day, the minimum required to live a healthy and productive life. Hunger is often connected to the concept of *food insecurity*, which incorporates concepts of food availability, access, and utilization. In 1990, the US Agency for International Development (USAID) defined *food security* in these terms: "When all people at all times have both physical and economic access to sufficient food to meet their dietary needs for a productive and healthy life."[6] Undernutrition, by contrast, tends to have more precise definitions and indicators. *Undernutrition* signifies deficiencies in macronutrients or micronutrients, or both, and should not be confused with *malnutrition*, which includes both under- and overnutrition problems. Anthropometric markers are often used to indicate undernutrition; these markers include the classifications *underweight*, *stunting*, and *wasting*.

Brief History

The concept of using multidisciplinary approaches in the field of undernutrition has been appreciated for many years. Since the early 1970s, efforts have been made to bring different sectors to the table in order to tackle the issues of global hunger and undernutrition. Agricultural and health disciplines in particular have been visible and active in many developing countries, though there have been others from the education, gender, and finance sectors. During this earlier period, the primary focus was on the problem of protein-energy malnutrition (PEM), with a consensus that PEM arose from many different socioeconomic and biological conditions. The international community also recognized that the response had to be multifaceted and comprehensive in order to be effective.[7] This was supported by growing evidence linking nutrition and development as mutually reinforcing conditions.

The desired multidisciplinary action, however, was not realized. The challenges and lessons learned during this time should inform TPS approaches moving forward. The multisectoral strategy quickly became cumbersome and too complicated to put into action. The goals were ambitious and the solutions radical and untested. Organizationally, the strategies were collaborative to the point where leadership was lacking and action oversight absent. Finally, there was a political and economic naïveté in the movement, a lack of awareness regarding national priorities and sources of power and wealth. In several countries, multisectoral planning units were created that were separate from mainstream ministries but that lacked sufficient political or regulatory clout. Some of these quasi-state agencies exist today, still with little leverage.

Beginning with the FAO's World Food Conference in 1974, the global community convened several high-profile summits and conferences to declare its commitment to eradicating the problems of hunger and undernutrition. Lofty goals and recommendations have resulted, and indeed, progress has been made, in large part related to the economic development of nations. At the turn of the millennium, world leaders gathered to agree on eight noble Millennium Development Goals (MDGs) to be attained by the year 2015. The first of these goals is to "eradicate extreme poverty and hunger," with the target to "halve, between 1990 and 2015, the proportion of people who suffer from hunger." After one decade, the UN released a report on the progress made toward attaining the MDGs.[8] It showed that from 1990 to 2002, the share of undernourished populations decreased from 20 percent to 16 percent globally, but unfortunately, progress was stalled by the recent food and financial crises.[1] The undernutrition problem in some countries has worsened, and in other countries has simply remained unchanged. There is a need to reenergize and rethink both the problem and the solution to these issues.

Conceptual Framework

In 1990, UNICEF published an important and enduring conceptual framework on the causes of undernutrition. This framework has been modified slightly and adapted over the last two decades, but remains similar to its original content (figure 12.1). Distal determinants are shown at the base, underlying the more proximal and immediate causes of the core problems of maternal and child undernutrition. Throughout the framework, one encounters factors ranging from cells to society and cutting across different disciplines. Solutions to the problem have, however, with only a few exceptions, focused on single factors. The underlying and basic causes are most often neglected or passively left for others to solve. Few nutrition programs have incorporated the spectrum of causes or proactively ensured multiple factors are addressed. This UNICEF conceptual framework may serve as the basis for problem-solution analyses but requires new thinking from a transdisciplinary perspective.

Hunger and undernutrition contribute significantly to the global burden of disease and mortality, exacerbated in recent years by the food and financial crises. While the international nutrition community has long acknowledged the importance of a *multisectoral* approach, there is a pressing need to further embrace transdisciplinary science for problem definition and solutions. The following sections of this chapter present a pedagogical approach to instructing public health graduate students on the application of TPS. Progress toward attaining the first MDG and alleviating hunger and undernutrition depends on training public health practitioners to use the TPS scaffolding to find appropriate solutions.

Content and Application of TPS Approaches

The remainder of this chapter presents a method of instruction for conveying and applying transdisciplinary problem solving core concepts to the issues of

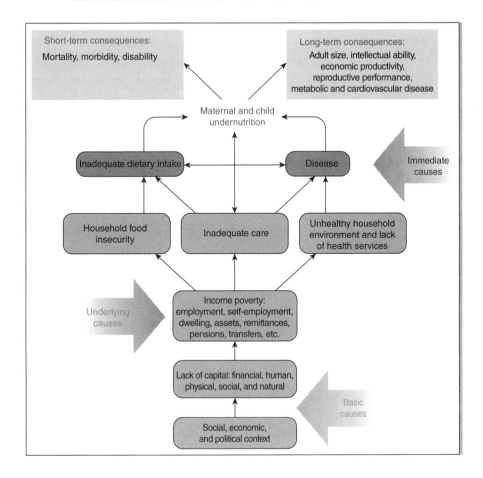

Figure 12.1. Maternal and child undernutrition
Source: R. E. Black et al., "Maternal and Child Undernutrition: Global and Regional Exposures and Health Consequences," *The Lancet*, 2008;371(9608):244.

global hunger and undernutrition. The course is designed to motivate novel ways of thinking about and characterizing the problem, and practical, creative approaches to solving it. The global aspect of the topic further justifies TPS and its nimble application in a variety of contexts and cultures.

Building on the processes described in chapter 1 by Stokols et al., this course addresses two domains of the problem-solution analysis cycle: the *disciplinary integration domain*, presented through a series of lectures and labs, and the *action translation domain*, embodied in student group work. Lectures cover foundational issues in undernutrition from biochemistry to infectious disease epidemiology to agronomy and the political economy of hunger and undernutrition. Each topic, however, is presented juxtaposed with other disciplines and overlaid with a matrix of vertically and horizontally integrated concepts. Vertically, issues are examined from molecular to intrapersonal, organizational to community, and ultimately, societal to global levels. Horizontally, traditional disciplines concerned with hunger and undernutrition are woven into the foundational topics. The fusion of methods and disciplines should elicit lively discussions and new ideas. Labs and case studies are interspersed throughout the course, as either in-class exercises or take-home activities, to reinforce concepts and the practical application of TPS, as emphasized in chapter 1 of this volume.

The group work on applying TPS, described in the second major part of this section, occurs throughout the course. Students self-select into one of three TPS working groups: a research group, a programming group, and a policy group. This decision may be made in consideration of career interests, capabilities, or practical reasons. Cross-cutting themes considered by the members of each group are the distinct role their group's domain plays in global hunger and undernutrition; the actual players in this domain; and the strategies and tools applied, including programming and policy models, funding resources, and communication and dissemination strategies. Periodically, plenary discussions are held, or students are mixed into groups other than their own to share ideas. Throughout the course, each group works through the phases of a TPS initiative—development, conceptualization, implementation, and translation. This work culminates in a group paper and presentation on using TPS to address global hunger and undernutrition.

Disciplinary Integration

A series of important issues and fundamental concepts pertaining to global hunger and malnutrition are covered—again, these are positioned horizontally in relation to various disciplines and vertically from molecular to societal and global levels. Each topic relates to both problem and solution analyses and may be covered using a variety of instruction techniques, including lectures, debates and discussions, case studies, labs, and field visits.

Biochemistry Basics of Nutrient Deficiencies

Nutrition has been defined as the process by which an organism uses food or anything ingested through digestion, absorption, transport, storage, or elimination for the purposes of growth, reproduction, and maintenance of health and normal functioning.[9] Beginning at the molecular and cellular levels, students are introduced to essential macro- and micronutrient nutrients and key pathways in nutrition metabolism.[10] Some basic anatomy and physiology of the digestive system is given as a prelude to the discussion of the pathology of particular nutrient deficiencies. Emphasis is placed on problem nutrients, those deficient in resource-poor populations, with discussion of the full spectrum of determinants. Macronutrients are briefly covered, in 3 groupings: (1) carbohydrates, energy, and PEM; (2) proteins and nitrogen balance; and (3) lipids, focusing particularly on risks associated with a dietary imbalance of linoleic and alpha-linolenic fatty acids.[11] In this session, a brief overview is offered of water- and fat-soluble vitamins, macro- and microminerals, and ultratrace elements, emphasizing those known to be deficient with health consequences around the world: Vitamin A, Vitamin B_{12}, folate, iodine, iron, and zinc.

Lab Idea 1: Hunger fast

This lab is suggested for early in the course. Students (those without health conditions that would preclude participation) are asked to skip meals or fast for 8 to 12 hours during a twenty-four-hour period. Students then reflect on and discuss in groups how they felt physically and mentally, what effects they observed in their own bodies, and which metabolic processes may have been perturbed. They will be asked to speculate on a more chronic deprivation of food and nutrients and the potential effects.

Evolution and the Genetics of Undernutrition

The last decade has seen rapid advances in the field of genetics with the sequencing of the human genome and launching of the International HapMap Project. Important insights into genetic variability across populations and gene-environment interactions have emerged. Nutrition is an important environmental exposure that is also influenced by differing genotypes. This interplay has yet to be studied extensively in developing countries despite the potentially important implications for intervening with sudden changes in nutrient intakes (with micronutrient supplementation, for example) or understanding the rapidly changing dietary trends across the globe. The thrifty genotype hypothesis is one area that is being explored carefully with regard to chronic disease and nutrition in developing countries.[12] Hemoglobinopathies are another example of a potentially important genetic issue related to nutrition, specifically iron metabolism.[13]

This session introduces students to the fields of nutrigenetics and nutrigenomics, with discussion of the health consequences arising from genetic variation in combination with changing nutrition exposures.[14] The session also discusses nutrition in the contexts of evolution and adaptation and of ideas proposed with regard to Paleolithic nutrition.[15]

Lab Idea 2: The musical rest metaphor

Students who can play musical instruments are asked to volunteer to prepare a short piece or segment of music. Then, in class, they are asked to play the music twice, once as written and once without any rests. Students then discuss the differences in the two versions, and ideally, come to the conclusion that the silences matter enormously for the overall musicality of the piece. The gaps, or "rests," in nutrition that can occur during particular "movements" in the life cycle and their consequences are then discussed. This music tempo metaphor might be extended to other aspects of nutrition biology, such as the rhythms of growth velocity.

Undernutrition in the Life Cycle

This session covers nutrition in various periods of the lifecycle: periconception and fetal, pregnancy and lactation, infancy and early childhood, school-age, adolescent, adult (people of reproductive age), and elderly. The *nutrition throughout the life cycle* framework commonly referenced in the international nutrition community serves as a basis for this session.[16] Key findings and evidence for the transdisciplinary causes and consequences of undernutrition in different periods is covered. For example, the Dutch Famine studies examine the different outcomes associated with starvation exposure in varying trimesters of pregnancy.[17,18] Other research points to the critical importance of maternal nutrition.[19,20] A seminal study produced by Shrimpton et al. and using data from around the world illustrates the timing of growth faltering during infancy; it has now been updated with the World Health Organization (WHO) Child Growth Standards from 2006 and new data.[21,22] The long-term consequences of early undernutrition exposure on attained adult height, schooling, income, and offspring birth weight are also reviewed.[23] Program models addressing undernutrition in different life cycle periods (table 12.1) are reviewed and critiqued using a TPS perspective.[24]

Nutrition Assessment and Surveillance

This session covers existing state-of-the-art and field-friendly markers of undernutrition but also extends further into discussion of new transdisciplinary indicators that might be introduced into nutrition surveillance efforts around the world. Three assessment types are presented: anthropometry, dietary intakes, and biomarkers. First, the WHO Child Growth Standards and their

Table 12.1. Examples of program types for addressing undernutrition

Program type	Brief description	Disciplines represented
Behavior change communication (BCC)	BCC is a form of nutrition education that involves communication, dialogue, and negotiation with caregivers to improve a health behavior, often an infant-feeding practice. Communication may occur at the interpersonal, group, or population level.	Communication Anthropology
Child survival (CS)	CS programs, originating from USAID, typically include a nutrition intervention, such as BCC or micronutrient supplementation, combined with one or two other child survival interventions, such as vaccinations, improved hygiene and sanitation, insecticide-treated bed nets, and so forth.	Public health Infectious disease
Conditional cash transfer (CCT)	CCT programs transfer cash or other resources as an incentive to modify behaviors such as use of preventative health care services (antenatal or well-baby care), school enrollment and attendance, or purchase of better-quality foods.	Economics Public health Education
Facility- and community-based management of severe acute malnutrition (SAM)	Facility-based care of SAM supplements the hospitalized malnourished individual, often with specially designed milks, and treats infections. Community-based care of SAM typically provides ready-to-use therapeutic foods (lipid-based supplements), rather than milks, until recovery.	Medicine
Food fortification	Foods are fortified with critical micronutrients found to be deficient in populations. Examples include salt iodization, sugar fortified with vitamin A, and wheat fortified with folic acid, iron, or other nutrients. Biofortification involves breeding plants to increase particular micronutrient content (for example, orange-fleshed sweet potatoes with Vitamin A).	Food industry Public health Agriculture

(Continued)

Table 12.1. (*Continued*)

Program type	Brief description	Disciplines represented
Growth monitoring and promotion (GMP)	GMP programs typically involve the monitoring over time of young children's growth, weight, and height. Health workers collect and plot measures on growth reference, or standard, curves. The promotion occurs as health workers provide feedback and advice to caregivers on their child's nutrition.	Public health Communication
Homestead food production	Village model farms (VMFs) are developed with gardening and small livestock production. Community members then draw on the VMFs for food they produce and nutrition education. BCC is becoming increasingly integral to this model.	Agriculture Economics Public health Communication
Micronutrient supplementation	Micronutrient supplements (Vitamin A, iron and folate, zinc, or multiple micronutrients) are provided to vulnerable populations in particular time intervals.	Public health Epidemiology
Positive deviance/ Hearth	PD/Hearth identifies children who are growing well in a community despite its poor conditions. Lessons are gleaned from their families about particular health practices and the child's diet, and these findings are then incorporated into a two-week-long hearth session for those mothers whose children are undernourished and not growing as well.	Anthropology Communication

history, rationale, and departure from the US National Center for Health Statistics/WHO growth reference curves is explained.[25] Students may be trained on how to measure height and length, weight, and mid-upper arm circumference (MUAC) in the measuring anthropometry lab (see Lab Idea 3).[26] There is a brief introduction to body composition markers, including the use of bio-electrical impedance and skinfold measures. Second, dietary intake measures are covered: twenty-four-hour recalls, food frequency questionnaires, household consumption surveys, and other markers of frequency of consumption and dietary diversity.[27] And finally, an overview of biomarkers for key micro-nutrients is given.[28] Some Vitamin A markers are serum retinol, breast milk retinol, night blindness, and relative dose response. For iron, some markers are serum ferritin, soluble transferrin receptor, hemoglobin concentration, hematocrit, and mean cell volume. Serum or plasma zinc concentration is checked for zinc, and urinary iodine for iodine. To conclude the lecture, the programming, policy, and research uses of nutrition assessment are discussed in terms of targeting, monitoring, and evaluation.

Lab Idea 3: Measuring anthropometry

Students planning to pursue careers in international public health are likely to encounter anthropometric concepts in the literature, programming, policy, or grant writing for that field. Nutrition is related to many important infectious and chronic diseases. Those intending to work directly in nutrition or hunger field positions will also be likely to require practical measurement skills. This lab introduces students to internationally recognized protocols for measuring height, weight, and MUAC.

The nine-step protocol for length and fifteen-step protocol for height measures are first reviewed, along with protocols for weight and MUAC. Students first practice using dolls and each other, and then young children might be brought in as available. Validation and reliability exercises may be applied. It is recommended that students be trained to use Shorr-Board® or similar stadiometers to the nearest millimeter; the Seca or similar digital scales, with instruction on the mother-child function and procedures; and circumference tapes for MUAC.

Epidemiology and Spatial Aspects of Undernutrition

Building on the previous assessment session, this session covers the epidemiology of hunger and undernutrition, drawing on such disciplines as environmental health, urban planning, and demography. Findings from the *Lancet* series on maternal and child undernutrition form the basis of this session (see, for example, Black et al.[3]). Students are introduced to methods applied by the global burden of disease project to calculate the disease burden imposed by nutrition factors. Estimations of risk for cause-specific mortality and population attributable fractions for calculating the proportional reductions in mortality and DALYs associated with addressing various nutrition conditions are presented. The Global Hunger Index is defined and critiqued,[5] along with methods for estimating global hunger prevalence by using food balance sheets produced by the FAO. The Famine Early Warning System Network (FEWS NET) of USAID and multiple tools for monitoring determinants of famine, such as agro-climate, markets, and livelihoods, are introduced. Finally, new technologies and methods using geographic information systems (GIS) for monitoring and surveillance are discussed.

Nutrition's Contribution to Infectious Disease

Pivotal findings linking undernutrition to child mortality were published in 1995 and led to important policy impacts.[29] The study showed that 53 percent of all childhood deaths in developing countries were attributable to undernutrition, and although this percentage has since been lowered to 35 percent, the study elevated the profile of nutrition internationally. Undernutrition leads to impaired immune functioning, primarily through cell-mediated immunity. Epidemiological studies reinforce this by showing that it is undernutrition that increases duration of illness and case fatality rates, rather than new or repeated infection episodes. This session presents the evidence base for the links between undernutrition and such major infectious diseases as diarrhea, respiratory infection, malaria, helminthes, HIV/AIDS, and tuberculosis. Diarrheal disease, or environmental enteropathy, is particularly emphasized due to the known synergies with infant feeding practices, growth, and zinc nutrition. The WHO recommends that zinc supplements be provided together with oral rehydration therapy (ORT) to shorten duration of diarrhea and increase stool volume. TPS solutions to the nutrition and infectious disease problem are especially important to highlight in this session. Hand washing, improved access to and use of toilets, and water treatment are examples of infectious disease preventive practices that might be promoted, together with nutrition strategies such as improving infant feeding practices.[30]

Community-Based Approaches to SAM

Severe acute malnutrition (SAM), defined as an extremely low weight-for-height z-score (WHZ) of < -3, can have a case fatality rate of 30 to 50 percent.[31] Globally, fifty-five million children are wasted, with WHZs of < -2. While this course places a higher priority on deriving public health solutions that prevent undernutrition, there is an unquestionable need to treat these children. Improved identification and management of SAM in hospitals and communities can reduce case fatality by over one-half. This session covers assessment and identification of different forms of SAM, including *marasmus* and *kwashiorkor*. It overviews inpatient and community-based care algorithms and the latest evidence for various therapeutic measures and feeding regimens. Community management of SAM is given special regard owing to the advent of ready-to-use therapeutic food (RUTF), though students should be challenged to think more broadly about interventions extending beyond the food. Discussion of the evidence base for these foods and the issues of patents and local production are also part of the session.

Anthropology and Food Culture

In the global context especially, an anthropological perspective is essential for addressing undernutrition and hunger. The large differences that exist among populations in food choice and diet often arise from cultural norms and practices. Without deep understanding of the ethnographic and ecological factors in play, positive change is unlikely to occur. In this session, the major work of nutritional anthropologists is covered, including evidence from the Marshall Islands and Nepal.[32–35] Methods for exploring cultural and anthropological factors are reviewed, such as in-depth interviews, focus groups, and participant observation. The information gathered should inform programs, policies, and, in particular, the communication strategies addressed in the subsequent session. In this session, examples of vertical integration may be particularly useful, where basic scientists and social scientists have actively collaborated in research, for instance.

Lab Idea 4: Culture and *Hungry Planet*

The photographic essay *Hungry Planet: What the World Eats*,[36] is viewed by the students. Groups debate and compile observations on the differences arising from culture, environment, economics, or other influences. Questions might be posed about aspects of the diet that might be learned and passed on. What is shared, symbolic, systematic, or patterned in the various diets? Finally, if any of the students speak other languages, they might provide insight into aspects of a country's diet that are embodied in its language.

Communicating for Improved Health Behaviors

There has been consensus since the 1990s in the international nutrition community that the program model known as behavior change communication (BCC) is an effective approach to improving infant and young child feeding practices (see figure 12.2).[37,38] The BCC model lays out a systematic process of formative research to, first, understand health behaviors and, second, identify the barriers and opportunities for change. Next, a strategy that incorporates appropriate messages, negotiation tactics, and various context-specific communication channels is designed, implemented, and evaluated. Other more general communication principles and theories[39] are presented in this session and also global experiences with social marketing for nutrition.[40] The Essential Nutrition Action (ENA) program model and strategy may be discussed, with emphasis on the effective use of multiple levels of communication and media types. At the interpersonal level, counseling and some more innovative approaches, such as use of video narratives and mobile phones, are examined. Mass media, including radio and television and social marketing, are reviewed at the population level. Various visual and audio examples of different forms of communication are integrated into the lecture. Examples from a Population Services International (PSI) project in Kenya or the Academy for Educational Development's LINKAGES Project in Ethiopia and Madagascar may be presented.

Lab idea 5: Nutributter® packaging

The France-based company Nutriset recently released new packaging for its Nutributter® product. This ready-to-eat supplemental food, containing peanut butter, milk powder, vegetable oil, sugar, and micronutrient fortificants, is intended for use in the prevention of undernutrition among children aged six to twenty-four months. Nutributter is packaged in 20 gram sachets, the usual daily dosage for children. It can be stored at room temperature and is generally resistant to microbial contamination if covered. The new packaging comes in an array of colors and with a variety of images of positive young child feeding practices, such as breast-feeding.

In small groups, students critique the new packaging from a TPS perspective. They should discuss the visual images, colors, and text for appropriate messaging about young child nutrition and use of the food.

Source: Adapted from the Nutriset website, www.nutriset.fr/en/product-range/produit-par-produit/nutributter.html.

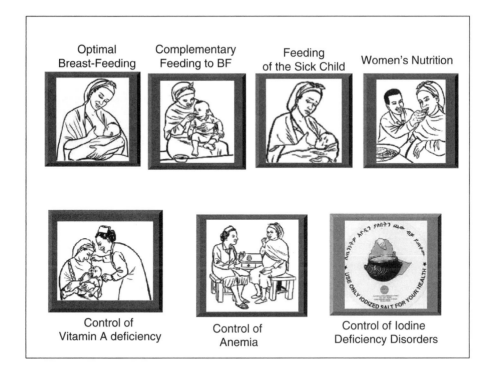

Figure 12.2. BCC messages
Source: LINKAGES/Ethiopia, *2003–2006 Final Report* (Washington, DC: Academy for Educational Development; n.d.). © by LINKAGES and JSI (John Snow Inc.).

New Models of Agriculture for Improved Nutrition

The agriculture sector should be closely linked to nutrition through the obvious connection of food production for consumption. In reality, these two sectors often display significant differences in objectives and approaches to hunger alleviation. Improving population nutrition often falls under the domain of ministries of health, with little or no interaction with the ministries of agriculture. In recent years, the food price crisis has directed more attention to the intersection of the two sectors. This session presents the history and evolution of the interplay between agriculture, hunger, and undernutrition. Frameworks and evidence emanating from a recent, high-level, international conference, *Leveraging Agriculture for Improving Nutrition and Health*, are given, including a framework from the impact evaluation of KickStart International's irrigation pump program in East Africa (figure 12.3).

Three key strategies that link agriculture and nutrition concerns are covered, highlighting TPS elements that could address gaps in each model:

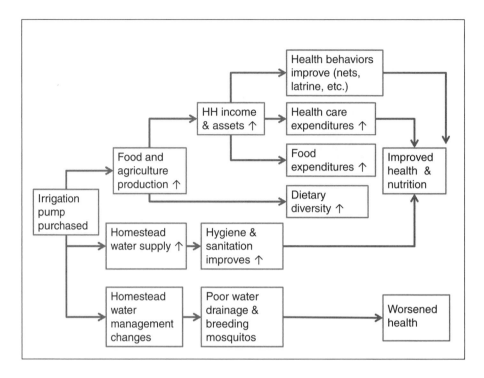

Figure 12.3. KickStart irrigation pump effects on nutrition and health

Note: HH = household.

Source: L. Iannotti, paper presented at "Health & Nutrition in the KickStart Impact Evaluation: Leveraging Agriculture to Improve Nutrition and Health," Ministerial International Conference sponsored by International Food Policy Research Institute and others; February 2011; New Delhi.

biofortification, homestead food production (HFP) programming, and food aid. Biofortification is the process of selecting and breeding crop varieties that have a high vitamin and mineral content and that also have valued agronomic qualities. Evidence now shows that biofortified orange-fleshed sweet potatoes positively affect Vitamin A nutrition.[41] HFP, the subject of a case study by the global Millions Fed research project,[42] and other forms of home gardening and small livestock promotion projects aimed at reducing undernutrition are covered. Finally, this session also reviews issues in food aid and the competing and overlapping agricultural and nutritional objectives that exist in this area.

Leveraging Political Economy for Household Nutrition

The UNICEF conceptual framework (see figure 12.1) illustrates the root cause of maternal and child undernutrition as the social, economic, and political context, which leads to income poverty. While the conditions forming this context are often part of the problem definition, solutions to undernutrition largely neglect these distal factors and leave them to other forces of change. In this session, a case is made for elevating and integrating both micro- and macroeconomic determinants and related political factors more systematically into TPS strategies for undernutrition. The debate in the international nutrition community has narrowly focused on how gross domestic product (GDP) per capita relates to nutrition indicators and how country outliers justify behavioral interventions.[43] In the economics literature, studies often center around the income-energy relationship, without regard to micronutrient nutrition and broader behavioral issues.[44] Recent work on the food price crisis is beginning to explore some of these impacts.[45] Finally, this session addresses the role of markets and distribution systems in driving nutrition inequities. International trade practices and country-level infrastructure and policies are discussed.

The limited repertoire of existing solutions is presented through discussion on the ways that TPS might expand the options for overcoming or even mobilizing the political economy of undernutrition and hunger. The mixed findings for conditional cash transfer programs (described in table 12.1) in Mexico, Colombia, Brazil, and other countries are covered.[46–48] Other strategies aimed at microenterprise development and increasing productive assets and wealth are also discussed.

Engineering a Safer Environment for Nutrition

Water is essential for human health and is a factor in many of the varied pathways to undernutrition: water is needed for agriculture and food production, water quality and quantity are related to infection, and even the energy expenditure to access water can be a factor. Sanitation and hygiene conditions are also closely linked to nutrition, primarily through infectious diseases associated with the fecal-oral route of transmission. Each year, 1.4 million children die from diarrhea.[49] Issues with the water source, storage, and sanitation conditions have been shown to increase the risk of height deficits and diarrheal episodes.[50,51] This session examines the problem and potential solutions for undernutrition as viewed from the engineering and environmental disciplines, integral to other disciplinary approaches: access to clean water, toilet type and sanitation facilities, and hygiene practices such as hand washing.

Action Translation

As described previously, throughout the course and in tandem with the disciplinary integration sessions, three "expert" TPS working groups, focusing on the domains of research, programming, and policy, put into operation the TPS phases of development, conceptualization, implementation, and translation.

These working groups mimic the real-life situation in which experts from multiple disciplines are convened to make recommendations about a particular public health problem. Students work within and across groups to issue a final paper outlining the problem and solution recommendations in a transdisciplinary framework. Because the students initially self-select into one of the three groups, it may become necessary to rearrange group membership to equalize and balance the working groups.

A particular issue within the larger hunger and undernutrition problem is selected by the instructor. For the sake of example, the problem of undernutrition during a young child's complementary feeding (CF) period is presented here. The *complementary feeding period*, generally occurring from six to twenty-four months of age, is the time when other foods are introduced into the child's diet, along with continued breast-feeding, to sustain health and growth. In developing countries, it is a highly vulnerable period when children are at greatest risk for infectious disease morbidities, growth faltering, micronutrient deficiencies, and developmental delays with lifelong consequences. The CF issue continues to be one of the most complicated and intractable of the undernutrition issues that exist globally. It is an ideal problem for sorting through with a transdisciplinary framework in that it demands consideration across the full spectrum of disciplines from molecular to societal levels and will remain unsolved without holistic, comprehensive approaches.

The title of this course, "TPS Global Hunger and Undernutrition," contains the word *global* because one of the course assumptions is that students will work or think beyond the borders of their home country. This aspect of the course makes practice in using TPS even more imperative so that students can in later years more fully understand and define problems and solutions across different societies. The global dimension may actually facilitate the use of TPS by encouraging and sometimes necessitating cross-fertilization and learning in different contexts. Further, practitioners often find a general openness to new ideas and approaches in international collaborative relationships. However, there is also tremendous complexity when individuals speaking different languages and coming from varied cultures and histories work together to derive solutions to the nutrition problem. Students in this course must consider these issues and develop processes to both take advantage of opportunities and overcome barriers in the global arena.

For the group work project, it is suggested that one country be selected for application of TPS—drawing on global programs, policies, and research. This is a common scenario in international nutrition work; countries plan and implement at the national level with inputs from the global level. In this example, the country selected is Tanzania, where the prevalence of stunting for children less than five years of age is 44 percent, of underweight 22 percent, and of wasting 4 percent.[24,25,52,53] The following subsections describe the efforts of each of the TPS working groups.

Research TPS Working Group

The students in this group take the role of the scientists whose task is to synthesize the existing evidence base and generate new knowledge. They are "thinkers," with translation as an important objective. In the community of individuals working on global undernutrition and hunger, these experts would represent universities, research institutions, and think tanks. The students in this group will become familiar with important research clusters specializing in hunger and undernutrition.

Various strategies and tools are explored and applied in this TPS working group. Meta-analyses and systematic reviews are examined first in the search for evidence relevant to the problem and solution of, in this case, CF. Next, students might compile findings from basic science, clinical trials, randomized controlled trials, and field-based effectiveness studies. Searches should be conducted across different disciplinary databases—health, anthropology, economics, politics, and so forth. Methodological pluralism (see chapter 1) is encouraged through application of TPS methods. In addition to the literature review, students develop causal theory frameworks reflecting TPS. Demographic and health surveys (DHS) and data may be downloaded from Measure DHS and explored carefully for risk factors of undernutrition.[54] Students are instructed on how to generate the HAZ (height-for-age z-score), WAZ (weight-for-age z-score), and WHZ. Depending on students' skill level in quantitative work, regression models may be built, with different transdisciplinary factors to demonstrate the greater explanatory power resulting from TPS. Qualitative methods such as in-depth interviews, focus group discussions, direct observations, and ethnographic studies may be examined as methods for better understanding contributing factors to undernutrition.

Like the other working groups, the research working group will attempt to identify possible funding sources for their work and will discuss communications and dissemination strategies. The primary international and national conferences where those working in undernutrition and hunger convene are identified as well as key peer-reviewed journals and other important places for publication of research findings.

Programming TPS Working Group

The students in this group take on the role of expert practitioners who plan, implement, and evaluate programs to address undernutrition and hunger. They are "doers," those committed to effecting change on the ground. In the world outside the classroom, the experts in this group would represent three broad groups of organizations. The first consists of nongovernmental organizations (NGOs) and nonprofit organizations, such as CARE, Catholic Relief Services, Helen Keller International, Save the Children, and World Vision. These NGOs and nonprofits have years of experience working on undernutrition by applying various models, though few of these models might be described as TPS. Second, the working group would also include representatives from private sector organizations involved in the food and nutrition industry, such as Nestlé, Procter & Gamble, and Cargill. The third and final set of experts would be representatives of social enterprise organizations, a relatively new category of endeavor that which blends the for-profit approach with an NGO agenda. These organizations might apply a market-driven business model to achieve social development objectives, for example. In this TPS course, several examples are given. The France-based company Nutriset is a successful social enterprise committed to work on undernutrition. Nutriset, along with its many franchises such as Meds and Food for Kids and Edesia, manufactures ready-to-use therapeutic and supplemental foods, such as Plumpy'Nut®, for treating and preventing undernutrition. Other social enterprise players cited in the class are KickStart International and Population Services International.

The programming TPS working group has several existing strategies and tools to incorporate into its transdisciplinary problem solving. To begin with, such expert groups commonly use a logic model approach (figure 12.4). Frameworks such as the log frame or theory of change may also be used, but their basic structure tends to be similar.[55] As described later, this programming group will overlay the TPS framework on the logic model to ensure that disciplines are represented and integrated through the various input, output, outcome, and impact pathways. Multiple program models are also available to draw on for TPS work (as outlined in table 12.1). Some of these models are more comprehensive than others, striving to address two or more determinants of undernutrition. For example, the HFP program in Bangladesh and other countries has incorporated food production, improved income, and more recently, health sector linkages.[42] USAID child survival programming generally addresses immunizations, nutrition, diarrheal disease, pneumonia, malaria, maternal and newborn care, HIV/AIDS, and tuberculosis, though grants are generally dispersed in a few selected technical areas.[56] Tanzania is a particularly interesting country in terms of nutrition programming. The Iringa Nutrition Project is a famous, large-scale community nutrition program often cited in the global nutrition community. The project was initiated in 1984 by the government of Tanzania and UNICEF and expanded from 168 to 620 villages over its lifespan. Over the years, its approaches and mediocre successes have been debated.[57]

Process components   Outcome components

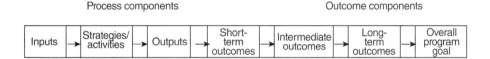

Figure 12.4. CDC logic model components
Source: Adapted from Centers for Disease Control and Prevention, "Logic Model Basics," *Evaluation Briefs*, December 2008; No. 2.

Students in this working group identify potential funding mechanisms for their TPS solutions and strategize about how best to communicate and disseminate their TPS program model and evaluation results for replication, sustainability, and scaling-up purposes. These purposes might be accomplished through conferences like the Global Health Conference, written materials, or media and online strategies such as websites or blogs.

Policy TPS Working Group

The students in this group take on the role of experts working on policies to address the problems of hunger and undernutrition. They are the stewards of nutrition planning, regulation, norms, and standards. In a working group outside the classroom, they would be policymakers in the public sector from multiple levels: national, state, and district. Ministries of agriculture, health, finance, and gender would be represented. Agencies or think tanks with policy agendas would also be represented. UN, multilateral, and bilateral agencies would be among the major policy players.

As is the case with the other two action domains, this expert group may draw on several existing policies and tools for building its TPS agenda. In the past two decades, several important international conferences have been held to set the stage and generate momentum and direction in policymaking for undernutrition and hunger. In 1992, the International Conference on Nutrition was held in Rome, Italy; representatives of the attending countries pledged to establish multisectoral working groups and National Plans of Action for Nutrition (NPANs). Students should consider successes and failures from this conference, using the TPS lens. The Millennium Development Goals in particular should be a focus of this expert working group, and especially the progress made toward attaining the first MDG—"eradicate extreme poverty and hunger"—and Target 1C—"halve between 1990 and 2015, the proportion of people who suffer from hunger."

Specific to the set TPS problem of nutrition during the complementary feeding period, students focus on international policies pertaining to young child feeding practices and nutrition. In 2003, the WHO and UNICEF released the report *Global Strategy for Infant and Young Child Feeding*.[24] The policy presented in this report arose from a two-year participatory process with experts from around the world. Other important strategies and information that should serve as the basis for future TPS policies can be found in the International Code of Marketing of Breast-Milk Substitutes; the Baby-Friendly Hospital Initiative (BFHI); the Innocenti Declaration, *On the Protection, Promotion and Support of Breastfeeding*; and *Codex Alimentarius: FAO/WHO Food Standards*. Finally, if the course is held in the fall, World Food Day, held annually on October 16, is an excellent opportunity for students in this group and others to practice developing a TPS campaign that mobilizes action and raises awareness of the problems of undernutrition and hunger.[58]

Students should also consider national-level policies with large-scale nutrition impacts, such as agriculture subsidies and trade policies, food price adjustments, and efforts to regulate food safety and fortification, among others. Policy action tools are available to be explored. Students can use the RAPID Outcome Mapping Approach of the Overseas Development Institute (ODI) to facilitate stakeholder identification and influence. They can plot individual policymakers identified as particularly influential on the Alignment, Interest and Influence Matrix (AIIM) to plan for policy impact.[59] The PROFILES project, launched in 1993 by the Academy for Educational Development, provides software for computer-based modeling to generate figures on the consequences of undernutrition in different country contexts and cost-benefit analyses of varying interventions.[38] The TPS approach might be introduced to PROFILES. As in the other working groups, identifying sources for funding policy action is necessary here; funding might potentially come from government financing mechanisms, bilateral agencies, multilateral agencies, or foundations. Communication and dissemination strategies are integral to policy impact from the outset and at all levels.

Evaluation Methods

Assessment methods selected for this TPS course should be designed to simultaneously help students achieve the learning objectives of the course and prepare for transdisciplinary problem solving in the real-world community of global hunger and undernutrition. The methods suggested in this section will assist in evaluating student performance with respect to both the class learning objectives and the TPS core concepts. Students should complete this TPS course uniquely trained to generate comparable products, often expected in global health work, with an innovative transdisciplinary angle. Grading criteria for the various TPS assignments may include features drawn from a TPS framework: terminology and language emanating from various disciplines, integrated theories, and combined methodologies and tools, among others.

Transdisciplinary Problem Analysis

Among the first steps in the application of TPS is a thorough analysis of the broad set of factors potentially influencing the public health problem. Literature reviews and primary data collection and analyses may be involved, the challenge being to search for evidence across multiple science and practice disciplines. This process should lead to the identification and weighing of factors, from cells to society, in the causal pathways to the public health problem. One evaluation method that might be used early in the "TPS Global Hunger and Undernutrition" course involves the problem analysis in which students individually begin to delve into a particular aspect of the problem using the TPS framework. For example, students may be asked to analyze the problem of undernutrition during the complementary feeding period of six to twenty-four months when children in developing countries are at highest risk for growth faltering and infectious disease with lifelong health and developmental consequences. This TPS problem analysis would describe the problem in terms of magnitude and severity and present a comprehensive analysis of risk factors and determinants across disciplines. Students would be expected to discuss the factors as operating independently or in interaction with others. As discussed above, the UNICEF conceptual framework (figure 12.1) could serve as a basis for new frameworks developed by the students during the TPS problem analysis that depict a broader array of factors. One country might be selected for in-depth analysis of the problem within its borders, but also examined in relation to the problem globally. In Tanzania, for example, key determinants of undernutrition in young children might be a low prevalence of exclusive breast-feeding due to strong cultural practices and limited awareness of its importance, poor quality complementary foods due to limited market access and high food prices, drought combined with dependence on rain-fed agriculture leading to reduced food production and income, a high prevalence of infectious disease morbidities, and the lack of access to safe drinking water.

Transdisciplinary Solution Analysis

Also among the TPS core concepts are capabilities related to developing public health solutions. These comprehensive, holistic solutions should reflect the transdisciplinary factor analysis described previously. Here, the challenge for students and practitioners is in finding TPS solutions that are also practical and feasible to implement. In this course, students may work toward developing solutions in their particular domain of research, programming, or policy. The solution analysis should integrate various disciplines and make the argument that application of TPS increases the likelihood of sustainability, replicability, and scaling up. Thus, continuing to use Tanzania as the selected country for problem analysis, students in the research working group might compile and summarize the evidence base in undernutrition research in Tanzania, from cells to society, and identify gaps in the TPS framework where there should be future research. Those in the programming working group might present an overview of past and present nutrition programs in Tanzania, identify deficits from a TPS perspective, and propose more optimal programming solutions. This group should incorporate a logic model reflecting strategies across different disciplines. Finally, students in the policy working group might discuss shortcomings and opportunities evident in the Tanzania National Plan of Action for Nutrition and in other policies in that country. These policies should be analyzed in relation to international norms and standards like those found in the BFHI, *Codex Alimentarius*, or the WHO Child Growth Standards. Students might also use the AIIM matrix to help with laying out a policy influence strategy. In all groups, key stakeholders are identified and communication and dissemination strategies outlined.

Consensus Building and Collaboration

The ability to communicate and collaborate with scientists and practitioners in different disciplines is pivotal to the success of TPS. The necessary skills may be enhanced in the classroom through a variety of approaches. Participation in plenary discussion and small-group work may be evaluated both by the instructor and by peers in the class. Working group evaluation forms have been used in TPS courses to allow students to evaluate other group members on preparation, contributions, respect for others' ideas, and flexibility. Reflections and written commentaries on assigned readings and take-home labs allow students to practice synthesizing material and better communicate ideas through writing.

In addition, group action projects may be used to further assess performance in the area of TPS consensus building and collaboration and also to evaluate problem and solution analyses. The research, programming, and policy working groups would collaborate to build on the individual TPS problem and solution efforts and produce a proposal for TPS action. Students would have to make a compelling case that the problem was inherently transdisciplinary and that the solution was comprehensive and integrative. The assignments and evaluation methods might take the form of papers and presentations that follow a typical proposal format: (1) background and rationale (the TPS problem analysis along with the new TPS conceptual framework), (2) goal and objectives, (3) strategies and activities, (4) monitoring and evaluation (the TPS solution analysis and the new logic model), and (5) conclusion and innovations. Key stakeholders, including scientists and practitioners, might be invited to participate and contribute to the evaluation of the group projects.

The evaluation methods for the course should ultimately aim to assess whether the student has understood and appropriately applied TPS core concepts, such as team building across disciplines; has proposed vertical and horizontal integration of disciplines; and has engaged in the development of new conceptual frameworks and TPS methods in relation to the assigned problem. The success of the course, the students, and ultimately TPS in operation relies on new standards of evaluation seeking integrative, imaginative ideas to solve the problems of hunger and undernutrition.

Summary

Hunger and undernutrition are leading risk factors in the global burden of disease and mortality; 925 million people around the world are food insecure, and nearly one-third of children less than five years old are stunted from undernutrition. Efforts to meet the first Millennium Development Goal, eradication of extreme poverty and hunger, have thus far been unsuccessful. As is the case with other public health challenges, undernutrition is a complex problem with an intricate web of causes. While there is consensus in the international nutrition community that multisectoral approaches are needed, transdisciplinary science and practice has yet to be embraced and applied by that community. This chapter has presented a pedagogical approach for instruction in transdisciplinary problem solving and the practical aspects of real-world application. With improved TPS capabilities across the domains of research, programming, and policy, students may be better equipped to combat this critical public health problem in the future.

Key Terms

anthropometry	The measurement of human body size and composition. The most common anthropometric measures are height (or length for children less than two years old), weight, mid-upper arm circumference (MUAC), waist circumference, and skinfold measures.
biofortification	The process of selecting and breeding crop varieties with high vitamin and mineral content that also have valued agronomic qualities.
macro- and micronutrients	Macronutrients are nutrients required in relatively large quantities and providing most of

the body's dietary energy: carbohydrates, proteins, and fats. Micronutrients are nutrients required in smaller quantities, including both vitamins and minerals.

protein-energy malnutrition (PEM)

Undernutrition arising from deficiencies in the macronutrients: carbohydrates, proteins, and fats. Globally, PEM is less prevalent than micronutrient deficiencies.

severe acute malnutrition (SAM)

Undernutrition characterized by an extremely low weight-for-height z-score (WHZ) of < -3. *Marasmus*, severe energy deficiency, and *kwashiorkor*, severe protein deficiency, are often associated with SAM.

stunting

A threshold indicator based on evidence for health effects in young children; defined as a height- or length-for-age z-score of < -2. Generally associated with chronic, long-term nutritional deprivation. In adult women, *short stature* is defined as a height of < 145 cm.

underweight

A threshold indicator based on evidence for health effects in young children; defined as a weight-for-age z-score of < -2. Associated with both short- and long-term nutritional deprivation.

wasting

A threshold indicator based on evidence for health effects in young children; defined as a weight-for-height or -length z-score of < -2. Generally an indicator of short-term, acute weight loss associated with illness, famine, or other crises. In adults, *thinness* or *acute undernutrition* is defined as a body mass index < 18.5 kg/m^2.

Review Questions

1. What does it mean to be hungry? Why do perspective and context matter in the definition? What are the consequences of gaps in nutrition during particular life cycle periods?

2. Why do the issues of hunger and undernutrition lend themselves to TPS? What is the magnitude and severity of the problem globally,

and how might the application of TPS change the trajectory of progress toward meeting the first Millennium Development Goal?

3. What features of the global perspective in this course can be leveraged in the application of TPS? Correspondingly, what challenges might be encountered when TPS is conducted at the global level?

4. How might the disciplines most relevant to global hunger and undernutrition be vertically and horizontally integrated to define the problem and develop solutions?

5. can the UNICEF framework for maternal and child undernutrition be improved to better reflect TPS and serve as a basis for developing new policies, programs, and research?

6. What processes are necessary to form effective, action-oriented transdisciplinary teams?

References

1. Food and Agriculture Organization of the United Nations. The State of Food Insecurity in the World: How Does International Price Volatility Affect Domestic Economies and Food Security? Rome: Food and Agriculture Organization of the United Nations; 2011.

2. World Health Organization. The World Health Report 2002—Reducing Risks, Promoting Healthy Life. Geneva: World Health Organization; 2002.

3. Black RE, Allen LH, Bhutta ZA, Caulfield LE, de Onis M, Ezzati M, et al. Maternal and child undernutrition: global and regional exposures and health consequences. The Lancet. 2008;371(9608):243–260.

4. Koplan JP, Bond TC, Merson MH, Reddy KS, Rodriguez MH, Sewankambo NK, et al. Towards a common definition of global health. The Lancet. 2009;373(9679):1993–1995.

5. von Grebmer K, Ruel M, Menon P, Nestorova B, Olofinbiyi T, Fritschel H, et al. Global Hunger Index: Focus on the Crisis of Child Undernutrition. 5th ed. Bonn, Washington, DC, Dublin: Welt Hunger Hilfe, International Food Policy Institute (IFPRI), and Concern Worldwide; 2010.

6. US Agency for International Development. Food and Food Security. Available at: transition.usaid.gov/policy/ads/200/foodsec/fs_foodsec.html [accessed July 25, 2012].

7. Field JO. Multisectoral nutrition planning: a post-mortem. Food Policy. 1987;12(1):15–28.

8. Inter-agency and Expert Group on MDGI. The Millennium Development Goals Report. New York: United Nations; 2010.

9. Stipanuk M. Biochemical and Physiological Aspects of Human Nutrition. Philadelphia, PA: W.B. Saunders; 2000.

10. Gropper S, Smith J, Groff J. Advanced Nutrition and Human Metabolism. Belmont, CA: Wadsworth/Thomson Learning; 2009.

11. Briend A, Dewey KG, Reinhart GA. Fatty acid status in early life in low-income countries—overview of the situation, policy and research priorities. Maternal & Child Nutrition. 2011;7(suppl 2):141–148.

12. Prentice AM, Rayco-Solon P, Moore SE. Insights from the developing world: thrifty genotypes and thrifty phenotypes. The Proceedings of the Nutrition Society. 2005;64(2):153–161.

13. Weatherall DJ. The inherited diseases of hemoglobin are an emerging global health burden. Blood. 2010;115(22):4331–4336.

14. Mutch DM, Wahli W, Williamson G. Nutrigenomics and nutrigenetics: the emerging faces of nutrition. FASEB Journal. 2005;19(12):1602–1616.

15. Konner M, Eaton SB. Paleolithic nutrition: twenty-five years later. Nutrition in Clinical Practice. 2010;25(6):594–602.

16. United Nations Administrative Committee on Coordination, Sub-Committee on Nutrition. 4th Report on The World Nutrition Situation: Nutrition Throughout the Life Cycle. Geneva: World Health Organization; 2000.

17. Stein AD, Zybert PA, van der Pal-de Bruin K, Lumey LH. Exposure to famine during gestation, size at birth, and blood pressure at age 59 y: evidence from the Dutch Famine. European Journal of Epidemiology. 2006;21(10):759–765.

18. Lumey LH, Stein AD, Kahn HS, van der Pal-de Bruin KM, Blauw GJ, Zybert PA, et al. Cohort profile: the Dutch Hunger Winter families study. International Journal of Epidemiology. 2007;36(6):1196–1204.

19. Iannotti LL, Zavaleta N, Leon Z, Shankar AH, Caulfield LE. Maternal zinc supplementation and growth in Peruvian infants. American Journal of Clinical Nutrition. 2008;88(1):154–160.

20. Ceesay SM, Prentice AM, Cole TJ, Foord F, Weaver LT, Poskitt EM, et al. Effects on birth weight and perinatal mortality of maternal dietary supplements in rural Gambia: 5 year randomised controlled trial. British Medical Journal. 1997;315(7111):786–790.

21. Shrimpton R, Victora CG, de Onis M, Lima RC, Blossner M, Clugston G. Worldwide timing of growth faltering: implications for nutritional interventions. Pediatrics. 2001;107(5):E75.

22. Victora CG, de Onis M, Hallal PC, Blossner M, Shrimpton R. Worldwide timing of growth faltering: revisiting implications for interventions. Pediatrics. 2010;125(3):e473–e480.

23. Victora CG, Adair L, Fall C, Hallal PC, Martorell R, Richter L, et al. Maternal and child undernutrition: consequences for adult health and human capital. The Lancet. 2008;371(9609):340–357.

24. World Health Organization, UNICEF. Global Strategy for Infant and Young Child Feeding. Geneva: World Health Organization; 2003.

25. World Health Organization. The WHO Child Growth Standards. Geneva: World Health Organization; 2006.

26. Cogill B. Anthropometric Indicators Measurement Guide. Washington, DC: Food and Nutrition Technical Assistance Project; 2001.

27. Willet W. Nutritional Epidemiology. New York: Oxford University Press; 1998.

28. Gibson RS. Principles of Nutrition Assessment. New York: Oxford University Press; 2005.

29. Pelletier DL, Frongillo EA, Jr., Schroeder DG, Habicht JP. The effects of malnutrition on child mortality in developing countries. Bulletin of the World Health Organization. 1995;73(4):443–448.

30. Dewey K, Mayers D. Early Child Growth: How Do Nutrition and Infection Interact? Washington, DC: Alive & Thrive, Academy for Educational Development; 2011.

31. World Health Organization. Nutrition Health Topics. Available at: www.who.int /nutrition/topics/en [accessed October 19, 2012].

32. Gittelsohn J, Haberle H, Vastine AE, Dyckman W, Palafox NA. Macro- and microlevel processes affect food choice and nutritional status in the Republic of the Marshall Islands. Journal of Nutrition. 2003;133(1):310S–313S.

33. Goodman A, Dufour D, Pelto G. Nutritional Anthropology: Biocultural Perspectives on Food and Nutrition, New York: McGraw-Hill; 1999.

34. Howard M, Millard A. Hunger and Shame: Child Malnutrition and Poverty on Mount Kilimanjaro. New York: Routledge; 1997.

35. Gittelsohn J. Opening the box: intrahousehold food allocation in rural Nepal. Social Science & Medicine. 1991[1982];33(10):1141–1154.

36. Menzel P, Aluisio F. Hungry Planet: What the World Eats. New York: Random House; 2007.

37. Academy for Educational Development, Center for Global Health Communication and Marketing. Behavior Change Communication. Available at: www .globalhealthcommunication.org/strategies/behavior_change_communication [accessed July 25, 2011].

38. Academy for Educational Development. PROFILES. Available at: http://www .aedprofiles.org [accessed July 25, 2011].

39. Heath C, Heath D. Made to Stick: Why Some Ideas Survive and Others Die. New York: Random House; 2008.

40. de Pee S, Bloem MW, Satoto, Yip R, Sukaton A, Tjiong R, et al. Impact of a social marketing campaign promoting dark-green leafy vegetables and eggs in central Java, Indonesia. International Journal for Vitamin and Nutrition Research. 1998;68(6):389–398.

41. Low JW, Arimond M, Osman N, Cunguara B, Zano F, Tschirley D. A food-based approach introducing orange-fleshed sweet potatoes increased vitamin A intake and serum retinol concentrations in young children in rural Mozambique. Journal of Nutrition. 2007;137(5):1320–1327.

42. Iannotti L, Cunningham K, Ruel M. Diversifying into healthy diets: homestead food production in Bangladesh. In: Spielman D, Pandya-Lorch R, eds. Millions Fed: Proven Successes in Agricultural Development. Washington, DC: International Food Policy Research Institute; 2009:145–151.

43. The World Bank. Repositioning Nutrition as Central to Development: A Strategy for Large-Scale Action. Washington, DC: The World Bank; 2006.

44. Subramanian S, Deaton A. The demand for food and calories. Journal of Political Economy. 1996;104(1):133–162.

45. Iannotti L, Robles M, Pachón H, Chiarella C. Food prices and poverty negatively affect micronutrient intakes in Guatemala. Journal of Nutrition. 2012;142(8):1568–1576.

46. Hoddinott J, Maluccio JA, Behrman JR, Flores R, Martorell R. Effect of a nutrition intervention during early childhood on economic productivity in Guatemalan adults. The Lancet. 2008;371(9610):411–416.

47. Soares F, Ribas RP, Osório RG. Evaluating the impact of Brazil's Bolsa Família. Latin American Research Review. 2010;45(2):173–190.

48. Attanasio O, Gomez L, Heredia P, Vera-Hernandez M. The Short-Term Impact of a Conditional Cash Subsidy on Child Health and Nutrition in Colombia. 2000 Report Summary: Familias 03. London: Institute of Fiscal Studies; 2000.

49. World Health Organization. World Health Statistics 2011. Available at: www.who.int/gho/publications/world_health_statistics/2011/en/index.html [accessed November 28, 2011].

50. Checkley W, Buckley G, Gilman RH, Assis AM, Guerrant RL, Morris SS, et al. Multi-country analysis of the effects of diarrhoea on childhood stunting. International Journal of Epidemiology. 2008;37(4):816–830.

51. Fink G, Gunther I, Hill K. The effect of water and sanitation on child health: evidence from the demographic and health surveys 1986–2007. International Journal of Epidemiology. 2011;40(5):196–204.

52. World Health Organization. Indicators for Assessing Infant and Young Child Feeding Practices, Part 1: Definitions. Geneva: World Health Organization; 2008.

53. de Benoist B, McLean E, Egli I, Cogswell, M, eds. Worldwide Prevalence of Anemia 1993–2005: WHO Global Database on Anemia. Geneva: World Health Organization; 2008.

54. Measure DHS. Demographic and Health Surveys. Available at: www.measuredhs.com [accessed July 25, 2011].

55. Centers for Disease Control and Prevention. Logic model basics. Evaluation Briefs. December 2008; No. 2.

56. US Agency for International Development. USAID Child Survival and Health Grants Program. Available at: transition.usaid.gov/our_work/global_health/home/Funding/cs_grants/cs_index.html [accessed July 25, 2011].

57. Pelletier DL, Shrimpton R. The role of information in the planning, management and evaluation of community nutrition programmes. Health Policy and Planning. 1994;9(2):171–184.

58. Food and Agriculture Organization of the United Nations. World Food Day. Available at: www.fao.org/getinvolved/worldfoodday [accessed October 16, 2011].

59. Mendizabal E. The Alignment, Interest and Influence Matrix (AIIM). London: Overseas Development Institute; 2011.

Chapter 13

Implementing Public Health Interventions in Developing Countries

A Transdisciplinary Solution for Safe Drinking Water in Rural India

Ramesh Raghavan
Ravikumar Chockalingam
Zeena Johar

Learning Objectives

- Understand how transdisciplinary problem solving can be applied to diarrheal disease in an international context.
- Describe the determinants of diarrheal disease in a global context.
- Identify transdisciplinary solutions directed at the determinants of diarrheal disease.
- Discuss the importance of social and political contexts in the solution of global public health problems.
- Explain what makes a transdisciplinary solution feasible in a given context.

•••

Public health can be thought of as the practice of medicine upon populations, involving as it does the use of various conceptualizations and instruments to safeguard population well-being.[1] Such attempts to safeguard the health of populations call for solving the public health challenges that beset them, a task that requires public health students and scholars to possess a robust conceptual framework in order to understand the determinants of a problem and then to deploy the best available evidence to address those determinants at a population level. However, extant models of solution analysis, briefly described later, tend to suggest solutions directed toward a particular disciplinary orientation (such as policy analysis), and require the analyst to conform the public health problem to fit the conceptual instrument of its putative solution. Public health professionals working in highly diverse contexts, such as developing countries, often face challenges in reconciling a particular disciplinary perspective to a highly specific and oftentimes contentious challenge. However, there appears to be little pedagogy reflecting how public health students and scholars can learn to develop solutions in diverse intellectual and cultural environments.

This perceived gap in pedagogy led to the development of content for this book addressing international concerns of undernutrition and hunger (chapter 12) and air pollution (chapter 14) and, in this chapter, diarrheal disease. The case study in this chapter describes how a group of graduate students in public health and social work spent six weeks in three villages in southern India, where they used a transdisciplinary framework for understanding the determinants of real-life problems facing rural communities, and for finding ways to assist these communities in overcoming these problems. The students worked on five assigned public health problems, developed in collaboration with a partner organization of the Brown School at Washington University in St. Louis, the IKP Centre for Technologies in Public Health (ICTPH). Each student was placed in an interdisciplinary team consisting of an instructor, representatives from ICTPH, and community health workers, and worked on the problem collaboratively over the duration of the course. (Key elements of the design of this course are listed in table 13.1.) Through this process, students learned to integrate insights from a variety of disciplines in solving public health challenges, learning the importance of social ecology in public health problem solving, and reconciling the differing worldviews of classical public health teaching and practice and the realities of life in the developing world.

This chapter summarizes this learning, first briefly reviewing the solution analysis, and then presenting a case study of diarrheal disease in one of the three villages, Alakudi. We analyze the determinants of diarrheal disease in this village to illustrate the diversity of intellectual disciplines that influence a public health challenge, and then discuss the solutions developed to address this challenge. We end with a summary of how transdisciplinary thinking can surmount not only disciplinary but also socioecological barriers and can develop solutions that are relevant to the community and to the client.

General Heuristic for Solution Analysis

Traditional approaches to the solving of public health problems are either drawn from a single discipline or are interdisciplinary.[2] These approaches tend to examine a determinant of a public health problem from the perspective of a single intellectual tradition. However, as we discuss later in this chapter, a transdisciplinary approach can provide the public health scholar with a richer set of conceptual frameworks to solve public health problems.

Unidisciplinary approaches to the solution of problems extant within communities range from the inclusive and qualitative to the technocratic and quantitative. On one hand, scholars have argued for an inductive, community approach to problem solving and have developed approaches used by a plurality of stakeholder groups.[3–6] Community-based participatory research is a widely accepted approach to the elicitation of particular and locally relevant problems and solutions, among other goals.[7–9]

On the other hand, there is a long history of quantitatively oriented approaches, stemming from applied economics and policy studies, that attempt to quantify preferences in some way and then to evaluate the consequent differences in these quantities.[10,11] These approaches emphasize identifying a defined set of metrics (usually initiated by the analyst) that can be used to quantify various outcomes resulting from interventions, choosing between these outcomes according to some predefined set of goals and intentions, and then deciding to adopt one particular alternative. Tools developed for purposes of program or policy evaluation—such as cost-benefit and cost-effectiveness analyses[12]—can also be conceptualized as tools of solution analysis, as they assist decision making in favor of one alternative over another. For this reason, other strategies such as meta-analysis or decision analysis are also useful for the analyst identifying solutions.[13]

These two types of approaches—qualitative and quantitative—can be complementary. For example, tools from operations research and applied mathematics, such as system dynamics, have been adapted to elicit community-preferred solutions,[14] and several research studies sited in communities but not fully involving communities in conceptualization and solution of problems are described as *community-placed* instead of *community-based*.[15]

The challenge for the public health student or scholar faced with this array of tools is to apply these tools to the solution of real-life problems that may not comport with the disciplinary foci or theoretical orientations of the tools. Just as patients present to physicians with problems, not with diagnoses, communities present to the public health professional with determinants that sometimes cannot be addressed using instruments derived from a particular intellectual tradition. The "diagnostic" and difficult challenge for the public health professional is to identify the disciplinary determinants that underlie these public health challenges and then to forge an understanding of the problem and its solution that is inherently transdisciplinary.

In the rest of this chapter, we outline one particular approach to transdisciplinary solution analysis that is grounded in a real-life problem. Our goal is illustrative, not prescriptive; over the course of this exercise, we have slowly come to the realization that the instruments of transdisciplinary inquiry have to be continually refined and reinvented to fit with the objects of our inquiry. In the case that follows, we provide one particular approach to a particular problem, along with the caveat that the solutions to different problems in different contexts may call for a different blend of disciplines and perspectives. In some ways, this case study is an operationalization within Indian villages of the concepts articulated by Stokols and colleagues in chapter 1 of this volume.

Case Study: Water Contamination in Alakudi

Alakudi is a village in Thanjavur district in Tamil Nadu, a state in southern India. Thanjavur district is located in the delta of the river Cauvery and is crisscrossed with water channels that irrigate its fields of paddy and sugarcane. Alakudi has a population of a little over 3,000 individuals, 49.6 percent of them female. (All data in this section are unpublished data from the IKP Centre for Technologies in Public Health in Thanjavur; www.ictph.org.in.) Alakudi is a farming village; nearly half of its residents own and work on agricultural lands and a third rear livestock: primarily cows, bulls, buffalo, or chickens. One in eight residents of Alakudi is reportedly below the poverty line, and over half of all the households (58 percent) are estimated to earn between `72,000 and `144,000 a year. (Amounts in rupees are indicated by `; 46 Indian rupees = US$1 at the time of this writing.) The average annual household income in Alakudi was reported to be `115,640, whereas the median household income was recorded at `76,800.

Most of the villages in Thanjavur district, including Alakudi, obtain their drinking water from underground aquifers. Groundwater is pumped up from bore wells (also called tube wells) and is stored in overhead tanks (OHTs). From the OHTs, water is supplied though a network of pipes to both the public standpipes (PSPs, or community pipes) and individual connections in homes. The only purification occurs in the OHT, through *blast chlorination* (or shock chlorination) at an intermittent frequency of one to three times a month. For the rest of the time, the water is pumped through the network untreated. Public tap water is the major source (92.2 percent) of drinking water. Only 9.3 percent of the households have drinking water facilities in their dwelling units; people in the remaining households walk a distance in order to fetch water. Virtually all (99.6 percent) of the water samples tested from the 732 households in Alakudi using the H_2S field-testing kits tested positive for bacterial contamination.

This contamination is due to the fact that most residents of Alakudi engage in open defecation, alongside pathways, in bushes, and in and around agricultural fields. Alakudi has a rudimentary drainage system, which is paved for the most part, and runs along the grid streets. It is, however, an open drainage system and filled with garbage and untreated sewage; it does not lead to a sewage treatment plant but ends in a septic tank, which is also poorly maintained. Anecdotal evidence suggests that Alakudi has a very high incidence of diarrheal diseases, with 5.3 percent of the residents seeking services for gastrointestinal disorders.

Figure 13.1 shows the structures through which water is procured for use by village residents. As described earlier, all of Alakudi's piped water comes from two overhead tanks, up to which groundwater is pumped from a bore well. We refer to these as point of source, or level 1. The village panchayat runs water pipes (level 2) from these overhead tanks; these pipes terminate in forty-nine community taps distributed throughout the village (figure 13.2).

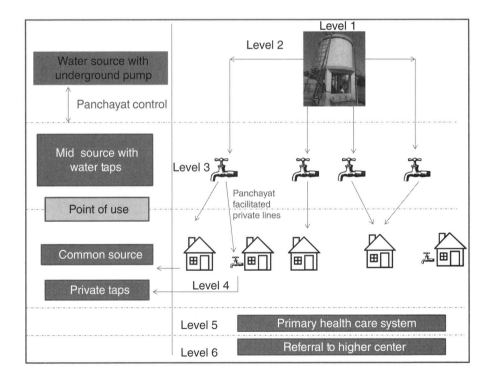

Figure 13.1. Water structures in Alakudi

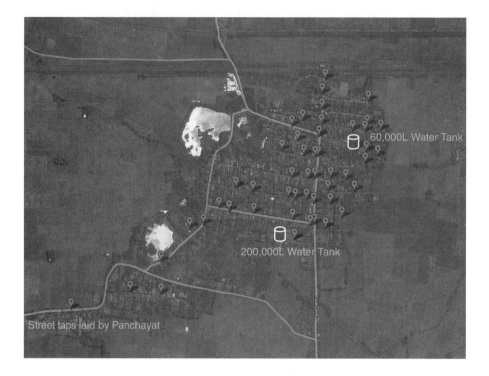

Figure 13.2. Water tap distribution in Alakudi

These community taps form the point of access for water for most village residents (level 3). For those who can afford to pay to have a tap installed inside their homes, the panchayat provides a line from the nearest pipe to their house for a fee of approximately `3,000. The use of water inside the house constitutes another focus for implementation of solutions (level 4). Solutions to the control of diarrheal disease can hence be mounted at any of these levels, in addition to delivering curative services at the primary health center (level 5) and the higher tertiary care centers (level 6).

The maintenance of this water distribution and purification system forms a substantial portion of total annual expenditures for Alakudi's village *panchayat*, which is a village-based, elected administrative unit that functions as a local institution of self-government and is headed by an elected panchayat president, who serves as the village equivalent of a mayor. All panchayats, including Alakudi's, are perpetually beset with financial problems. The panchayat's annual water-related expenditures in fiscal year 2006–2007 amounted to approximately `231,765, whereas its annual collection of water taxes amounted to `65,380. This deficit is routinely subsidized by the state of Tamil

Nadu through a regulatory body called the State Finance Commission, which results in village panchayats becoming dependent on state general revenues for their functioning.[16] This subsidy, and inefficiencies in tax collection, produces resource constraints for the panchayat. The difficulty of tax collections is further compounded by the fact that the panchayat clerk is expected to collect all monthly dues (including water charges) by personally going to all households in the village. For villages with over 700 households this is an extremely challenging proposition.

The problem of poor water quality in Alakudi is typical of India, where even the largest and most cosmopolitan cities cannot ensure the safety of the water flowing through municipal taps. Additionally, Alakudi suffers from a lack of sanitation, which is one of most fundamental health and infrastructure issues facing rural India. Penetration of toilets in Indian villages is relatively low, with only 10 to 20 percent of residents in Alakudi using toilets. Alakudi has one large public toilet complex, with a local septic tank maintained erratically by the panchayat. This complex is very poorly maintained, and is not currently in use.

Current Approach to Solving the Problem

The accepted approach to the treatment of diarrhea involves the use of low-osmolarity oral rehydration solution, which is a combination of sterile (boiled) water, sugar, and salt in a specified formulation.[17] That this combination is useful in the treatment of diarrheal disease has been recognized for millennia—the classical textbook of Ayurvedic medicine, the *Sushruta Samhita*, written c. 1500 BCE, recommends the use of an oral solution composed of tepid water, molasses, and rock salt as a treatment for diarrhea (Book III, Verse II).[18] The rediscovery and refinement of oral rehydration solution into its current formulation, and its widespread use as a public health intervention, occurred in the aftermath of a massive diarrheal disease outbreak in Bangladesh in 1971, and is credited with saving the lives of several hundred thousand refugee children.[19] Today, the World Health Organization makes available a precisely formulated sachet of oral rehydration salts (ORS), meant to be dissolved in one liter of drinkable water in the home of a patient with diarrheal disease, and administered to the patient until signs of dehydration are no longer evident. These sachets are available free of charge from primary health centers in India, including the one in Alakudi, and anecdotal evidence reveals that residents of Alakudi seem very aware that ORS is the appropriate treatment whenever a child has diarrhea.

The distribution and use of ORS is a curative approach; it has certainly reduced the sequelae of diarrheal disease, but it can do little to mitigate disease incidence and prevalence. Alakudi still continues to experience episodes of diarrhea partly because of contamination of the water used for drinking by village residents, a contamination caused by a variety of upstream determinants, including the widespread problem of open defecation, described in the earlier section. Finding a solution to these determinants of diarrheal disease has proven to be far harder than deploying a treatment for diarrhea, and requires the use of disciplinary approaches and their integration into transdisciplinary solutions.

The solution is not necessarily as simple as informing village residents about the dangers of open defecation. Panchayat leaders in Alakudi are well aware of the dangers of open defecation, and Alakudi has a public toilet for residents' use. However, the panchayat sees it as an imperfect solution to the problem. Alakudi does not have a piped sewage system, and solid wastes are stored in a septic tank. For a variety of financial, administrative, and manpower reasons, this septic tank is rarely cleaned. Regular overflows of raw sewage into surrounding areas are a common feature of this public toilet. This toilet is also situated very close to the overhead tank that supplies Alakudi with drinking water, increasing the probability of water contamination. The panchayat hence perceives that both open and closed defecation seem to result in identical outcomes, and is unwilling to allocate additional resources to maintenance of the toilet or its septic tank.

Even were the panchayat to invest in the toilet, considerable demand-side barriers to its use exist. From a user perspective, closed defecation is problematic given the design of Indian toilets, in which solid wastes are not contained in a water body as they are in Western toilets. This causes defecation to be associated with fecal smells; open defecation is preferred due to the dissemination of these odors. Absent adequate toilet ventilation, closed defecation presents considerable, and insurmountable, olfactory challenges. Open defecation is also a traditional practice in agrarian communities and is reportedly resistant to change,[20] making it a difficult target for a public health interventionist working in Alakudi.

Constructing Transdisciplinary Teams

A key element of the master of public health (MPH) program at the Brown School is a series of required courses in transdisciplinary problem solving. While the content of these courses varies (recent topics include tobacco control, obesity, and health reform), they all share common structural characteristics related to attempting to solve problems using a transdisciplinary approach. We developed a new course for this series, called "Implementing Public Health Interventions in Developing Countries" (table 13.1), and enrolled students from both the MPH and the master of social work (MSW) programs at the Brown School. All enrolled students received a travel subsidy toward their airfare, and the Brown School's International Programs office coordinated visas and other necessary paperwork.

Table 13.1. Key course elements

Element	Details and purpose
Predeparture briefing	A general orientation to the field environment and field partner, personal safety, and disease risk mitigation.
Establishment of an instructional calendar	A supplement to a syllabus, the instructional calendar allowed us to link didactic and field training so as to build connections between the two.
Field calendar for field rotations	A calendar containing information on the site of rotation, supplemented by e-mails to student field teams about who would be part of each field team. Each field team included students, an instructor (when feasible), a representative from our partner organization, and a community health worker (where applicable).
Multidisciplinary team (MDT) meeting	Meetings attended by partner organization representatives where students presented preliminary intervention and implementation designs. Meetings were designed to solicit partner organization feedback on the design of interventions.
Skills lab	An opportunity for all students to be cross-trained in practical skills for the practice of public health in field environments. For example, they received Basic Life Support certification and learned about measurement of blood pressure, water chlorination and testing, oral cavity examinations, and identification of heart sounds.
Problem analysis	Students identified and described a problem confronting village residents and its determinants. They then identified practical and feasible public health interventions relevant to the local context and available health resources.
Solution analysis	Students described the intervention, its implementation, and its evaluation. Key expectations included transdisciplinarity, feasibility, cost effectiveness, and sustainability of the intervention.
Formal presentations	A set of three team presentations built student skills in presenting solutions to a "client" organization.

Prior to departure we divided students into three-person or (in one case) two-person teams. Each team had at least one MSW and one MPH student; as outlined in chapter 1, the goal was that working intensively with a person from a different discipline would challenge traditional disciplinary perspectives and help students to transcend them while in the field.

Our partner organization, ICTPH, organized all in-country travel, including the train journey from the nearest international airport to Thanjavur, arranged housing in two-person dormitory-style accommodations, provided field personnel to act as translators and community health workers, and transported students to and from field sites. ICTPH also provided three meals a day to students in an attempt to reduce their risk of contracting enteric illness.

We maintained the integrity of these student teams while on field visits. Instructors rotated between student teams on field visits, and on such visits, each student team had at least one community health worker and one ICTPH employee to serve as translator and coordinator. A total of five such *field teams* were constructed, each field team focusing on a particular public health challenge. This chapter examines the work of a field team focused on diarrheal disease.

Transdisciplinary Approach to Problem Solving: Decomposing Solutions by Location

The first step in identifying alternative solutions is a systematic search for all the determinants of the condition, and then finding solutions to those determinants that appear feasible to deploy given available resources and a given field practice area. Box 13.1 outlines the steps undertaken by the students (led by the instructors) to identify transdisciplinary solutions. Even though open defecation is a known determinant of water contamination, and even though

---

Box 13.1: Steps in transdisciplinary problem solving

1. Identify the public health problem.
2. Identify the determinants of this problem at the personal, household, and community levels.
3. Understand the social and political ecology of the field practice area (the village).
4. Identify strategies to address these determinants from diverse literatures.
5. Isolate a set of candidate strategies, based on the evidence.
6. Integrate strategies into a single intervention, based on your knowledge of the field practice area.
7. Seek feedback from field partners on the feasibility and acceptability of the intervention. If necessary, repeat step 4.
8. Identify implementation approaches for this intervention.
9. Identify evaluation approaches for this intervention.

hygiene promotion has been advanced as a cost-effective public health intervention,[21] we did not target change in defecation behaviors in Alakudi given the challenges described previously. Instead, we began to examine locational aspects of water contamination that might lend themselves to transdisciplinary solutions. For each of the two locations discussed below, we undertook the steps listed in the text box. The final result of this exercise was the identification of a public health intervention that might be feasibly implemented (the *what*), of a place to deliver this intervention (the *where*), and of a plan to implement and evaluate this intervention (the *how*).

From Water Source to Point of Access

The traditional approach to solving the problem of water contamination in Alakudi involves the use of chlorination. Approximately 2.5 grams of bleaching powder for every 1,000 liters of tank capacity is mixed with water in a non-metal bucket to form a thick solution, this is sedimented, and the supernatant chlorine solution is lowered into a tank containing water whose turbidity and acidity have been ascertained. The bucket is violently agitated, which results in the solution dispersing throughout the water tank. Water is then tested, and is safe for use within an hour.[22] Water chlorination, hence, is a task requiring insights from fields as diverse as community medicine (preventive medicine), medical microbiology, and environmental health.

Other solutions we considered to enhance the quality of water in the tank stemmed from tank construction, usually the domain of civil engineering.[23] How can tanks be designed for optimal control of pathogens? One solution that sprang immediately to mind was the location of the tank, situated as it was close to the village toilet. As mentioned earlier, the maintenance of this septic tank is unsatisfactory, leading to leakage of untreated human waste. The potential problem with locating sources of groundwater (such as the water accessed by the tube well that feeds the tank) close to sources of pollution is well known in the engineering literature.[24] Our concerns with the quality of the tank and its construction uncovered a monograph on the construction of joints in water tanks,[25] which, as public health practitioners (not engineers), we attempted to apply to the tank in question. We also found that the cover of the tank fit poorly, allowing for potential contamination from animal droppings and other waste, which led us to work in disciplines ranging from ornithology to public health to learn about bird droppings, the pathogenic bacteria they carry, and their impact on human health.[26–29] Even this brief foray into disciplines outside public health suggested to us that several of these disciplines were essentially preventive in orientation; in engineering, for example, one uses structural tools to solve problems that may arise with time and with use.

Even if the design and construction of the tank had been impeccable, several dangers lay in wait downstream. Our focus on what we called level 2 problems—determinants of loss of water quality in the conduits between the tank and community taps—brought other disciplines to bear. An immediate focus of study was the problem of open defecation. Even though the practice itself seemed unhygienic, its chief sequelae in this case seemed likely to be related to precisely where this defecation was occurring. When people defecated in close proximity to buried pipes, the water in those pipes could be contaminated by pathogens in the excreta—especially if the pipes were old or had been poorly manufactured.

This led to research on the causal factors for diarrheal disease—the associated bacteria, viruses, and protozoa—in disciplines such as microbiology[30] and parasitology.[31] We scoured the literature for guidance on survival times for these pathogens and discovered, for example, that one of the strains of the cholera bacterium associated with disease could survive for nearly three weeks under favorable atmospheric conditions.[32] Clearly, soil could retain the bacterium for a period of time adequate for reinfection, as could the irrigation canals that were plentiful in the district in which Alakudi is located.[33]

Civil engineers working in the field of water distribution systems had studied differential rates of decay of chlorine as it made its way through water pipes made of high-reactivity (for example, iron) or low-reactivity (for example, PVC) materials.[34] A study in Uzbekistan found higher rates of diarrheal disease among individuals who received chlorinated water piped to their homes than among those who practiced home chlorination, which suggested the presence of leaky pipes and acquired contamination.[35] In fact, soft pipeline deposits that accumulate in water distribution pipes are known reservoirs of a range of bacterial and fungal pathogens that can compromise drinking water.[36] Although what we learned was suggestive of the need for careful manufacturing and maintenance, the feasibility of a water distribution system–directed solution was low in Alakudi, which led the team to switch its areas of intervention emphasis.

If the problem was locational, perhaps a solution could be geographical—perhaps the intervention could simply be to encourage village residents to shift their preferred locations of open defecation, without making any attempts to change the practice, away from areas where pipes ran underground. This thinking led the team to the geographic information system and environmental science literature, where the problem of water pipe breaks is well studied.[37,38] We were impressed at the availability of specialist applications for geo-mapping water resources.[39] Because we were unable to obtain the plans showing water pipe locations from the panchayat office, we resorted to using a free iPhone application that allowed us to geo-tag each water pipe. These bits of geographical information were then mapped onto the village of Alakudi, as shown in figure 13.2. The results seemed to suggest that the water taps were well distributed throughout Alakudi, and there did not seem to be a place that could be reserved for human waste. Alternative solutions like the pour-flush toilets developed by companies like Sulabh were also considered but were not explored owing to financial concerns.[40]

From Point of Access to Point of Use

Alternative solutions focused on the point of access—the village taps from which a majority of Alakudi's residents procure their water. A solution focused on village taps seemed to be an ideal supply-side strategy, requiring few behavioral changes other than prevention of contamination within the home after the water had been collected from the tap. So we began to explore filtration systems that could be feasibly mounted onto the forty-nine village taps, and we encountered a wealth of literature focused on this topic.[41-48] Several of these approaches emphasized mechanical filtration (using activated carbon or ceramic filters, for example), with or without an impregnated chemical disinfectant. The challenge with most commercially available filtration systems was the cost—most commercial systems were unobtainable in rural Tamil Nadu and, even if we procured them from the state capital, Chennai, the ongoing maintenance of these systems was open to question. Given the village's experience with the public toilet, we were not convinced that the sustainability of a commercial tap-based filter system could be assured.

Our attempts to devise cheap water filtration systems led us into an unexpected field—that of water purification systems used in aquariums. Fish, we discovered, are fastidious about water quality, and poor water quality in home aquariums is a leading cause of fish death. The aquarium enthusiast literature is filled with ideas for homemade, inexpensive filtration devices that could easily be adapted to Alakudi's water taps and that met our other requirements as well, being locally available, inexpensive to replace, and with few moving parts requiring servicing or assembly. A search for aquarium filtration systems on YouTube resulted in several videos demonstrating the use of several types of filters, and we narrowed our explorations to canister filters as a filtration solution. A canister filter is made up of several layers, through which water must successively pass, and during which it is progressively cleaned. A canister filter that seemed particularly well designed was the one used by the British Antarctic Survey, which consisted of a biological filter layer, a mechanical filtration layer, and a foam stripper.[49] Such a design, especially when coupled with chlorination immediately prior to water use (introducing chlorine into the device may destroy the biological filter), seemed to address all the challenges involved with providing a tap-based approach.

The challenge was sustainability. While many of the components of the filter could be locally sourced—sand and gravel, for example—foam requires regular replacement and is available only from commercial vendors. We thus began to identify Indian companies that manufacture filter components, and we intended to contact the village panchayat office to determine the availability of local resources to support ongoing maintenance of the filters. Although the panchayat would likely pay for filters attached to community taps, households with in-home taps would be responsible for the filtration systems on those taps. These households were wealthier than the households using community taps, and several were reportedly already boiling their water and then filtering it using muslin cloth. They reserved the use of this boiled and filtered water for their children, however, preferring to use untreated tap water for adult consumption.

Finally, point-of-use strategies involved improving the quality of water and its storage in the home. For several years, the local not-for-profit and the primary health center community agencies had been distributing chlorine tablets that households were asked to drop into filtered water and that would make the water drinkable for twenty-four hours. The readily available brand in Alakudi is Aquatabs®, and despite a community health worker–led informational campaign, there seemed to be little uptake of the tablets among village residents. The problem, it was discovered, was the change that chlorination made to the taste of the water, especially when treated water had been brought to a boil for cooking purposes. Residents complained of foul-tasting *sambar* and *rasam* (watery, lentil-based stews mixed with rice before being eaten). Foregoing chlorination of water that is going to be boiled is an option, but this requires water separation strategies, which were not universally established. These issues, combined with fact that the water available in Alakudi is not turbid and so to the eye it looks potable, meant that residents simply did not see the need to chlorinate their domestic water on a routine basis. Given that in-home chlorination programs were likely to be short lived, we felt that moving chlorination upstream and deploying other contamination prevention interventions at the household level—such as the use of narrow-mouthed containers for water storage[50,51]—might be a more feasible and sustainable option.

Valuing the Outcomes of Proposed Solutions

As the previous discussion illustrates, not all transdisciplinary solutions can be feasibly implemented in a given field practice area. Part of the problem is the lack of availability of resources that can be deployed toward the implementation of the intervention. But the greater problem, in our experience, is the variance between scientific and stakeholder perspectives—the fact that what is desired by public health professionals is not always desired by the community; when decisions are made without sufficient knowledge of community perspectives, resources are often left unutilized, as the case of Alakudi's public toilet illustrates. Assessing preferences in the field, therefore, is critical to the success of public health interventions (see box 13.2).

Standard policy approaches tend to compare outcomes using relatively standardized metrics, such as quality-adjusted life-years (QALYs), in cost-utility analyses.[52,53] These utilities, or preferences, are elicited using other instruments,[54] and often vary widely depending upon the stakeholder whose preference it is that is being assessed.[55] These differences are magnified in field-based settings in developing country contexts for two principal reasons. First, we found some of our preference elicitations to be contaminated by response biases, whether caused by social desirability, acquiescence, or extremity.[56] Second, considerable linguistic barriers exist, even when interviewers and respondents are speaking the same language; this is due to variations in dialect across many Indian languages, which make accurate assessments difficult.

Field-based focus groups are a relatively quick way to obtain preferences.[57] We had success in recruiting participants for informal group discussions moderated around a set of questions. Recording is often a challenge in field settings, and even when recording was done, it needed to be translated prior to analysis, because currently available qualitative software packages do not work in Tamil, the language spoken in Alakudi. We found relatively brief (twenty-minute) sessions to be most effective, with a heterogeneous group of participants that allowed us to capture diverse outcomes and perspectives on their valuation.

Box 13.2: Challenges in preference assessment for transdisciplinary solutions

1. Communities may not value the outcomes that public health professionals value.

2. Communities vote with their behaviors, ignoring solutions they do not value.

3. Standardized approaches to preference assessment may not be well understood due to cultural norms and values.

4. Social desirability and linguistic differences pose further challenges to preference assessment.

5. Field-based qualitative strategies (focus groups and interviews) may help disentangle the sometimes diverse outcomes resulting from transdisciplinary solutions.

Key informant interviews are another way to elicit preferences.[58] We solicited information from a diverse array of informants, most usefully from community health workers, who are often excellent key informants, with deep knowledge of the community and substantive knowledge of the health issues facing community members. Other stakeholders, such as panchayat presidents, may wield considerable power in village circles but may not be as accessible as village residents or community health workers. But as the continuation of open defecation in Alakudi illustrates, not taking preferences of village residents into account is incompatible with success of public health programs.

Lessons Learned

This course was designed to introduce students to transdisciplinary thinking by engaging them in transdisciplinary problem solving. Our method of approaching a substantive area through pedagogy revealed several insights that we did not possess prior to constructing this course, and these are summarized here.

First, we found the greatest value of a transdisciplinary approach to be its utility for solving a public health challenge confronting a community. Using transdisciplinary thinking instrumentally in this manner, instead of discussing it substantively, seemed to heighten the applicability and salience of such an approach. Second, many of the challenges in public health practice lie in contexts rather than in content. The literature is invariably clear regarding what needs to be done in order to affect population health; the challenge lies in finding out what needs to be done in a given context that can be sustainably implemented. The value of transdisciplinarity lies, in our experience, in its focus on context, in its embrace of intellectual traditions that are rooted in local realities, and in its ability to address population concerns in ways that are culturally sensitive and feasible. Third, we have now become convinced that the best way to teach transdisciplinary thinking is via immersion; by minimizing classroom activities and increasing field experiences. A pedagogical transdisciplinary approach predicated on doing rather than thinking or reflecting seems critical for assisting students to see the value of this approach. Finally, a transdisciplinary approach is not only intellectual but also experiential. All experiences are grist for the mill of a transdisciplinary approach, whether they derive from the literature or simply from being coparticipants in a village milieu. The best solutions, in our view, come from the serendipity that is engendered by being open to all learning experiences.

Our six-week stay in the three villages was insufficient for us to see the actual implementation of our ideas into practice. The mandate of this course was to provide information to our field partner, ICTPH, on the best way to solve the problem of diarrheal disease in its practice areas. In subsequent visits to Thanjavur we hope to learn how ICTPH is working with its community health workers in deploying these student interventions in Alakudi.

Summary

Communities present with public health problems that do not recognize disciplinary boundaries; these problems often require solutions that cannot be contained within a single discipline or intellectual tradition. Transdisciplinary problem solving in such circumstances can be both a blessing and a curse. It is a blessing in the sense that it expands individual disciplinary boundaries, allowing for the expansion of methodologies, permitting a fuller understanding of the problem, and resulting in a more comprehensive set of solutions. It is a curse in the sense that it expands the workload as well as likelihood of a workable solution. It imposes conceptual, methodological, and procedural challenges, all of which need to be examined by the public health professional and many of which will require careful choices if sustainable solutions to health challenges are to be deployed successfully in field settings.

Key Terms

panchayat	A village-based elected body responsible for all village-level administrative tasks.
panchayat president	The chief executive officer of a panchayat.

Review Questions

1. Why does the village of Alakudi have a high prevalence of diarrheal disease?
2. At what levels can the problem of water contamination be addressed? At which of these levels can the most sustainable solution be deployed? Why?
3. How would you describe problem analysis as it is applied to specific public health problems?
4. How would you describe solution analysis as it is applied to specific public health problems?
5. What disciplines inform the solution proposed in this chapter?
6. Why are many public health solutions unsustainable? How can we increase their sustainability?

References

1. Mann JM. Medicine and public health, ethics and human rights. The Hastings Center Report. 1997;27:6–13.
2. Mitchell PH. What's in a name?: multidisciplinary, interdisciplinary, and transdisciplinary. Journal of Professional Nursing. 2005;21:332–334.
3. Roussos ST, Fawcett SB. A review of collaborative partnerships as a strategy for improving community health. Annual Review of Public Health. 2000;21:369–402.
4. Shortell SM, Zukoski AP, Alexander JA, Bazzoli GJ, Conrad DA, Hasnain-Wynia R, et al. Evaluating partnerships for community health improvement: tracking the footprints. Journal of Health Politics, Policy and Law. 2002;27:49.
5. Lasker R, Weiss E. Broadening participation in community problem solving: a multidisciplinary model to support collaborative practice and research. Journal of Urban Health. 2003;80:14–47.
6. Zakocs RC, Edwards EM. What explains community coalition effectiveness? a review of the literature. American Journal of Preventive Medicine. 2006;30:351–361.
7. Israel BA, Schulz AJ, Parker EA, Becker AB. Review of community-based research: assessing partnership approaches to improve public health. Annual Review of Public Health. 1998;19:173–202.
8. Israel BA, Schulz AJ, Parker EA, Becker AB. Community-based participatory research: policy recommendations for promoting a partnership approach in health research. Education for Health. 2001;14:182–197.
9. Minkler M, Wallerstein N. Community-based Participatory Research for Health. San Francisco: Jossey-Bass; 2003.
10. Weimer DL, Vining AR. Policy Analysis: Concepts and Practice, 4th ed. Upper Saddle River, NJ: Pearson Prentice Hall; 2004.
11. Stokey E, Zeckhauser R. A Primer for Policy Analysis. New York: W.W. Norton; 1978.
12. Drummond MF, Sculpher MJ, Torrance GW. Methods for the Economic Evaluation of Health Care Programmes. 3rd ed. New York: Oxford University Press, USA; 2005.
13. Petitti DB. Meta-analysis, Decision Analysis, and Cost-effectiveness Analysis: Methods for Quantitative Synthesis in Medicine. New York: Oxford University Press, USA; 2000.
14. Homer J, Hirsch G, Minniti M, Pierson M. Models for collaboration: how system dynamics helped a community organize cost-effective care for chronic illness. System Dynamics Review. 2004;20:199–222.
15. O'Toole TP, Aaron KF, Chin MH, Horowitz C, Tyson F. Community-based participatory research. Journal of General Internal Medicine. 2003;18:592–594.
16. Sahasranaman A. Panchayat finances and the need for devolutions from the state government. Economic & Political Weekly. 2012;47(4).
17. Hahn S, Kim YJ, Garner P. Reduced osmolarity oral rehydration solution for treating dehydration due to diarrhoea in children: systematic review. British Medical Journal. 2001;323:81–85.

18. Ruxin JN. Magic bullet: the history of oral rehydration therapy. Medical History. 1994;38:363–397.

19. Mahalanabis D, Choudhuri AB, Bagchi NG, Bhattacharya AK, Simpson TW. Oral fluid therapy of cholera among Bangladesh refugees. Johns Hopkins Medical Journal. 1973;132:197–205.

20. Banda K, Sarkar R, Gopal S, Govindarajan J, Harijan BB, Jeyakumar MB, et al. Water handling, sanitation and defecation practices in rural southern India: a knowledge, attitudes and practices study. Transactions of the Royal Society of Tropical Medicine and Hygiene. 2007;101:1124–1130.

21. Cairncross S, Shordt K, Zacharia S, Govindan BK. What causes sustainable changes in hygiene behaviour? a cross-sectional study from Kerala, India. Social Science & Medicine. 2005;61:2212–2220.

22. Park JE, Park K. Textbook of Preventive and Social Medicine. Jabalpur, India: Banarsidas Bhanot; 2009.

23. Linsley RK, Franzini JB. Water-Resources Engineering. 3rd ed. New York: McGraw-Hill; 1979.

24. Canter LW, Knox RC. Septic Tank System Effects on Ground Water Quality. Chelsea, MI: Lewis Publications; 1985.

25. Xue-chun LI. The construction of construction joint in water tank engineering. Shanxi Architecture. 2007;28:159–160.

26. Amon JJ, Drobeniuc J, Bower WA, Magaña JC, Escobedo MA, Williams IT, et al. Locally acquired hepatitis E virus infection, El Paso, Texas. Journal of Medical Virology. 2006;78:741–746.

27. Dodge HJ, Ajello L, Engelke OK. The association of a bird-roosting site with infection of school children by *Histoplasma capsulatum*. American Journal of Public Health. 1965;55:1203–1211.

28. Kapperud G, Espeland G, Wahl E, Walde A, Herikstad H, Gustavsen S, et al. Factors associated with increased and decreased risk of *Campylobacter* infection: a prospective case-control study in Norway. American Journal of Epidemiology. 2003;158:234–242.

29. Lopez-Martinez R, Castanon-Olivares LR. Isolation of *Cryptococcus neoformans* var. neoformans from bird droppings, fruits and vegetables in Mexico City. Mycopathologia. 1995;129:25–28.

30. Murray PR, Rosenthal KS, Pfaller MA. Medical Microbiology. 4th ed. St. Louis, MO: Mosby; 2002.

31. Garcia LS, Bruckner DA. Diagnostic Medical Parasitology. Washington, DC: American Society for Microbiology; 1997.

32. Felsenfeld O. Notes on food, beverages and fomites contaminated with *Vibrio cholerae*. Bulletin of the World Health Organization. 1965;33:725–734.

33. Hood MA, Ness GE. Survival of *Vibrio cholerae* and *Escherichia coli* in estuarine waters and sediments. Applied and Environmental Microbiology. 1982;43:578–584.

34. Hallam NB, West JR, Forster CF, Powell JC, Spencer I. The decay of chlorine associated with the pipe wall in water distribution systems. Water Research. 2002;36:3479–3488.

35. Semenza JC, Roberts L, Henderson A, Bogan J, Rubin CH. Water distribution system and diarrheal disease transmission: a case study in Uzbekistan. American Journal of Tropical Medicine and Hygiene. 1998;59:941–946.

36. Zacheus OM, Lehtola MJ, Korhonen LK, Martikainen PJ. Soft deposits, the key site for microbial growth in drinking water distribution networks. Water Research. 2001;35:1757–1765.

37. DanXia F, Ming C. Spatial analysis of the influencing factor of water pipe break based on GIS technology. Urban Geotechnical Investigation & Surveying. 2007;2:30–32.

38. Pelletier G, Mailhot A, Villeneuve JP. Modeling water pipe breaks—three case studies. Journal of Water Resources Planning and Management. 2003;129:115–123.

39. Maidment DR. Arc Hydro: GIS for Water Resources. Redlands, CA: Esri Press; 2002.

40. Jha PK. Health and social benefits from improving community hygiene and sanitation: an Indian experience. International Journal of Environmental Health Research. 2003;13:133–140.

41. Addiss DG, Pond RS, Remshak M, Juranek DD, Stokes S, Davis JP. Reduction of risk of watery diarrhea with point-of-use water filters during a massive outbreak of waterborne *Cryptosporidium* infection in Milwaukee, Wisconsin, 1993. American Journal of Tropical Medicine and Hygiene. 1996;54:549–553.

42. Chaudhuri M, Sattar SA. Enteric virus removal from water by coal-based sorbents: development of low-cost water filters. Water Science & Technology. 1986;18:77–82.

43. Jain P, Pradeep T. Potential of silver nanoparticle-coated polyurethane foam as an antibacterial water filter. Biotechnology and Bioengineering. 2005; 90:59–63.

44. Jalan J, Somanathan E, Choudhuri S. Awareness and the Demand for Environmental Quality: Drinking Water in Urban India. Kathmandu, Nepal: SANDEE; 2003.

45. Rao VC, Waghmare SV, Lakhe SB. Detection of viruses in drinking water by concentration on magnetic iron oxide. Applied and Environmental Microbiology. 1981;42:421–426.

46. Salvatorelli G, Medici S, Finzi G, De Lorenzi S, Quarti C. Effectiveness of installing an antibacterial filter at water taps to prevent *Legionella* infections. Journal of Hospital Infection. 2005;61:270–271.

47. Vonberg RP, Eckmanns T, Bruderek J, Rüden H, Gastmeier P. Use of terminal tap water filter systems for prevention of nosocomial legionellosis. Journal of Hospital Infection. 2005;60:159–162.

48. Wallis C, Stagg CH, Melnick JL. The hazards of incorporating charcoal filters into domestic water systems. Water Research. 1974;8:111–113.

49. Ward LS, Peck JP. The coldwater marine aquarium at the British Antarctic Survey. Aquarium Sciences and Conservation. 1997;1:53–63.

50. Quick RE, Venczel LV, Gonzalez O, Mintz ED, Highsmith AK, Espada A, et al. Narrow-mouthed water storage vessels and in situ chlorination in a Bolivian

community: a simple method to improve drinking water quality. American Journal of Tropical Medicine and Hygiene. 1996;54:511–516.

51. Roberts L, Chartier Y, Chartier O, Malenga G, Toole M, Rodka H. Keeping clean water clean in a Malawi refugee camp: a randomized intervention trial. Bulletin of the World Health Organization. 2001;79:280–287.

52. Dolan P, Shaw R, Tsuchiya A, Williams A. QALY maximisation and people's preferences: a methodological review of the literature. Health Economics. 2005;14:197–208.

53. La Puma J, Lawlor EF. Quality-adjusted life-years. JAMA. 1990;263:2917–2921.

54. McHorney CA. Health status assessment methods for adults: past accomplishments and future challenges. Annual Review of Public Health. 1999;20:309–335.

55. Shumway M, Saunders T, Shern D, Pines E, Downs A, Burbine T, et al. Preferences for schizophrenia treatment outcomes among public policy makers, consumers, families, and providers. Psychiatric Services. 2003;54:1124–1128.

56. Paulhus DL. Measurement and control of response bias. In: Robinson JP, Shaver PR, Wrightsman LS, eds. Measures of Personality and Social Psychological Attitudes. San Diego, CA: Academic Press; 1991:17–60.

57. Stewart DW, Shamdasani PN, Rook DW. Focus Groups: Theory and Practice. Thousand Oaks, CA: Sage Publications; 2007.

58. Marshall MN. The key informant technique. Family Practice. 1996;13:92–97.

Chapter 14

Indoor Air Pollution and Respiratory Health

A Transdisciplinary Vision

Gautam Yadama   Mario Castro
Kenneth B. Schechtman   Nishesh Chalise
Pratim Biswas

Learning Objectives

- Demonstrate an understanding of household air pollution, the scope of the problem, its toll on the lives of the poor, and its complex social, economic, cultural, and ecological causes.

- Recognize that public health problems which persist over time are embedded in complex social and cultural systems.

- Develop an appreciation for household air pollution as a transdisciplinary public health problem requiring more than a technical fix.

- Understand and recognize barriers to and enablers of evidence-based interventions to improve household air pollution.

- Identify relevant disciplines for addressing a given complex public health challenge, and combine various methods to improve our understanding of that transdisciplinary public health problem.

● ● ●

Three billion people live in millions of households in developing countries that depend on solid fuels—wood, crop waste, coal—to meet their daily household energy needs for cooking and heating. Daily burning of solid fuels in primitive and inefficient stoves increases household air pollution, a leading cause of chronic obstructive pulmonary disease and other respiratory diseases. Exposure to indoor air pollution is responsible for a number of respiratory health issues and contributes significantly to the global burden of disease. This is a leading public health challenge in rural and urban poor households around the world, particularly for women and children, who are the most exposed to smoke and emissions from burning solid fuels. Black soot from inefficient combustion of solid fuels also adversely affects the environment.

Improved cookstoves have been introduced around the world by governments and nongovernmental organizations. However, their sustained uptake has been disappointing, and there is scant empirical evidence of their effectiveness under real-world conditions. Uptake and sustained use of improved cookstoves is complex and is embedded in the social, cultural, and ecological realities of the rural poor. Ignoring the context of the rural households and their behaviors has resulted in ineffective dissemination and implementation of interventions to improve household air quality through improved stove programs. A transdisciplinary approach focused on the problem, and less on the perspective and methods of a particular discipline, is critical for advancing a solution to this public health challenge. In this chapter, we propose a way of conceptualizing indoor air pollution as a transdisciplinary challenge. In this new perspective, we emphasize understanding and amplifying the voice of the actors who are embedded in the problem of burning solid fuels, and understanding their preferences for interventions that they deem viable. We also describe our approach of combining the study of emissions and lung function with participatory community-based approaches in order to model the barriers and enablers of improved stove use and their impact on health of rural households.

Access to clean air is paramount for ensuring the health, productivity, and overall well-being of billions of poor individuals around the globe. A decline in air quality affects people's ability to maintain healthy and disease-free lives irrespective of personal wealth and resources. The impact of a deleterious environment affects all people globally, irrespective of national boundaries, race, and economic status. The impact of low environmental quality in indoor air, however, is overwhelmingly borne by the poor.

The global disease burden due to household air pollution, or indoor air pollution (the terms are used interchangeably in this chapter), measured in disability-adjusted life-years, is estimated to be 4 percent of the total burden.[1] A significant source of household air pollution is the biomass combustion used by three billion people around the globe for cooking, heating, and carrying out daily household livelihood functions.[2,3] Negative health outcomes associated with exposure to solid biomass burning include chronic bronchitis; chronic obstructive pulmonary disease (COPD) and asthma; acute respiratory infections; decreased lung function; tuberculosis; and nasopharyngeal, laryngeal, and lung cancer.[1,4–7]

In this chapter, we will articulate this problem of biomass combustion by several billion poor people as a significant global health problem that is complex and that demands transdisciplinary research, practice interventions, and education (see chapter 1 regarding the need for cross-disciplinary approaches to solving complex social problems). Our objective in this chapter is threefold: (1) to motivate and deepen the understanding of indoor air pollution as an outcome of social, economic, cultural, and ecological drivers that enable rural households to move up the energy ladder to sustained use of clean fuels or clean combustion technologies; (2) to underscore the significance of transdisciplinary research and education in addressing this global health challenge; and (3) to provide a window into the opportunity this public health challenge presents to strengthen transdisciplinary research, education, and practice interventions with rural households of India that routinely use biomass fuels to meet their energy needs.

Household Air Pollution: A Complex Challenge

Biomass in the form of fuelwood, agricultural residue, and animal waste is among the most prevalent sources of energy in rural India and South Asia and indeed throughout the developing world. Combustion of biomass, however, has adverse impacts on public health, economic development, and local ecology. Approximately three billion people globally depend on biomass to meet daily cooking and heating needs and the estimates are that a significant portion of the global rural populations will remain dependent on biomass in 2030.[8] In India alone, two billion kilograms of biomass are burned every day, accounting for 90 percent of rural energy consumption.[9] Biomass combustion is responsible for a significant proportion of fine particulate matter emissions (such as carbonaceous aerosols) that result in the formation of *brown clouds* over the subcontinent.[10] Black carbon aerosols from biomass combustion are not only a health risk but also constitute a significant climate change agent, potentially more potent than carbon dioxide in terms of warming.[11] Emissions from biomass combustion contain dangerous levels of fine particulate matter ($PM_{2.5}$, PM_1, and smaller sizes) and carbon monoxide (CO), causing life-threatening and debilitating illnesses in its users, especially women and children.

Biomass burning has significant health effects on children, including increased infant and perinatal mortality and low birth weight.[1] Recent studies suggest that biomass combustion is an even greater risk factor for COPD than smoking. Exposure to unprocessed fuels nearly doubles the risk of pneumonia in children.[12] In 2008, 36 million deaths worldwide were attributed to noncommunicable diseases, of which 4.3 million (12 percent) were due to chronic respiratory diseases. The National Institutes of Health has called for studies to examine the spectrum of health impacts from household air pollution,[2] and the World Bank in a recent report identifies environmental pollution, including indoor air pollution, as one of the priority intervention areas for improving the health of the poor globally.[13] As mentioned previously, negative health outcomes associated with biomass burning include chronic bronchitis,[14] chronic obstructive pulmonary disease,[1,7] acute respiratory infections,[6] decreased lung function,[5] and tuberculosis.[4] The following health concerns resulting from biomass burning have been identified for children specifically: increased infant and perinatal mortality, low birth weight, pulmonary tuberculosis, and nasopharyngeal, laryngeal, and lung cancer.[1]

Ineffective and Failed Interventions: Explanations and Challenges

The continuing dependence on biomass as a primary energy source and the inefficient manner of its use is having devastating effects on both people and the environment. The extraction of fuelwood from forests is among the most significant ongoing driver of deforestation in South Asia.[15] This dependence drives fuelwood scarcity and increases opportunity costs due to the time required to collect fuelwood.[16,17] Worldwide, millions of "improved" stoves have been disseminated to the poor in the last three decades, but their rates of uptake and prolonged use has been disappointing. Much of the effort expended on improved stoves has been devoted to design work in the laboratory, with limited systematic attention being given to understanding the actual process of stove adoption and use.[18] In India, thirty-five million improved *chulhas* (stoves) were distributed from 1985 to 2000, as part of the National Program on Improved Chulhas (NPIC). Although millions of improved stoves were distributed, evaluations have shown that only 24 percent of the installed stoves were present in households at the time of the evaluation, and many of those that were present were not in use.[19] The absence of 76 percent of the improved stoves from households and the nonuse of many of the remaining 24 percent underscores the importance of knowing more about factors that influence sustained use of new more efficient cookstoves in rural India. Others have estimated that 85 percent of stoves were in disuse by 2002, declaring NPIC a failed initiative.[20]

Although more efficient and emissions-reducing technologies can be produced in the laboratory, designing them to meet the needs of users in various sociocultural contexts and at different scales (household to community) has proved challenging. Improved stove technology programs have often been unsuccessful in that (1) households are likely not to adopt the improved technologies at all, or (2) if they do adopt them they implement them in a way that does not achieve the sought-after levels of reduction in fuelwood used and harmful emissions.[16,20] *Adoption* in this context refers to the household decision to acquire new combustion technology, and *implementation* refers to the household's actual use in an appropriate and designed manner of the new combustion technology.[21] Hence the challenge of ensuring successful uptake and proper use of improved combustion technologies in rural households stems from the twin failures of adoption and implementation. The failure of these interventions stems from a misunderstanding of household decision-making processes regarding household energy choices that go beyond the narrow decision to adopt an improved cookstove.

Household decisions have to be understood within the context of the livelihoods of the rural poor: the social, political, cultural, economic, and ecological dimensions of energy security as well as the question of access to alternative sources of energy and having household strategies to meet fluctuating energy supply and demand.[16,22,23] We need substantial advancement in our understanding of energy transition, of the behavioral drivers of decisions to shift to new stoves, and of prevailing social and cultural norms that affect adoption and implementation of alternative energy technologies.[22]

In order to understand critical environmental, social, and economic factors that influence the adoption of clean energy technologies that are beneficial, it is necessary to assess what households and communities deem to be the key social, economic, cultural, and technological factors driving the adoption of new energy solutions that reduce household air pollution. The behavioral response to new energy solutions will depend on livelihood strategies of rural communities, household characteristics, and local ecology—whether solid biomass availability is abundant or scarce—household and community engagement in the use and management of local natural resources, culture-based preferences around food preparation, and the cost of obtaining traditional fuels.[22-25] The decision to adopt improved biomass-based energy solutions stems from how these factors influence a community or household's perception, as well as from the actual scarcity of traditional sources of energy—primarily fuelwood, crop waste, or animal waste. Where traditional biomass fuels are not scarce, households are less likely to adopt new and cleaner energy solutions.[16,26,27]

There is also evidence that types of community-level variables—social and economic institutions—predict a household's use of and access to alternate fuels rather than the traditional fuels for meeting daily needs.[28] The *energy ladder* theory of energy transition posits that as household income increases, preference for more modern sources of energy develop, leading households to adopt newer fuels and discard traditional, or older, forms of fuel.[29,30] This theory orders fuels from traditional to more modern. From least to most modern, the fuels are crop residues and animal wastes, fuelwood, charcoal, kerosene, bottled gas (LPG), and electricity.[30] The energy ladder theory has been applied to energy transition in both urban and rural areas, although urban households are thought to climb much more quickly due to their increased access to more modern fuels, higher incomes, and information on other energy sources.[30]

Although the energy ladder theory has held significant sway in the development and energy research communities, there are alternative conceptualizations of household energy transition. One argument holds that households' energy demand, and not preference, rises with income.[31] Another argument is that households do not move linearly up the energy ladder by replacing older fuels with more modern ones, but instead, as household income increases and new sources of energy are adopted, the use of older fuels is maintained to a significant degree in order to meet the increasing demand that follows increased income.[22] Energy stacking is also evident when households are given new stove technologies, in that they may retain older, inefficient stoves alongside the newer devices, undermining the goal of reducing air emissions. The drivers of energy stacking are energy insecurity and deeply entrenched household strategies to avert risk in the event that a new stove breaks down. This is understandable given that the household did not participate in the development of that new technology and is only peripherally knowledgeable about the workings of that technology.

Moreover, households that repeatedly experience shocks to their livelihoods will naturally limit their risk (albeit at the margins), and so they do not completely abandon reliable cookstoves for newer technology that they may not be able to sustain given the ubiquity of risk in their lives. The natural decision is to stack new technology along with older technology, in the process undermining potential gains in reducing harmful emissions. The trajectory of poor households along the clean energy continuum is not straightforward as households do not move entirely from one energy source to the next, leaving the former behind. This argument is further bolstered by the notion that households do not always see fuelwood or other plant biomass as inferior fuel because it may seem better suited for particular household uses, so it may be chosen even when income is sufficient and there is access to more modern fuels.[22]

Greater attention to the interactions between local ecosystems and household energy strategies, particularly in dryland communities around the world and in India, reveal another set of dynamics that is central to understanding the complexities of intervening in household air pollution. The very poor in the drylands of India survive because of vital ecosystem services from forests, which include biomass for household energy. The dynamic between household poverty and natural resource commons such as dryland forest ecosystems is intensified by economic and environmental uncertainties, institutional variations governing ecosystems, and the productivity of dryland cultivation. Drylands constitute 40 percent of the world's land and support 33 percent of the world's population.[32] An estimated two billion people live in arid and semiarid regions of the world, of which 410 million are in the drylands of India.[33] Local climatic variations in risk-prone drylands conspire to generate individual and collective responses that over time can exert severe pressures on critical forest resources. In the absence of options generated by state or market interventions or by informal institutional responses to the poor, overharvesting of vital natural resources might be a reasonable outcome.

In resource-poor communities, these interactions give rise to extreme conditions in both the ecological and human systems, despite local participants' full knowledge about the longer-term effects of overextracting behaviors. Three important characteristics of the ways in which biomass is accessed from commons play a significant role in the uptake and sustained use of improved cookstoves or other clean energy technologies that reduce household air pollution. First, the sheer availability of fuelwood, irrespective of quality, significantly reduces the opportunity cost of collecting that fuelwood, which further decreases the incentives to shift to cleaner cookstoves. Rural poor routinely collect fuelwood from the commons, and such availability negatively influences the relative advantage of an improved stove technology (see figure 14.1). Second, the reality that collection from the commons of fuelwood and other forms of biomass used for cooking falls on women and children is a barrier to shifting to alternative, clean-combusting stoves. Insofar as households undervalue women and children's labor, the perceived cost of collecting freely available biomass from commons is also seen as low, and households discount economic and health gains from shifting to either efficient and cleaner-burning woodstoves or to other technologies such as biogas. Third, in an attempt to reduce their burdens in collecting biomass fuel from great distances, women can begin to substitute plant biomass from proliferating invasive species. A widely observed trend in India is the abundant availability of kindling from proliferating invasive species such as *Lantana camara*.[34] Lantana, while profoundly altering local ecosystems including Indian forests, has been a welcome boon for the poor as a substitute for fuelwood in cookstoves. This is illustrative of how households experiencing scarcity and few alternatives continue to overharvest plant species, reinforcing the crisis in the biological system to such an extent that fundamental shifts in the biological system limit future possibilities in the social system, in turn leading to fundamental limits on program interventions.

Decisions around household energy and cooking technologies are subtle, complex, and nonlinear. Household decisions to adopt new technologies and alternative energy sources are motivated by factors both endogenous and exogenous to the household, predicated on the technology itself, driven in part by the distressed state of local environments and biomass availability, and reinforced by intrahousehold gender inequalities. Heterogeneous time preferences also are a factor in driving different classes of households to behave differently when they are choosing whether or not to invest in new technology. Analysis and modeling of the household dynamics of improved stoves will do well to heed these time preferences and the discount rates that the poor apply to their own health and well-being. The complexity only increases as we take household preferences for environmental outcomes into account.[35-39]

A central message is that the uptake of new, clean-combusting stoves is more complex than just utility maximization, that attributes and knowledge of an innovation and the sociocultural system in which it diffuses and the advantage of a new technology over other options are all important for sustained use of new technologies.[40,41] Key attributes discussed in studies by Pandey and Yadama[40] and by Blumenthal et al.[41] are synthesized in figure 14.1. If we overlook cultural, social, economic, and ecological factors driving stove use and improper use, we compromise not only the careful design and implementation of clean stove technologies but also our understanding of their

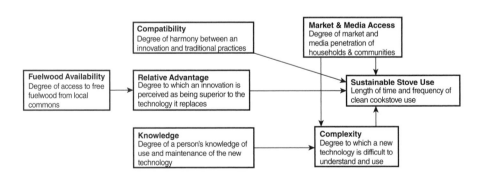

Figure 14.1. Conceptual model of sociocultural, technological, market, and ecological drivers influencing sustained use of clean cookstove technologies
Source: Adapted from S. Pandey and G. N. Yadama, "Community Development Programs in Nepal: A Test of Diffusion of Innovation Theory," *Social Service Review,* 1992;66(4):582–597.

prolonged impact on indoor air pollution and the subsequent health outcomes in women and children.[2, 13]

Household Air Pollution and Health Effects:
A Transdisciplinary Approach

Our review makes four dimensions abundantly clear: (1) the overwhelming evidence of adverse health and complex climate consequences from combustion aerosol emissions, (2) the dynamic complexity of the decisions and behaviors of poor households that are energy insecure and dependent on fragile and risk-prone ecological and agricultural systems, (3) the failure of previous efforts to develop effective biomass-based energy solutions that recognize the complexities of local livelihoods, and (4) the case for bringing key stakeholders together across the people, technology, and science divides to engage in developing shared pools of transdisciplinary intelligence to design effective and sustainable energy solutions that can reduce household air pollution and improve health of three billion people.

Failed or ineffective interventions are a result of the disjunction between, on the one hand, the normative frameworks explaining household energy use and associated pollution and health outcomes and, on the other hand, the subjective mental models that shape people's beliefs, behaviors, and household energy decisions and that are predicated on a very different understanding of the systems that are central to people's daily living. Normative explanations of real-world problems reflect disciplinary allegiance, which reduces the possibility that anyone using those explanations will strike on innovative and effective interventions to complex transdisciplinary problems. Disciplinary expertise is critical for explaining a facet of a complex problem, but disciplinary allegiance produces attenuated explanations.

Our case argues for mounting transdisciplinary research that leverages aerosol science, social science, and medical science together with practitioners to address household air pollution from solid fuel combustion. Our approach is to embark on research, education, and practice that overcome the disciplinary myopia of prior approaches to household air pollution and interventions to curb emissions. As urged by Stokols, Hall, and Vogel in chapter 1 in this book, our approach is to transcend preexisting disciplinary boundaries. We emphasize the embeddedness of the choice of energy sources and the logic for their justification in human-nature interactions. Our transdisciplinary approach gives prominence to understanding these interactions in the way they shape household energy choices and in their impact on indoor emissions and environment and on the likelihood of sustaining clean combustion interventions. In contrast to most prior dissemination projects, we focus systematically and theoretically on disentangling factors that drive the sustainable use of new

TRANSDISCIPLINARY PUBLIC HEALTH

and more efficient cookstove systems. The investigators on our team come from medicine, biostatistics, engineering, and social science and have a strong transdisciplinary approach to examining barriers to improved cookstove use and also substantial experience in doing research in rural India. In integrating disciplines, we will be able to disentangle technological barriers to sustained use of clean cookstoves from barriers that concern social, economic, cultural, and health.

Critical to our efforts at understanding and intervening in household air pollution is our long-standing collaboration with an influential nongovernmental organization, the Foundation for Ecological Security (FES), that works in over two thousand rural communities spread across seven states of India to increase biomass production to meet the energy and other needs of villagers. In collaborating with FES, we are able to keep the focus on the transdisciplinary nature of household air pollution (rather than retracting into the comfort of our respective disciplinary silos) and increase our ability to translate our findings into approaches that will be used by real-world communities (chapter 1 emphasizes translation as one of the hallmarks of TD approach). FES, with considerable experience in program implementation, transforms the team's ability to translate research findings into practical interventions, which is a key aspect of transdisciplinary research.[42] FES has also collaborated with us in conducting a graduate training workshop for our students on the theme of energy, environment, and sustainability in India, ideas that are central to the research proposed herein. FES is unique in its commitment to use systematic science to inform its interventions in order to improve the livelihoods, health, and well-being of rural households.

Transdisciplinary Framework for Examining Respiratory Health Outcomes from Clean Cookstoves

Our framework exemplifies the notion of transdisciplinary research by synthesizing and going beyond each individual discipline (recall that the description of the transdisciplinary approach in chapter 1 of this book includes the creation of new conceptual frameworks). It starts with a systematic examination of the mental models at the household level that concern energy system decisions; decisions about fuel and stove preference, decisions about shifting to cleaner combustion, and maintenance of new stove technologies (figure 14.2). People's mental models of what constitutes a sustainable energy system and available energy options shape household energy preferences. Mental models are themselves a consequence of household livelihood strategies, prior experiences, and knowledge of energy use, environmental quality, and local ecosystem interrelations. Individual and collective decisions predicated on these functional mental models accumulate over time to produce household energy preferences and

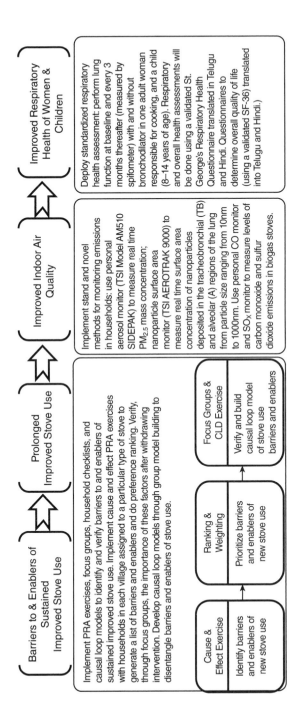

Figure 14.2. A framework for studying respiratory health outcomes from clean cookstove use

induce changes in the use of biomass fuels or other cleaner fuels, which, in turn, shape the future energy choices of rural households. In unpacking these intrahousehold energy decisions, with specific attention to social, economic, cultural, community, and ecosystem forces on these decisions, we identify a set of factors to track in understanding the sustainability of clean energy interventions, that is, improved cookstoves.

Our principal method for understanding household preferences and decisions is a combination of participatory rural appraisal (PRA) techniques[43] and participatory causal loop modeling[44] that allows us to arrive at qualitative models that explain the key drivers of household energy decisions. Improved cookstoves have previously been designed in labs and then distributed to rural villagers. We believe that food and cooking touch a deep sociocultural aspect of people's lives. It is thus important to involve people embedded in the problem if we are to develop effective solutions. We have decided to use participatory methods because we believe that participation of the end users in the research process will yield cookstove designs that are grounded in the reality of their lives.[45]

PRA is a set of methods through which local people share their perceptions and knowledge regarding their lives. We will be using two types of PRA exercises: cause-and-effect (CE) diagrams and preference ranking. In using CE diagrams with each village, we first elicit factors critical for sustained use of improved cookstove technology. The goal of a cause-and-effect exercise with households is to identify possible enablers and barriers (causes) to the effect that most concerns us—sustained use of improved stoves. We can anticipate reductions in emissions and in subsequent adverse respiratory health outcomes only when improved stoves are used sustainably. CE diagrams visually depict various barriers to sustained use, generate discussions, and enable an understanding of the context for these barriers and enablers of stove use. The CE exercise is followed by another qualitative PRA exercise, a preference ranking exercise with the same group of households to prioritize and weigh the preferences as to how they enable or hinder sustained use of improved stoves. Women identified as community liaisons will collaborate with the research team in implementing the CE and preference ranking exercises. In building the capacity of a community liaison, we ensure community embedded tracking of enablers and barriers to new stove use. As we intervene, we will track a list of enablers and barriers in each of the households.

We use participatory causal loop modeling,[46,47] which will enable us to elicit causal linkages between the various barriers and enablers listed in the CE diagrams, resulting in a causal loop diagram (CLD). Systems science approaches such as CLD are essential to understanding and solving the complex implementation problems that result from a structure of feedback mechanisms among technologies, social and cultural norms, and livelihood options that are nonlinear, dynamic, and replete with adaptation, self-organization, and emergence.[48] Systems science embraces such structural complexity and takes a holistic view compared to traditional approaches where the system is reduced to its component parts. Systems science approaches generate practice-based evidence and emphasize permeability between research and practice in population and public health where the approach is to meld beneficiaries, practitioners, and researchers.[48] Using the CLD, we will be able to go beyond a list of factors to a dynamic theory that disentangles and explicates how barriers and enablers of sustained use of improved cookstoves relate.

An important aspect in transdisciplinary studies is in the use of appropriate tools and metrics. We provide one example here. Although there have been innumerable studies on cookstove aerosol emissions, very few studies have relied on the development of appropriate metrics based on relevant measurements. Further strengthening our innovative transdisciplinary approach is our ability to deploy state-of-the-art aerosol measurement instruments. An example is the quantification in real time of the surface area concentration of particles that deposit in the lungs from different models of stoves, both traditional and improved. In collaboration with FES, the Aerosols and Air Quality Research Lab (AAQRL) at Washington University in St. Louis developed new indices for measures of particle concentration.[49] Such studies not only provide more appropriate measures of potential health effects (in contrast to the traditionally used PM mass concentration measurements) but also help in the development of relevant indices that can be used in transdisciplinary studies. These indices have elucidated the importance of aerosol metrics and their utility as a quantitative tool for correlating with other social and cultural metrics as well as respiratory health measures. Surface area has not been studied as a dose metric for biomass cookstove particle emissions in the past due to the unavailability of appropriate instruments. We will quantify emission levels of fine particulate matter and other harmful gases such as carbon monoxide (CO) and sulfur dioxide (SO_X). We also measure mass concentrations as $PM_{2.5}$ and PM_1 (using the TSI Sidepak Personal Aerosol Monitor; TSI, St. Paul, MN, USA). We will train field research staff in measuring real-time surface area concentration of particles deposited in the tracheobronchial (TB) and alveolar (A) regions of the lung using a nanoparticle aerosol monitor (TSI AEROTRAKTM 9000; TSI, St. Paul, Minnesota, USA), and we will monitor CO and SO_X levels. CO will be measured using a Langan Model T15n monitor (Langan products, San Francisco, USA). Regarding health outcomes, we will perform spirometry tests and administer surveys to understand the change in health outcomes from using an improved cookstove. Using a spirometer, we will measure the forced expiratory volume in one second (FEV_1) and forced vital capacity (FVC) at baseline and every three months. People with obstructive pulmonary disease tend to have lower values of FEV_1 and FVC. We will also use validated surveys such as the World Health Organization's Quality of Life (WHO-QOL) survey, St. George's Respiratory Questionnaire (SGRQ), and the Pediatric Quality of Life Inventory (PEDsQL) to measure the general quality of life of the participants. Our effort to systematically link sustained use of new energy systems to changes in household emissions and subsequent health outcomes is only possible because of our transdisciplinary integration of social, aerosol, and medical sciences.

The strength of our team is in its span of represented disciplines and experience as it brings researchers, students, and practitioners together to work on transdisciplinary problems that transcend human, ecological, and energy systems. By transdisciplinary we mean, "a process whereby team members representing different fields work together over extended periods to develop shared conceptual and methodological frameworks that not only integrate but also transcend their respective disciplinary perspectives."[42] Creating transdisciplinary knowledge is a process of eroding disciplinary walls in the service of a deeper understanding of a societal problem and in such a way that "a shift occurs from solely 'reliable scientific knowledge' to inclusion of 'socially robust knowledge' that dismantles the expert/lay dichotomy while fostering new partnerships between the academy and society."[50]

As stated earlier, our focus is on co-evolving trajectories of household energy choices, local ecologies, and rural livelihoods that can serve as a practical laboratory for transdisciplinary training of the next generation of public health practitioners who will address environmental issues affecting the very poor. Our overarching question is grounded in the reality of rural households, their ability to meet energy needs from biomass under emerging human and local ecosystem changes, and is ideal for exploiting knowledge at the intersections of combustion and aerosol science, systems science, social science, and ecological science. In grounding our work in a real-world problem, we "necessarily integrate heterogeneous knowledge bases, whether these are gathered under the institutional cover of a discipline or not."[51] Our real-world challenge provides a platform for students to train and learn across disciplines, providing them with meta-cognitive and meta-disciplinary tools to navigate a variety of knowledge landscapes.

Our transdisciplinary educational strategy is to form several combinations of groups of faculty, students, and practitioners from India and the United States and from different disciplines to accomplish the following:

1. Create new learning environments that transcend disciplines and focus on the core problem of human, ecosystem, and household energy interactions.
2. Build learning or educational scaffolding, so to speak, to enable members of our team to climb out of their chosen discipline and into

another to understand the problem through a different lens and to realize the attenuated perspective of any single discipline.

3. Enable all members of a team—students, faculty, and practitioners alike—to transcend and step out of their discipline and visualize the problem in all its complexity.

4. Design educational and research processes to integrate methodologies that are cross-disciplinary in order to develop new insights into human, ecosystem, and energy system interactions and their effects on sustainable energy choices.

Summary

Disuse of new stove technology is quickly attributed to the social, economic, and cultural constraints that the rural poor face in the maintenance and use of a technology designed by outsiders. Another commonly proffered answer is incompatibility of the technology with household practices or difficulties in understanding the proper use and maintenance of new stove technology. However, we must also answer an equally important question: why are the poor unable to properly maintain technology that is deemed superior, and why do they find it incompatible with their livelihoods? We must answer this deeper question before the next round of technologies is implemented and then declared a failure in addressing harmful health and climate effects. Given the renewed emphasis on promoting more efficient stoves for the billions of poor in South Asia and sub-Saharan Africa, we cannot afford to remain satisfied with unfocused general answers. We must probe deeper into the micro- and macrodrivers of the sustainability of new technologies and of their wider uptake in rural societies. We must seek systematic answers to redress previous failures and elevate the voices and preferences of the poor in this global health and climate problem.

How does one listen to and collaborate with the rural poor to enable sustained use of clean stoves, and not dictate "appropriate" technologies? Participation in development programs is a promise of inclusion and of eventual improvement in quality of life. Participation and collaboration are a way to shift the axis of power and enable new actors to gain greater influence on outcomes related to their development and human condition. It is a path away from the language of target groups and beneficiaries and toward citizenship, agency, governance, and rights.[52–54] When participatory processes tend to emphasize consensus, even well-intentioned participatory institutions can exacerbate existing forms of exclusion, silencing dissidence and masking dissent.[55] Indeed, the voices of the marginal may not even be raised in such institutional spaces, thereby undermining the project of inclusiveness in health, social, and economic development efforts.[52,56] The marginalization of women and of the very poor is not one-dimensional; that is, caused only by gender or poverty. Rather, it is an outcome of the intersection of multiple forms of subordination, and especially so in Indian villages, which are highly stratified by caste, class, ethnicity, and gender. So how does one consider the poor and collaborate to obtain and share knowledge toward the common purpose of designing effective stove technologies to mitigate black carbon emissions from biomass combustion and ensuring their sustained use toward better health outcomes?

Perhaps equitable collaboration across disciplines and across stakeholders who are in different informational spaces will lead to such effective combustion technologies and to sustained household use. Our goal is to create those respectful trading zones of knowledge that will result in shared mental models of the problem at hand, instead of imposing predetermined solutions on the poor.[57] If new stove technologies are to make a difference in the lives of the poor and in the climate, then we must aim for research paradigms that reflect a deeper understanding of the societal dimensions shared by those experiencing harmful emissions. This requires engineers working on combustion and aerosols, medical practitioners concerned about respiratory health, biostatisticians concerned about research design, and social scientists working at the nexus of energy, environment, and poverty.[58] Such shared mental models, according to Gorman, Groves, and Shrager,[58] result in a moral imagination that transforms multidisciplinary collaborators to true transdisciplinary collaborators. Our approach of participatory, community-based causal loop modeling techniques transcends discipline and focuses on addressing the problem in all its complexity. Our approach is to build teams of engineering, social, and medical science faculty and students to engage in group model building with poor households in the field. This approach structures and increases the likelihood of transdisciplinary collaboration in which all stakeholders contribute to understanding the most likely stove technologies that will address the reduction of black carbon emissions in poor households.

The tendency for certain stakeholders to dominate in the process of innovation has been the history of previous improved stove efforts. Kirk Smith[59] classifies the history of improved stoves into phases—first focusing on smoke exposure and then on improving fuel efficiency, and then producing a *phoenix phase* that combines the experiences of past failures, but even this phase fails to consider the context and the local circumstances and priorities. In all three phases, it is the outsiders determining what is required and what the next phase is in the innovation. Our approach of using transdisciplinary teams of faculty and students to explore the key dimensions of viable technologies to mitigate black carbon and to conduct group model building on the problem of viable technologies is, out of respect and value for shared meanings, defining a common problem space and integrating combustion and aerosol science with the public health goal of affecting the lives of a few billion people. Successful models of such transdisciplinary work can be transformative not only in affecting real-world problems but also in changing the worldview of engineering, medicine, public health, and social science students alike. In creating citizen scientists with deep public engagement and an awareness of the dynamic processes involved in addressing the needs of biomass-dependent households, we hope to arrive at a point of doing things differently than they were done before.[60]

Key Terms

biomass	In an energy context, biomass is organic matter such as wood, crop waste, and other plant material that can be burned to produce energy.
chronic obstructive pulmonary disease (COPD)	The American Thoracic Society defines COPD as, "a preventable and treatable disease characterized by airflow limitation that is not fully reversible. The airflow limitation is usually progressive and is associated with an abnormal inflammatory response of the lungs to noxious particles or gases, primarily caused by cigarette smoking. Although COPD affects the lungs, it also produces significant systemic consequences."
complex problem	A problem that has multiple interrelated factors at different levels and the causes and effects are not easily discernible. Such interactions underlying complex problems give rise to unexpected patterns of behavior.
disability-adjusted life-years (DALYs)	The number of years of life lost because of a disease or a disability. It is a widely used metric of disease burden.
improved cookstoves	Cookstoves designed to increase the combustion efficiency of biomass and consequently reduce harmful emissions and lower the consumption of wood.
incomplete combustion	The incomplete conversion of a fuel's carbon and hydrogen into carbon dioxide and water. Incomplete combustion produces carbon

	monoxide and other toxic pollutants and also a high concentration of particles that often result in environmental and health problems.
indoor air pollution (IAP)	The chemical, biological, and physical contamination of household air, resulting in adverse health outcomes.
particulate matter	Solid or liquid particles suspended in air and produced by a combustion system. They are typically of submicrometer size, have a long lifetime, and can be carried long distances.

Review Questions

1. What are the health-related impacts of exposure to indoor air pollution?

2. What are the environmental problems arising from inefficient combustion of biomass?

3. Why have multiple efforts to disseminate improved cookstoves failed?

4. What is the difference between a disciplinary and a transdisciplinary approach to a public health problem?

5. Why do we need a transdisciplinary approach to understand and solve the problem of sustained use of improved cookstoves?

6. What are mental models, and how can we understand them?

References

1. Bruce N, Perez-Padilla R, Albalak R. Indoor air pollution in developing countries: a major environmental and public health challenge. Bulletin of the World Health Organization. 2000;78(9):1078–1092.
2. Martin WJ, Glass RI, Balbus JM, Collins FS. A major environmental cause of death. Science. 2011;334(6053):180–181.
3. World Health Organization. World Health Statistics 2008. Geneva: World Health Organization; 2008.
4. Pérez-Padilla R, Pérez-Guzmán C, Báez-Saldaña R, Torres-Cruz A. Cooking with biomass stoves and tuberculosis: a case control study. International Journal of Tuberculosis and Lung Disease. 2001;5(5):441–447.
5. Regalado J, Pérez-Padilla R, Sansores R, Páramo Ramirez JI, Brauer M, Paré P. The effect of biomass burning on respiratory symptoms and lung function in rural Mexican women. American Journal of Respiratory and Critical Care Medicine. 2006;174(8):901–905.

6. Mishra V. Indoor air pollution from biomass combustion and acute respiratory illness in preschool age children in Zimbabwe. International Journal of Epidemiology. 2003;32(5):847–853.

7. Chapman RS, He X, Blair AE, Lan Q. Improvement in household stoves and risk of chronic obstructive pulmonary disease in Xuanwei, China: retrospective cohort study. British Medical Journal. 2005;331(7524):1050.

8. International Energy Agency. World Energy Outlook 2006. Paris: OECD/IEA; 2006.

9. Balakrishnan K, Sankar S, Parikh J, Padmavathi R, Srividya K, Venugopal V, et al. Daily average exposures to respirable particulate matter from combustion of biomass fuels in rural households of southern India. Environmental Health Perspectives. 2002;110(11):1069–1075.

10. Gustafsson O, Kruså M, Zencak Z, Sheesley RJ, Granat L, Engström E, et al. Brown clouds over South Asia: biomass or fossil fuel combustion? Science. 2009;323(5913):495–498.

11. Schmidt CW. Black carbon: the dark horse of climate change drivers. Environmental Health Perspectives. 2011;119(4):A172.

12. Dherani M, Pope D, Mascarenhas M, Smith KR, Weber M, Bruce N. Indoor air pollution from unprocessed solid fuel use and pneumonia risk in children aged under five years: a systematic review and meta-analysis. Bulletin of the World Health Organization. 2008;86(5):390–398.

13. Bank W. Household Cookstoves, Environment, Health, and Climate Change: A New Look at an Old Problem. Washington, DC: The World Bank, Environment Department; 2011.

14. Akhtar T, Ullah Z, Khan MH, Nazli R. Chronic bronchitis in women using solid biomass fuel in rural Peshawar, Pakistan. Chest. 2007;132(5):1472–1475.

15. Kohlin G, Parks PJ. Spatial variability and disincentives to harvest: deforestation and fuelwood collection in South Asia. Land Economics. 2001;77(2):206–218.

16. Barnes DF, Openshaw K, Smith KR, van der Plas R. What Makes People Cook with Improved Biomass Stoves?: A Comparative International Review of Stove Programs. Washington, DC: The World Bank; 1994.

17. Amacher GS, Hyde WF, Kanel KR. Household fuelwood demand and supply in Nepal's Tarai and Mid-hills: choice between cash outlays and labor opportunity. World Development. 1996;24:1725–1736.

18. Ruiz-Mercado I, Masera O, Zamora H, Smith KR. Adoption and sustained use of improved cookstoves. Energy Policy. 2011;39(12):7557–7566.

19. National Council of Applied Economic Research. Annual Report: 2002–2003. New Delhi: National Council of Applied Economic Research; 2003.

20. Kishore VVN, Ramana PV. Improved cookstoves in rural India: how improved are they?: a critique of the perceived benefits from the National Programme on Improved Chulhas (NPIC). Energy. 2002;27:47–63.

21. Klein KJ, Knight, AP. Innovation implementation—overcoming the challenge. Current Directions in Psychological Science. 2005;14(5):243–246.

22. Hiemstra-van der Horst G, Hovorka AJ. Reassessing the "energy ladder": household energy use in Maun, Botswana. Energy Policy. 2008;36:3333–3344.

23. Masera OA, Saatkamp BD, Kammen DM. From linear fuel switching to multiple cooking strategies: a critique and alternative to the energy ladder model. World Development. 2000;28:2083–2103.

24. Duflo E, Greenstone M, Hanna, R. Indoor air pollution, health and economic well-being. SAPIENS. 2008;1:7–16.

25. Bandi M, Kumar VMR, Reddy MG, Reddy MS, Reddy VR, Springate-Baginski O. Participatory forest management in Andhra Pradesh: implementation, outcomes, and livelihood impacts. In: Springate-Baginski O, Blaikie P, eds. Forests, People, and Power: The Political Ecology of Reform in South Asia. London: Earthscan; 2007:302–334.

26. Cooke P, Kohlin G, Hyde WF. Fuelwood, forests, and community management— evidence from household studies. Environment and Development Economics. 2008;13:103–135.

27. Amacher GS, Hyde WF, Joshee BR. The adoption of consumption technologies under uncertainty: the case of improved stoves in Nepal. Journal of Economic Development. 1992;17(2):93–105.

28. Macht C, Axinn WG, Ghimire D. Household Energy Consumption: Community Context and the Fuelwood Transition. Population Studies Center Research Report 07-629. Ann Arbor: University of Michigan, Institute for Social Research; 2007.

29. Leach GA. Residential energy in the Third World. Annual Review of Energy. 1988;13(1):47–65.

30. Leach G. The energy transition. Energy Policy. 1992;20(2):116–123.

31. Foley G. Photovoltaic Applications in Rural Areas of the Developing World. World Bank Technical Paper No. 304. Washington, DC: The World Bank; 1995.

32. Adeel Z, King C, Schaaf T, Thomas R, Schuster B. People in Marginal Drylands: Managing Natural Resources to Improve Human Well-Being. A policy brief based on the Sustainable Management of Marginal Drylands (SUMAMAD) project. Hamilton, ON: United Nations University International Network on Water, Environment and Health; 2008.

33. Dobie P. Poverty and the Drylands. Challenge Paper Series. Nairobi: UNDP Drylands Centre; 2001.

34. Hiremath AJ, Agrawal M. Plant invasion and environmental pollution: causes of concern. Tropical Ecology. 2010;51(2):303–304.

35. Chapman GB, Coups EJ. Time preferences and preventive health behavior: acceptance of the influenza vaccine. Medical Decision Making. 1999;19(3):307–314.

36. Chesson HW, Viscusi WK. Commonalities in time and ambiguity aversion for long-term risks. Theory and Decision. 2003;54(1):57–71.

37. Green L, Fry AF, Myerson J. Discounting of delayed rewards: a life-span comparison. Psychological Science. 1994;5(1):33–36.

38. Komlos J, Smith PK, Bogin B. Obesity and the rate of time preference: is there a connection? Journal of Biosocial Science. 2004;36(2):209–219.

39. Picone GF, Sloan F, Taylor D. Effects of risk and time preference and expected longevity on demand for medical tests. Journal of Risk and Uncertainty. 2004;28(1):39–53.

40. Pandey S, Yadama GN. Community development programs in Nepal: a test of diffusion of innovation theory. Social Service Review. 1992;66(4): 582–597.

41. Blumenthal D, Weissman JS, Wachterman M, Weil E, Stafford RS, Perrin JM, et al. The who, what, and why of risk adjustment: a technology on the cusp of adoption. Journal of Health Politics, Policy and Law. 2005;30: 453–474.

42. Stokols D, Hall KL, Moser RP, Feng AX, Misra S, Taylor B. Cross-disciplinary team science initiatives: research, training, and translation. In: Frodeman R, Klein JT, Mitcham C, eds. The Oxford Handbook of Interdisciplinarity. Oxford, UK: Oxford University Press; 2010:471–493.

43. Kumar S. Methods for Community Participation: A Complete Guide for Practitioners. Rugby, Warwickshire, UK: ITDG Publishing; 2002.

44. Sterman JD. Business Dynamics: Systems Thinking and Modeling for a Complex World. Boston: Irwin McGraw-Hill; 2000.

45. Smithson J. Focus groups. In: Alasuutari P, Bickman L, Brannen J, eds. The Sage Handbook of Social Research Methods. Thousand Oaks, CA: Sage Publications; 2008.

46. Andersen DF, Richardson GP, Vennix, JAM. Group model building: adding more science to the craft. System Dynamics Review. 1997;13(2):187–201.

47. Vennix JAM. Group model-building: tackling messy problems. System Dynamics Review. 1999;15(4):379–401.

48. Holmes BJ, Finegood DT, Riley BL, Best A. Systems thinking in dissemination and implementation research. In: Brownson RC, Colditz GA, Proctor EK, eds. Implementation Research in Health: Translating Science to Practice. Oxford, UK: Oxford University Press; 2012:175–191.

49. Sahu M, Peipert J, Singhal V, Yadama GN, Biswas P. Evaluation of mass and surface area concentration of particle emissions and development of emissions indices for cookstoves in rural India. Environmental Science & Technology. 2011;45:2428–2434.

50. Klein JT. A taxonomy of interdisciplinarity. In: Frodeman R, Klein JT, Micham C, eds. The Oxford Handbook of Interdisciplinarity. Oxford, UK: Oxford University Press; 2010:15–30.

51. Krohn W. Interdisciplinary cases and disciplinary knowledge. In: Frodeman R, Klein JT, Mitcham C, eds. The Oxford Handbook of Interdisciplinarity. Oxford, UK: Oxford University Press; 2010:31–49.

52. Cornwall A. Whose voices? Whose choices? Reflections on gender and participatory development. World Development. 2003;31(8):1325–1342.

53. Gaventa J. Towards participatory governance: assessing the transformative possibilities. In Hickey S, Mohan G, eds. Participation: From Tyranny to Transformation?: Exploring New Approaches to Participation in Development. London: Zed Books; 2004:25–41.

54. Nussbaum M. Women's capabilities and social justice. In: Molyneux M, Razavi S, eds. Gender, Justice, Development, and Rights. New York: Oxford University Press; 2001:45–77.

55. Mouffe C. Feminism, citizenship, and radical democratic politics. In: Butler J, Scott J, eds. Feminists Theorize the Political. New York: Routledge; 1992:369–384.

56. Meinzen-Dick R, Zwarteveen M. Gendered participation in water management: issues and illustrations from water users' associations in South Asia. Agriculture and Human Values. 1998;15(4):337–345.

57. Gorman ME. Collaborating on convergent technologies: education and practice. Annals of the New York Academy of Sciences. 2004;1013:1–13.

58. Gorman ME, Groves JF, Shrager J. Societal dimensions of nanotechnology as a trading zone: results from a pilot project. In: Baird D, Nordmann A, Schummer J, eds. Discovering the Nanoscale. Amsterdam: IOS Press; 2004:63–73.

59. Smith KR. Dialectics of improved stoves. Economic and Political Weekly. March 11, 1989:517–522.

60. Fisher E, Mahajan RL, Mitcham C. Midstream modulation of technology: governance from within. Bulletin of Science, Technology & Society. 2006;26(6):485–496.

Name Index

Subject Index

Page numbers in italics refer to figures and tables.

engineering a safer environment for, 283; evidence on, 269; gross domestic product and, 283; new models of agriculture for improving, 281–282; school-based, 164; social marketing for, 280; throughout the life cycle, 274. *See also* Diet; Undernutrition

O

Obesity: and the Affordable Care Act, 117; applying solutions to, 204; cancer linked with, 35; child development and, 198–199; childhood, case addressing, 189–208; complexity of, 56; conceptual framework for, 193–194; defined, 207; economics of, 201–202; epidemiological perspective of, 194–196; evidence on, 159; genetic influences of, 196–197; governmental role in prevention and control of, 202; incidental laws and, 131, 132; and income inequality, 108; and the interpersonal environment, 198; and the intrapersonal environment, 196; and metabolic abnormalities, 197–198; and other environmental influences, 199–201; and parental modeling, 199; policies and, 201–203; prevention of, effective approaches to, 156; risk for, 194; and school setting, 202–203; strategy for, 104; systems approach to, 203–204; training and education working on, 39; translating what works to address, 204

Objectives and goals, developing, 174

Occupational health programs, triangulation of evidence on, 161

Office of Portfolio Analysis and Strategic Initiatives, 48

Olin Business School, 253

On the Protection, Promotion and Support of Breastfeeding, 288

Opportunity costs, 105, 106, 107, 108, 156, 322, 325

Oral rehydration salts (ORS), 303

Oregon Department of Transportation, 253

Oregon Office of Innovative Partnerships and Alternative Funding, 262

Oregon Solar Highway project, 253

Organisation for Economic Co-operation and Development, 37, 49

Organizational behavior, learning about, 252, 253, 254

Organizational factors, influence of, on TD initiatives, 12–13, 18, 19

Organizational variables, 159, *160*

Ornithology, 307

Osteoarthritis, 164

Osteoporosis, 164

Ottawa Charter for Health Promotion, 123

Outcomes evaluation: challenges in, 21, 94; lessons for, 20–21, 45, 81, 82, 86; in a logic model, *83*; planning for, 165

Outcomes valuation, 310–312

Outcomes variance, 147

Overseas Development Institute (ODI), 288

Overweight, defined, 207

P

Paleolithic nutrition, 273

Panchayat presidents: defined, 313; described, 302

Panchayats: accessibility of, for assessment, 312; control of water by, 301, 302, 310; defined, 302, 313; status of, 302; and taxes, 303; view of, 304

Paradoxes, 108, 135

Parasitology, 308

Parent education, injury prevention and, 230–231

Parental capacity, 224, 225, 226

Parental modeling: defined, 199, 207; and obesity, 199

Parental supervision, 222, 224

Parents as Teachers, Inc. (PAT), 191, 203, 205, 208

Participatory action research, 147, 148